T0275640

CAMBRIDGE LIBRARY COLLECTION

Books of enduring scholarly value

History of Medicine

It is sobering to realise that as recently as the year in which On the Origin of Species was published, learned opinion was that diseases such as typhus and cholera were spread by a 'miasma', and suggestions that doctors should wash their hands before examining patients were greeted with mockery by the profession. The Cambridge Library Collection reissues milestone publications in the history of Western medicine as well as studies of other medical traditions. Its coverage ranges from Galen on anatomical procedures to Florence Nightingale's common-sense advice to nurses, and includes early research into genetics and mental health, colonial reports on tropical diseases, documents on public health and military medicine, and publications on spa culture and medicinal plants.

Historical Sketch of
the Progress of Pharmacy in Great Britain

The pharmacist Jacob Bell (1810–59) spent much of his career working to raise the standards and reputation of his profession. A founder in 1841 of the Pharmaceutical Society of Great Britain, he sought to improve scientific education for practitioners as well as protect the profession through legislation. Although he served briefly in Parliament, Bell exerted his greatest influence through editing the *Pharmaceutical Journal*. An extended piece that he produced for the journal in 1842 forms the first part of the present work. He traces the development of pharmaceutical practice and legislation from the sixteenth century to the birth of the Pharmaceutical Society. At the behest of the society's council, Theophilus Redwood (1806–92) continued the narrative after Bell's death, concluding with the 1868 Pharmacy Act. Published in 1880, the book provides a thorough account of the gradual establishment of British pharmacy as a separate and respected profession.

Cambridge University Press has long been a pioneer in the reissuing of out-of-print titles from its own backlist, producing digital reprints of books that are still sought after by scholars and students but could not be reprinted economically using traditional technology. The Cambridge Library Collection extends this activity to a wider range of books which are still of importance to researchers and professionals, either for the source material they contain, or as landmarks in the history of their academic discipline.

Drawing from the world-renowned collections in the Cambridge University Library and other partner libraries, and guided by the advice of experts in each subject area, Cambridge University Press is using state-of-the-art scanning machines in its own Printing House to capture the content of each book selected for inclusion. The files are processed to give a consistently clear, crisp image, and the books finished to the high quality standard for which the Press is recognised around the world. The latest print-on-demand technology ensures that the books will remain available indefinitely, and that orders for single or multiple copies can quickly be supplied.

The Cambridge Library Collection brings back to life books of enduring scholarly value (including out-of-copyright works originally issued by other publishers) across a wide range of disciplines in the humanities and social sciences and in science and technology.

Historical Sketch of
the Progress of Pharmacy
in Great Britain

JACOB BELL
THEOPHILUS REDWOOD

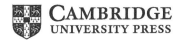

CAMBRIDGE
UNIVERSITY PRESS

CAMBRIDGE
UNIVERSITY PRESS

University Printing House, Cambridge, CB2 8BS, United Kingdom

Published in the United States of America by Cambridge University Press, New York

Cambridge University Press is part of the University of Cambridge.
It furthers the University's mission by disseminating knowledge in the pursuit of
education, learning and research at the highest international levels of excellence.

www.cambridge.org
Information on this title: www.cambridge.org/9781108070027

© in this compilation Cambridge University Press 2014

This edition first published 1880
This digitally printed version 2014

ISBN 978-1-108-07002-7 Paperback

HISTORICAL SKETCH

OF THE

PROGRESS OF PHARMACY

IN

GREAT BRITAIN.

BY

JACOB BELL

AND

THEOPHILUS REDWOOD.

LONDON:

PRINTED FOR THE

PHARMACEUTICAL SOCIETY OF GREAT BRITAIN,

17, BLOOMSBURY SQUARE.

1880.

BUTLER AND TANNER,
THE SELWOOD PRINTING WORKS,
FROME, AND LONDON.

PREFACE.

THE first part of this Historical Sketch was written by Mr. Jacob Bell in 1842, as an introduction to the *Pharmaceutical Journal*. It contains an account of the early but unsuccessful attempts made to separate pharmacy from the practice of medicine in this country, and of the efforts which at a later period were successfully made to found an institution with the object of raising up a race of qualified men devoted to the practice of pharmacy as a distinct occupation.

The latter part of the work has been produced by desire of the Pharmaceutical Council as a record of events and the results of operations which have taken place from the founding of the Pharmaceutical Society until the passing of the Pharmacy Act of 1868. In the collection of facts which are embodied in this narrative the author has received valuable assistance from members of the Pharmaceutical Council, from the Secretary, and especially from Mr. Joseph Ince.

June, 1880.   T. R.

HISTORICAL SKETCH

OF THE PROGRESS OF

PHARMACY IN GREAT BRITAIN.

AT the period at which our history commences, Pharmacy was
in the hands of the Physicians, who professed the healing art
in all its branches, and prepared their medicines themselves,
or superintended the preparation of them. The science of
medicine was so little understood, and so imperfectly cultivated, that it was in general practised empirically, and was
often confounded with sorcery and witchcraft. The Greek
word, φαρμακεύω, signifies either to practise witchcraft or to
use medicine, and this acceptation of the term was acted upon
in our own country as late as the 16th century. There were,
therefore, persons of various classes, both men and women,
who professed to cure disease, some by incantations; others,
who considered that by their genius they were "cut out and
configurated for it;" and others, again, who had obtained a
kind of traditional education from recognised Physicians, and
who therefore constituted the medical profession.

But no laws existed for the protection of the public from
ignorant practitioners. Indeed, it was difficult to discriminate
between the different degrees of ignorance which prevailed:
so much so, that it was not uncommon for patients to be
placed in public thoroughfares, in the hope that some of the
persons who happened to pass might be able to recommend a
remedy from the result of their own experience, when afflicted
with similar symptoms. The first Act of Parliament relating
to the medical profession was passed in the year 1511, and is
entitled "*An* ACT *for the appointing of* PHYSICIANS *and* SUR-
GEONS."

The preamble is worded thus:—

B

* " Forasmuch as the science and cunning of Physick and Surgery (to the perfect knowledge of which be requisite both great learning and ripe experience) is daily within this realm exercised by a great multitude of ignorant persons, of whom the greater part have no manner of insight in the same, nor in any other kind of learning ; some also can read no letters on the book, so far forth that common artificers, as smiths, weavers, and women, boldly and accustomably take upon them great cures, and things of great difficulty, in the which they partly use sorcery and witchcraft, partly apply such medicines unto the disease as be very noxious, and nothing meet therefore, to the high displeasure of God, great infamy to the faculty, and the grievous hurt, damage, and destruction of many of the king's liege people; most especially of them that cannot discern the uncunning from the cunning. Be it therefore (to the surety and comfort of all manner of people) by the authority of this present Parliament enacted :—That no person within the city of London, nor within seven miles of the same, take upon him to exercise and occupy as a Physician or Surgeon, except he be first examined, approved, and admitted by the Bishop of London, or by the Dean of St. Paul's, for the time being, calling to him or them four Doctors of Physic, and for Surgery, other expert persons in that faculty : and for the first examination such as they shall think convenient, and afterward alway four of them that have been so approved. . . .

" That no person out of the said city and precinct of seven miles of the same, except he have been (as is aforesaid) approved in the same, take upon him to exercise and occupy as a Physician or Surgeon, in any diocese within this realm, but if he be first examined and approved by the Bishop of the same diocese, or, he being out of the diocese, by his vicar-general: either of them calling to them such expert persons in the said faculties, as their discretion shall think convenient.† . . . ."

By this Act the faculty of medicine was vested in one body of practitioners, who practised Medicine, Surgery, and Pharmacy. The Physicians' assistants were styled Apothecaries,

---

* 3 Henry VIII., c. 9.

† Dr. Goodall's " History of the College of Physicians."

and they, gradually acquiring information respecting the properties of drugs, began to transact business on their own account.

In the year 1518, Thomas Linacre, the Physician of Henry the Eighth, proposed the establishment of a College of Physicians, which was accomplished on the 23rd of September of that year. The powers of this body were extended in the year 1540 : the Physicians were exonerated from the necessity of attendance on juries and parochial offices,* and were empowered to enter the houses of Apothecaries in London, " to search, view, and see the Apothecary-wares, drugs, and stuffs," and to destroy such as they found corrupt or unfit for use. In the same year the Barbers and Surgeons were united into one company, but the Surgeons were prohibited from shaving, and the Barbers were restricted from performing any surgical operations, except drawing teeth. The Physicians, however, were allowed to practise surgery.

The Surgeons having abused their privileges, an Act was passed, in the year 1542, of which the following is the substance :—

Whereas in the Parliament holden at Westminster, in the third year of the King's Most Gracious Reign, amongst other things, for the avoiding of sorceries, witchcrafts, and other inconveniences, it was enacted, That no person within the City of London, nor within seven miles of the same, should take upon him to exercise and occupy as Physician and Surgeon, except he be first examined, admitted, and approved by the Bishop of London, etc. . .: Sithence the making of which said Act, the Company and Fellowship of Surgeons of London, minding onely their owne lucres, and nothing the profit or ease of the diseased or patient, have sued, troubled, and vexed divers honest persons, as well men as women, whom God hath endued with the knowledge of the nature, kind, and operation of certain herbs, roots, and waters, and the using and ministering of them, to such as have been pained with customable diseases, as women's breasts being sore, a pin and the web in the eye, uncomes of the hands, scaldings, burnings, sore mouths, the stone, stranguary,

---

* The Surgeons had been exonerated from these duties in the year 1513.

saucelin, and morphew, and such other like diseases. . . .
And yet the said persons have not taken anything for their
pains or cunning. . . In consideration whereof, and for
the ease, comfort, succour, help, relief, and health of the
King's poor subjects, inhabitants of this his realm, now
pained or diseased, or that hereafter shall be pained or
diseased, Be it ordained, etc., that at all time from henceforth
it shall be lawful to every person being the King's subject,
having knowledge and experience of the nature of herbs,
roots, and waters, etc., to use and minister . . according to
their cunning, experience, and knowledge . . the aforesaid
statute . . or any other Act notwithstanding."

This Act is understood to apply to the practice of medicine
without remuneration, and accordingly it was not uncommon
for empirics to evade the law by pretending to practise gratuitously. This, however, was not always successful; and
Dr. Goodall's *History of the* PROCEEDINGS *against* EMPIRICS
(published in 1684) contains an account of numerous prosecutions, in which the law was put in force in a summary
manner.

In the year 1552, *Grig*, a poulterer, in Surrey, "taken
among the people for a prophet, in curing divers diseases by
words and prayers, and saying he would take no money,"
was set on a scaffold in the town of Croydon, with a paper
on his breast, declaring him to be an impostor. He was
afterwards set on a pillory in Southwark.

In the reign of Queen Mary, a great number of empirical
impostors were prosecuted and punished, not only in London
but in other parts of the country; and during the reign of
Queen Elizabeth, these prosecutions continued, the delinquents
being fined various sums from £5 to £20, and in many cases
being imprisoned. Some of these quacks were patronised by
persons of rank, who wrote to the President of the College on
their behalf. Sir Francis Walsingham, Secretary of State,
interceded on behalf of "*Margaret Kenniæ,* an outlandish
ignorant sorry woman," but the College refused to remit the
sentence (1581).

John Booffeat (1583) was liberated from prison on the in-
tercession of a person of quality, upon condition that he
would submit to any penalty the College might inflict, if he
ever practised again.

Paul Fairfax (1588) was prosecuted for cheating the people by puffing the pretended virtues of a water which he called *Aqua Cœlestis*. He was fined £5 and imprisoned. The Lord Chamberlain addressed the College on his behalf, but to no purpose.

Paul Buck (1593), having been imprisoned for illegal practice, obtained letters of recommendation from Sir Francis Walsingham, the Lord High Admiral Howard, and Lord Essex.

John Lumkin, a surgeon (1593), being convicted of *mala praxis* on several patients, and being committed to prison, *propter malam praxin, et immodestos mores*, obtained letters from the Archbishop of Canterbury and the Dean of Rochester, and was released on bail.

In the year 1552 the question was argued before the Lord Mayor, whether Surgeons might give inward medicines, and the President of the College of Physicians was summoned to give his opinion, in accordance with which, the Lord Mayor decided that it was illegal for Surgeons to practise medicine. The College of Physicians issued a letter in 1595, prohibiting their interference with medical practice.

The question was again tried in the cases of *Read* and *Jenkins*, in 1595, when the Chief Justice decided, "That no Surgeon, as a Surgeon, might practise physic for any disease;" and that "no man, though never so learned a Physician or Doctour, might practise in London, or within seven miles, without the college licence."

In the year 1553, the College of Physicians obtained a new Act,* in which their former powers † were confirmed and enlarged, and in which it is stated that "the four censors, or any three of them, shall have authority to examine, survey, govern, correct, and punish all and singular Physicians and practisers in the faculty of physic, Apothecaries, Druggists, Distillers, and sellers of waters and oils, and preparers of chemical medicines," "according as the nature of his or their offences may seem to require."

In 1602, *Francis Anthony* was fined several times and imprisoned, for persisting in the administration of his *Aurum Potabile*, with which he occasioned the death of many patients.

---

* 1 Mary, c. 9.   † 32 Henry VIII., c. 40 (1540).

Dr. Alexander Leighton (1627) was interdicted from practice, being found unqualified, on examination by the president
and censors; he persisted in practice, was arrested, and censured in the Star Chamber and lost his ears. *Ellin Rix* undertook to cure a boy of consumption in fourteen days for £3.
" She gave him purging drinks once a day for seven days
together, and twice a day for 14 days more." The boy died
a fortnight after. She was fined £5 and imprisoned 14 days.

Mr. Briscoe, an apothecary (1634), appeared before the
president and censors, being accused of "falsifying a bill,"
having administered 2 drachms of *troch. alkakengi cum opio*
instead of *troch. gordonii*, as prescribed by Dr. Johnson, without asking the Doctor's opinion, for which offence he was
fined 5 marques and expelled the company.

It is uncertain at what period the Physicians gave up the
practice of preparing their own medicines; we are informed,
in a work entitled " *Short Answers to Tentamen Medicinale* "
(1704):

" 'Tis very well known there was no such thing as a Company of Apothecaries in the beginning of King James the
First's reign, but what drugs and medicines were then in use,
were sold in common by the grocers; and as for the preparing and compounding of them, that the Physicians principally
took care of themselves. But this growing too servile and
laborious a business, and no other means being likely to be
found out for easing themselves of it, but by lopping off a
considerable number of grocers who had mostly been brought
up that way, and constituting them a company by themselves,
wholly to be employed in the business of pharmacy, in selling
of drugs and preparing and compounding of medicines, according to the Physicians' orders and directions; in order to
this they obtained a charter for them to the number of a
hundred and fourteen."

This number coincides with the number of Physicians who
were then in practice in London.

The Apothecaries (who had been incorporated with the
Grocers into one company in the year 1606) were separated,
and obtained the charter above mentioned in 1617. It was
enacted at the same time that no grocer should keep an
Apothecary's shop, and that no Surgeon should sell medicines.
The power of searching the shops of Apothecaries within

seven miles of London, and examining their drugs, was also vested in the chartered body.

Soon after the Apothecaries were formed into a Society, they took into their serious consideration the frauds and artifices practised by the Grocers and Druggists from whom they obtained their drugs; and in order to remedy this evil, they established a dispensary in the year 1623, for the purpose of making some of the most important preparations for the use of their own members. This institution was placed under the inspection and superintendence of a Committee of Apothecaries, and was conducted, in the first instance, on a small scale, being confined to the manufacture of a limited number of preparations.

The first Pharmacopœia was published by the College of Physicians in the year 1618. This was the first step towards reducing the processes of Pharmacy to a regular standard for the guidance of dispensers of medicine. It was, however, a very imperfect production. Subsequent editions have been published by the College in 1621, 1632, 1639, 1650, 1677, 1721, 1746, 1788, 1809, 1815, 1824, and 1836.

The medicinal compounds formerly employed were chiefly empirical nostrums, or heterogeneous mixtures of substances, some of which neutralized others, and which were selected without any reference to scientific principles. One of the most striking instances of this practice is to be found in the Mithridate, which was a compound of seventy-two ingredients; and in looking over the ancient works on Pharmacy, a great variety of ridiculous formulæ present the same peculiarity. The science of Chemistry was so little advanced, that the real composition of ordinary remedies was seldom understood, and in many cases different virtues were attributed to the same substance, according to the source from whence it was obtained. Thus crab's eyes, prepared pearls, oystershells, and burnt hartshorn, were severally recommended as specifics in certain cases, the qualities of these remedies being supposed to be essentially different. Snails, vipers, the urine of men and animals, calculous concretions, various portions of criminals, as the thigh bone of a hanged man, and many other equally absurd remedies, were extolled as specifics for a variety of disorders.

Culpeper, in his translation of the Pharmacopœia (1653),

ridicules the catalogue of remedies derived from the animal kingdom, which were at that time enumerated in the Pharmacopœia of the college. The following is a portion of a list which will serve as a specimen, with Culpeper's remarks in parentheses :

"*The fat, grease, or suet of a duck, goose, eel, bore, heron, thymallos* (if you know where to get it), *dog, capon, bever, wild cat, stork, hedgehog, hen, man, lyon, hare, kite, or jack* (if they have any fat, I am persuaded 'tis worth twelve-pence the grain), *wolf, mouse of the mountains* (if you can catch them), *pardal, hog, serpent, badger, bear, fox, vultur* (if you can catch them), *album Grœcum, east and west benzoar, stone taken out of a man's bladder, viper's flesh, the brain of hares and sparrows, the rennet of a lamb, kid, hare, and a calf and a horse too* (quoth the colledg.) [They should have put the rennet of an ass to make medicine for their addle brains.] *The excrement of a goose, of a dog, of a goat, of pidgeons, of a stone horse, of swallows, of men, of women, of mice, of peacocks,*" &c. &c.

Although Culpeper abuses the college for inserting this absurd catalogue of remedies in their Pharmacopœia, he is not free from superstition himself, as he tells us, that " bees being burnt to ashes, and a ly made with the ashes, trimly decks a bald head, being washed with it." He also extols snails, as a cure for consumption, but blames the college for directing the slime to be separated from them with salt or bran before they are used, and supports his opinion by saying, that " Man being made of the slime of the earth, the slimy substance recovers him when he is wasted."

In describing *verbena* he says, " It is hot and dry, a great opener, cleanser, and healer, it helps the yellow jaundice, defects in the reins and ·bladder, and pains in the head, if it be but bruised and hung about the neck."

Of scammony, he says, " *Scammony*, or *diagridium*, call it by which name you please, is a desperate purge, hurtful to the body by reason of its heat, windiness, corroding or knawing, and violence of working. I should advise my country to let it alone ; 'twill gnaw their bodyes as fast as doctors gnaw their purses."

Culpeper says, that " the head of a cole-black cat being burnt to ashes in a new pot, and some of the ashes blown into the eye every day, helps such as have a skin growing over their sight. If there happen any inflammation, moisten an oak leaf in water and lay it over the eye.''

The compound waters, syrups, electuaries, and other pre-parations used at that time contain a vast number of herbs, flowers, juices, roots, etc., which are now obsolete, being found to be quite inert, and the properties ascribed to these remedies had reference, in many instances, to superstitious notions which belonged to the age. Culpeper, in the title-page of his Pharmacopœia, styles himself "*Nich. Culpeper, Gent., Student in Physick and Astrology,*" and in reading the work it is difficult to determine which science preponderates.

Notwithstanding the superstitious prejudices which prevail in the work, we see nevertheless in many passages an evidence of a close observance of nature, and just reasoning; for instance, in the translator's preface, we are told that "the time to gather all roots is before the herbs run up to seed." "Herbs are to be gathered when they are fullest of juice, which is before they run up to seed : and if you gather them in a hot sunshine day, they will not be so subject to putrifie. The best way to dry them is in the sun, according to Dr. REASON, though not according to Dr. TRADITION. Let flowers be gathered when they are in their prime, in a sunshine day, and dried in the sun. Let the seeds be perfectly ripe before they are gathered."

"In boyling syrups," Culpeper says, "have a great care of their just consistence, for if you boyl them too much they will candy, if too little, they will sour."

The Materia Medica was divided into two classes, Chymicals and Galenicals. The "Chymical Medicins" were of mineral origin, and prepared by fire; the Galenicals comprised the herbs, roots, and other vegetable or animal substances. The trade in these articles was also distinct, and Chymists are alluded to in works of the date now under consideration, as being a class of men who prepared these mineral compounds for the use of the Apothecaries.

THE TRIUMPHANT CHARIOT OF ANTIMONY, by Bazil Valen-tine, a work published in 1678, contains a curious account of that metal, with a great variety of processes for reducing it into a proper state for medicinal use. "This unlocking and preparing of mineral antimony," the author observes, "is per-formed by divers methods and ways, by the disposure and governance of the fire, with manifold labour of the hands, whence proceeds the operation, virtue, power, and colour of the medicine itself."

Antimony had hitherto been considered a poison, destitute of any utility, and was generally denounced by the profession; but Bazil Valentine undertook to prove that it is "more than any one simple of nature able to subdue and expel infinite diseases." He says, "The life of no one man is sufficient for him to learn all the mysteries thereof;" and that "when it is rightly prepared, its medicinal virtue consumes all noxious humours, purifies the blood in the highest degree, and performs all that may be effected by *aurum potabile*."

In tracing the origin of customs which are involved in the mist of antiquity, we are sometimes enabled to draw inferences, in cases where there is no very definite record of facts. In this respect, the following extracts from a pamphlet, published in the year 1671, entitled "*The Wisdom of the Nation is Foolishness*," serve to throw some light upon the subject:—

"Dr. Merret, a collegiate physician of London, and a practiser thirty years with Apothecaries, gives this account of them in his book lately put forth (page 8): They use medicines quite contrary to the prescriptions—myrtle leaves for senna, &c. . . They falsify the grand compositions of the London Dispensatory . . (page 9). 'Tis very common for them to load medicines with honey, and other cheaper ingredients, and to leave out in whole or in part those of greater value . . Such CHYMISTS which sell preparations honestly made, complain that few Apothecaries will go to the price of them . . All the drugs imported into England sooner or later are sold or made into medicines, although they have lain by years, with the MERCHANT, DRUGGIST, and APOTHECARY, before they are used."

Chemists are alluded to in a quaint poem, published in the year 1680, of which one stanza will serve as a specimen:

> " 'Mongst all professions in the town,
>   Held most in renown,
>   From th' sword to the gown,
> The upstart Chymist rules the roast;
>   For he with his pill,
>   Does ev'n what he will,

Employing his skill
Good subjects to kill,
That he of his dangerous art may boast.
O 'tis the Chymist, that man of the fire,
Who, by his black art,
Does soul and body part;
He smokes us, and choaks us,
And leaves us like Dun in the mire."

The following is an extract from an advertisement pub. lished in the year 1686 :

"GAZA CHYMICA.

" A magazine or storehouse of choice chymical medicines, faithfully prepared in my laboratory, at the sign of Hermes Trismegistus, in Watlin Street, London—by me, George Wilson, Philo-Chym.".

A house and shop, with a laboratory, were built on the Bedford estate, in the year 1706, by Ambrose Godfrey Hanckwitz, who had carried on business as a Chymist in the neighbourhood since 1680. He was a maker of phosphorus and other chymicals, which were rare at that period, and which he sold in different parts of the country during his travels. His laboratory was a fashionable resort in the afternoon, on certain occasions, when he performed popular experiments for the amusement of his friends. It opened with glass doors into a garden, which extended as far as the Strand, but which is now built upon. Four curious old prints of the laboratory in its former state are in the possession of its present proprietors, Messrs. Godfrey and Cooke, of Southampton Street, Covent Garden, also a portrait of Ambrose Godfrey Hanckwitz, engraved by George Vertue (1718), which he distributed among his customers as a keepsake.

The merchants and druggists, being a section of the Grocers' Company, merely sold articles in the raw or unprepared state, and the Chemists (who were not incorporated) took upon themselves the duty of preparing those medicines which required the aid of fire, and which were chiefly, if not entirely, minerals, earths, or preparations of the metals; and it is probable that the class alluded to derived their origin from the alchymists. It is unnecessary here to enter fully into the history of the alchymists, which would lead us into a series of details too voluminous for our present purpose. We need only observe, that their lives were devoted to the most persevering and laborious researches, undertaken in the hope of discovering an imaginary treasure, the *elixir vitæ* or *philosopher's stone*, from which they expected to obtain the power of transmuting the baser metals into gold, and also to prolong life.

M. Dumas gives the following as the process recommended by Raymond Lulle, who was born in 1235 :—"To make *the elixir of the sages*, or *the philosopher's stone* (and by this word *stone* the alchemists did not mean literally a stone, but a certain compound having the power of multiplying gold, and to which they almost always attributed a red colour), to make *the elixir of the sages*, take the *mercury of philosophers* (lead), calcine it until it is transformed into a *green lion* (massicot) ; after it has undergone this change, calcine it again, until it becomes a *red lion* (minium). Digest in a sand-bath this *red lion* with *acid spirit of grapes* (vinegar), evaporate this product, and the mercury will be converted into a kind of *gum* (acetate of lead) which may be cut with a knife : put this gummy matter into a luted cucurbit and distil it with heat. You will obtain an insipid phlegm, then spirit, and red drops. Cymmerian shades will cover the cucurbit with their sombre veil, and you will find in the interior a true dragon, for he eats his tail (*i.e.* the distilled liquor dissolves the residuum). Take this black dragon, break him on a stone, and touch him with red charcoal : he will burn, and assuming a glorious yellow colour, he will reproduce the *green lion*. Make him swallow his tail and distil this product again. Lastly, rectify carefully, and you will see appear *burning water* (pyro-acetic spirit) and *human blood*."*

This substance, called by the alchymist *human blood*, is a reddish-brown oil, which is formed during the distillation of the acetic acid in the above process. This oil has the property of precipitating gold, in the metallic state, from solu-

---

* *Leçons sur la Philosophie Chimique.* Par M. Dumas, 1837. For an outline of the History of Alchemy and the Alchemists, see *Histoire de la Chimie depuis les temps les plus reculés jusqu'à notre époque.* Par Le Dr. Ferd Hoefer. Tome Premier, 1842.

tions containing that metal; which property probably gave rise to an idea that it possessed the virtues which were so much desired. It wants, however, one very important property; namely, that of precipitating gold when there is none of that metal in the solution.

The Society of Apothecaries, which was formed in '1617, continued to prosper; and in the year 1671 they added a Chemical Laboratory to the Dispensary, which had been instituted in 1623. This was done by subscription, and the object contemplated in it was the preparation of chemicals for the use of the subscribers. It had been found no less difficult to obtain this class of substances in a state of purity than the ordinary drugs which were sold by the merchants and grocers, and by thus uniting in one establishment the preparations of " Chemicals " and " Galenicals," the Apothecaries opened out a new field of research to the members of their body, from which important results have arisen. The institution was, in the first instance, conducted on a small scale, commensurate with the limited means and the purpose for which it was designed; but the superior quality of the articles prepared by this Company of Apothecaries, led to an application (in 1682) on the part of other persons for a participation in the advantage.

We are not informed how soon this request was complied with, but within a few years the Company became a trading body and supplied any customers who came in their way.

About this period, Prince George of Denmark, the Lord High Admiral, contracted with the Company to furnish the Royal Navy with drugs and chemicals; and the increase in the demand rendered a considerable extension of premises and apparatus necessary, which was done by fresh subscriptions of large amount. By this means, the establishment became converted into a wholesale drug warehouse and manufactory, and although the original subscribers did not at first realize much, if any pecuniary advantage, they laid the foundation for a very lucrative concern.

Bate's Dispensatory, or, as it is usually termed, the *Pharma-copœia Bateana*, was published in 1691. It is arranged in three divisions: 1. Compound Chymick Internals; 2. Compound Galenick Internals; 3. Compound Externals. This work is curious on account of the mixture which it displays of laborious research and superstitious ignorance peculiar to the age.

In Quincey's "New Dispensatory," which enjoyed great celebrity, a different arrangement is adopted; the preparations being generally classified according to their effects, and the author enters at some length into the subject of therapeutics. The tenth edition was published in 1736.

In the year 1694, Apothecaries were exempted from serving the offices of constable, scavenger, and other parish duties, and from attendance on juries. By this time we are informed that their number had increased from 114 to nearly 1000. They had become a very influential body; and by practising medicine as well as Pharmacy, they excited the jealousy of the Physicians, who suffered materially from this encroachment, and endeavoured to reduce their rivals to their original condition, of grocers or vendors of drugs. The contest rose to a great height; on one side it was alleged that the improvement which had taken place among the Apothecaries was a great benefit to the public, and that the Physicians, by endeavouring to restrain them, were undoing what the labour of their predecessors had accomplished; while the other party animadverted on the extortionate charges of the Apothecaries, and the loss which the public sustained in being deprived of the advantage of the best advice in many cases, for which it was impossible to pay both the Physician and the Apothecary.

The evil was felt especially by the poor, and in order to meet the emergency, some of the Physicians united together in the establishment of dispensaries, where they supplied medicines on reasonable terms, employing assistants to dispense them under their own superintendence.

The following is a copy of an instrument subscribed by the president, censors, most of the elects, senior fellows, candidates, &c., of the College of Physicians, in relation to the sick poor :—

" Whereas the several orders of the College of Physicians, London, for prescribing medicines gratis to the poor sick of the cities of London and Westminster, and parts adjacent, as also the proposals made by the said College to the Lord Mayor, Court of Aldermen, and Common Council of London, in pursuance thereof, have hitherto been ineffectual, for that no method hath been taken to furnish the poor with medicines at low and reasonable rates : we, therefore, whose names are hereunder written, Fellows or Members of the said College, being willing effectually to promote so great a charity, by the counsel and good liking of the President and College, declared in their Comitia, hereby (to wit, each of us severally and apart, and not the one for the other of us) do oblige ourselves to pay to Dr. Thomas Burwell, Fellow and Elect of the said College, the sum of Ten Pounds a-piece of lawful money of England, by such proportions, and at such times, as to the major part of the Subscribers here shall seem most convenient ; which money, when received by the said Dr. Thomas Burwell, is to be by him expended in preparing and delivering medicines to the poor at their intrinsic value, in such manner, and at such times, and by such orders and directions, as by the major part of the Subscribers hereto in writing shall be hereafter appointed and directed for that purpose. In witness whereof we have hereunto set our hands and seals, this twenty-second day of December, 1696."

This document was published with fifty-three signatures and the following note :—

" The design of printing the Subscribers' names is to show that the late undertaking has the sanction of a College act ; and that it is not a project carried on by five or six Members, as those that oppose it would unjustly insinuate."

Three dispensaries were established, one at the Physicians' College in Warwick Lane ; another in St. Martin's Lane, Westminster ; and a third in St. Peter's Alley, Cornhill. They came into operation about the beginning of February, 1697, and were soon very generally resorted to for the preparation of Physicians' prescriptions, or " bills," as they were then termed, and also for the sale of medicines by retail.

The establishment of these institutions gave great offence to the Apothecaries, whose feelings on the occasion are thus expressed in the words of Garth, in his " Dispensary " :—

" Our manufactures now the Doctors sell,
And their intrinsick value meanly tell ;
Nay, they discover too (their spite is such)
That health, than crowns more valued, costs not much ;
Whilst we must shape our conduct by these rules,
To cheat as tradesmen, or to starve as fools."

A violent contest arose, and pamphlets were published on both sides of the question. It was asserted by the Apothecaries that the assistants employed at the dispensaries were unqualified, that the drugs were of bad quality, and the management in other respects defective. As a contrast to these abuses, the education and usefulness of the Apothecaries were insisted on in terms like the following :—

"Every Apothecary has eight years in his apprenticeship, by his own observation, to acquaint himself with drugs and plants, by the frequent use of them in the shops, besides often visiting the markets and physic-gardens ; and several set days in the summer, the Company have to go into the country on purpose to make acquaintance with all the vegetable tribes, the seniors, and more experienced, instructing the juniors. Then there is an elaboratory at their hall, open to all the Company, where they may see all the necessary processes of the chemical preparations, by which the different natures, &c., of bodies are laid open."

The following are the "*reasons*" which the Physicians gave '*for sending their wealthy patients, as well as the poor, to the dispensaries for their medicines* : "'

"First. Because the Physicians, prescribing for them, were assured that the medicines there were undoubtedly the best.

"Secondly. Because many excellent remedies are there deposited, which have never yet been trusted in the Apothecaries' shops.

"Thirdly. Because the Physician was not obliged to prostitute his honour and conscience by overloading his patient, to oblige a craving Apothecary, or run the risk of being undermined in his reputation by slanderous suggestions, for not submitting to be the Apothecaries' under-pickpocket.

"Lastly. Because he could serve his patient, quantity for quantity, and quality for quality, fifteen shillings in the pound cheaper than anywhere else : which is a thrift the greatest man that does not love to be cheated need not be ashamed of."

In corroboration of the justice of these allegations, with reference to the charges of Apothecaries, and the quantity of medicine they administered, an instance is quoted in the pamphlet above mentioned ("*The Wisdom of the Nation is Foolishness*"), and some of the items are enumerated.

"Apothecary's bill for attending Mr. Dalby, of Ludgate Hill, five days, total amount, £17 2s. 10d."

The following are the items of medicines for *one day* :

August 12th.	*s.*	*d.*		*s.*	*d.*
An emulsion . . .	4	6	Another bolus . . .	2	6
A mucilage	3	4	Another draught . .	2	4
Gelly of hartshorn . .	4	0	A glass of cordial spirits	3	6
Plaster to dress blister	1	0	Blistering plaster to the		
An emollient glister .	2	6	arms	5	0
An ivory pipe armed .	1	0	The same to the wrists	5	0
A cordial bolus . . ,	2	6	Two boluses again .	5	0
The same again . .	2	6	Two draughts again .	4	8
A cordial draught . .	2	4	Another emulsion . .	4	6
The same again . .	2	4	Another pearl julep .	4	6

This is quoted, not as an isolated case, but as an illustration of the practice of Apothecaries when attending patients of the higher classes.

Dr. Pitt, in a book entitled "*The Craft and Frauds of Physic exposed*" (1703), states,

"The *Dispensary* at the *College*, where all the preparations are made, and distributed to its now two branches, in *St. Martin's Lane, Westminster,* and *St. Peter's Alley, in Cornhill*, may probably make up yearly twenty thousand prescriptions. The doses of the electuaries, juleps, pills, etc., one with the other, may be about a penny a piece, though every the most useful drug, though of the highest prices, is in every composition. There never was, or ever will be, the least profit, beyond the necessary expense of servants, etc."

Dr. Pitt observes, in his preface, that when the abuses in the profession are complained of,

"The old usually answer, that they are ashamed to own the villany of their long former bills, by reforming their practice now. Others tell you that they'll leave physic as they found it, and not give themselves the trouble to treat the sick more faithfully. There are of the confederates who have said, that their scandalous profession would not last above four years, being every day more and more suspected, that they must make haste by venturing largely, to secure something by that time.

"But the affair is now laid clearly before you: in your

c

judgment of it, you are not capable of any error or fallacy. You see by the prices of the Dispensary, which are the just prices of the best medicines of the shop. You may observe by their practice and more certain success, that two or three medicines every day, at the value of as many shillings, overcome those diseases, which the more numerous aggravate to the death of the patient in all the difficult and dangerous cases. You may conclude from the whole, that this is the greatest instance and degree of madness, to rely on any advice, when the fee is procured by the multitude of medicines obtruded on all the diseases in all the constitutions."

" We know an Apothecary who over night appointed his servant to make ready twenty boles out of one pot, and twenty draughts out of one glass. These he conveyed to his customers the next morning, to the old and young, to the male and female, without distinction, and promised a new supply in the afternoon."

Another argument advanced by Dr. Pitt in favour of the Dispensaries is this :

"When the Apothecary deserts his station, is always abroad, and leaves the compounding part to his young unexperienced apprentice, who cannot avoid sometimes misusing one thing for another, by which errors very many are known to have lost their lives, you will allow that the people and the College shall reasonably provide for the safety of themselves and their patients."

Dr. Pitt exposes the absurd notions which at that time prevailed respecting the supposed virtues of many inert substances ; as, for instance, the Bezoar stone, which, he says, "has held its name and reputation almost sacred with us, though exploded long since in almost all other parts of Europe."

His observations on the " *Chymical medicins* " would almost apply to the homœopathic doses now in fashion.

" Their uses are very considerable to amuse the minds of the people with an assured expectation of releif from the magnify'd pretended powers of the preparations by fire * against all the feebleness of the spirits, and the last concluding coldness of death. And their titles are very necessary to

---

* Homœopathically, *for* "fire" *read* "friction in a mortar." See p. 125.

keep up the fallacy of the dearness of medicins : every chymi-cal grain or drop are the bezoar and the pearl, to deceiv the people into an opinion of their value."

" The profession has sunk into the craft of deceiving and amusing and making profit by new medicines, or preparations brought into fashion, and highly esteemed, as long as the mode of crying them up shall last."

These assertions of Dr. Pitt, and other allegations of a simi-lar nature against the Apothecaries, were answered by an Apothecary, in a small work above alluded to, entitled TEN-TAMEN MEDICINALE, *or an Enquiry into the Differences between* DISPENSARIANS *and* APOTHECARIES, *wherein the latter are proved capable of a skilful composition of Medicines, and a rational practice of Physick, to which are added some* PROPOSALS *to pre-vent their future increase.* (1704.)

Among other arguments, it is said, that

"The Physicians' directions in their bills, or dispensatory are not sufficient to instruct any one in the true composition of medicines there prescribed, unless he first be thoroughly acquainted with the nature and qualities of simple bodys, and qualify'd with most parts of knowledge necessary to one as a Physician. From whence it may justly be infer'd that he who is accomplished for a good Apothecary, is upon the bor-ders of making a good Physician."

In answer to the four " *Reasons* " above quoted, in favour of the Dispensaries, it is stated, that it is absurd to suppose that the Physicians can make their medicines better than the Apothecaries, since they devote so much less time to this pur-suit; that "when a Physician has got a guinea for his visit, it seldom much concerns his honour or conscience, how the Apothecary shall get a shilling for his medicines : " and that the assertions respecting the sophistication of drugs by Apo-thecaries are unjust and unfounded exaggerations.

The plan for preventing the further increase of Apothe-caries consisted in the institution of a strict examination of apprentices in Latin and Greek, public lectures at the hall, instruction in practical Pharmacy, and an examination at the close of apprenticeship, prior to the granting of a licence to practise as an Apothecary.

In another pamphlet, entitled " *The Necessity and Useful-ness of the* DISPENSARIES, *lately set up by the College of Physi-*

cians in London, for the use of the SICK POOR, *together with an Answer to all the objections rais'd against them by the* APOTHE-CARIES, *or others"* (1702), it is stated, that the Physicians were obliged to send their wealthy patients to the dispensaries in self-defence, because the Apothecaries entered into a combination to denounce all those who had subscribed to those institutions, and recommend others in their stead; that they purposely sent "ill-prepar'd medecins," in order "to make the patients question the Physicians' skill," and that they sometimes continued to keep patients in their own hands, even when labouring under dangerous disorders; and that, therefore, they required some check. It is also said, that the patients complained of the dearness of medicines sold by Apothecaries; as, for instance, when an ounce of a powder, value less than a shilling, was ordered in half-drachm doses, "yet the Apothecary, by officiously dividing it into sixteen papers, would make 8*s.* of it, viz. 6*d.* a paper." Another fact is mentioned, namely, that some "persons of condition" attended the dispensaries in *formâ pauperum,* and thus imposed upon the Physicians. (In this respect human nature still displays the same peculiarities, as we hear occasionally of patients leaving their carriages round the corner, while they call for the advice of a Physician who prescribes *gratis.*)

The author of the above pamphlet answers the argument "that Physicians ought not to sell physic, but only to prescribe it," by saying, "that Apothecaries ought not to give advice, but only to sell medicines."

Among the conflicting statements published on the subject of this controversy, it is not easy to arrive at the truth, but we may infer the prevalence of considerable exaggeration on both sides. It is clear, however, that the dispensaries prospered and enjoyed the patronage of the public; and we have reason to believe that the Assistants employed and instructed by the Physicians at these institutions, became dispensing Chemists on their own account; and that some of the Apothecaries, who found their craft in danger, followed the example, *from which source we may date the origin of the* CHEMISTS *and* DRUGGISTS.

It was not likely that the College of Physicians, or a section of the College, would for any length of time continue to conduct or superintend shops of this description. They had

commenced the undertaking from the double motive of enabling the public to obtain drugs at a reasonable rate, and at
the same time of gaining for themselves an advantage over
the Apothecaries, who had become formidable rivals. Having
succeeded in these objects, and a class of men having been
raised up to perform the drudgery of the business, it might
naturally be expected that they would be glad to be relieved
from any further mercantile responsibility ; and that the
parties whom they had employed as dispensers would be no
less anxious to assume the position of masters.

In the year 1723, the College of Physicians was again empowered by Act of Parliament* to visit and examine the shops
of Apothecaries, attended by the Master and Wardens of the
Company of Grocers, or one of them.

This Act was entitled, "*An Act for the better viewing, searching, and examining all Drugs, Medicines, Waters, Oils, Compositions, used or to be used for Medicines, in all Places where the
same shall be exposed to Sale, or kept for that Purpose, within
the City of London, and suburbs thereof, or within seven miles
circuit of the said city.*"

Some of the circumstances relating to this Act are rather
curious. James Goodwin, a Chemist and Apothecary, whose
business had for many years been extensive, made overtures,
in the year 1721, to the Royal African Company, to supply
them with drugs. Two Apothecaries (Markham, of Paternos-
ter Row, and Matthews, of the Poultry), who had been in
the habit of supplying the society, by the recommendation of
Dr. Levit, applied to the doctor to assist them in opposing
this inroad on their privilege. Dr. Levit, therefore, " undertook to destroy Goodwin, and to prove that he was an ignorant, illiterate person ; and that he neither knew a drug when
he saw it, nor what drugs were put into a composition." But
Goodwin being summoned before the company, so fully proved
the doctor's ignorance and his own integrity, that he obtained
the order for the supply of drugs. On this, Dr. Levit and
the Apothecaries vowed vengeance, and excited other Physicians to unite with them in applying for an Act of Parliament, conferring upon them additional powers in searching
shops. Among other Physicians, Dr. Shadwell joined with

* 10 George I., c. 22.

much spirit in this enterprise, having taken offence at Goodwin for applying to him for the payment of a debt due for
medicines.

On the 10th of June, 1724 (after the Act had passed), Dr.
Arbuthnot, Dr. Bale, and Dr. Plumtree, called at the shop of
Goodwin, and having ascertained that he was not at home,
they commenced the destruction of his goods, turning out one
drug after another, and burning them in the street.   Having
found a parcel of old plasters and other things, which had
returned from a voyage, in a chest sent to be re-filled, these
they sealed up, and sent to the College.   They then went to
another shop, belonging to Goodwin, in Charles Street, Westminster, and condemned every article which came into their
hands.   On the 13th, 14th, 15th, and 16th of June, paragraphs
were inserted in several public papers, of which the following
is a copy :—

"On Wednesday last, the four *Censors* of the *College of
Physicians*, and the two Wardens of the *Apothecaries'* Company, visited several *Chymists*, *Druggists*, and *Apothecaries'*
shops, pursuant to the authority granted them by a late Act
of Parliament, and we hear they burnt several drugs and
other things in the *Medicinal* Faculty, before the doors of Mr.
Goodwin, chymist, facing the *Haymarket*, the corner of *Pall
Mall*," etc.

It is stated as a remarkable circumstance, that Goodwin
was the only person whose drugs were condemned on this
occasion, although he, being in a large way of business, was in
the habit of supplying many other Druggists and Apothecaries
with a great proportion of their stock : in some articles he had
introduced considerable improvements, which gave him the
advantage of a very extensive trade.   Goodwin being summoned before the president and censors of the College, challenged all present to prove any of his drugs faulty, and offered
to compound on the spot any preparation, to compare with
those which had been condemned.   But he was ordered to
leave the room, and on being recalled was told that all the
articles were pronounced bad.   Having collected the evidence
of his servants, who had assisted in compounding the medicines,
he appealed again to the censors, and called on Dr. Arbuthnot,
who assured him that his drugs should not again be burnt before his house : but two days afterwards, when he was out on

business, the censors came before his door with a coach-load of faggots, made a great fire, and burnt the goods, to the great terror of Mrs. Goodwin, who happened to be at home. This event was also published in the papers.

In the year 1727, a bill was introduced, entitled "An Act* for continuing the Laws therein mentioned, relating to Copper Bars exported, and for better preventing Frauds committed by Bankrupts, and for searching Drugs and Compositions for Medicines." The Apothecaries petitioned the House of Commons against this Act, and were heard by their counsel, Mr. Fitzakerly and Mr. Lingard: who urged, with much earnestness, the objections against the bill. But when the Apothecaries were called upon to state whether any of them had suffered any of those hardships which had been mentioned, they remained silent, on which Goodwin came forward and stated his case. This annoyed the Apothecaries, because Goodwin was not a member of their company, on which account they had not called him as a witness, and were unwilling to be under any obligation to him. Dr. Friend and Dr. Shadwell spoke in prejudice of Goodwin, and would not allow him to reply; but Mr. Hungerford pleaded in his behalf. It was determined by the Committee that the Act should continue in force three years.

Goodwin being thus foiled, petitioned the House of Lords against the bill for continuing an Act entitled "*An Act* for the better viewing, searching, and examining all Drugs," etc., and was heard before the Committee on the 13th of May; but, notwithstanding the case which he made out, he could not succeed in gaining his point, and the bill was passed. It is said, however, that he gained £600 damages for the injury he had sustained.

The author of a pamphlet, entitled "Reasons against the Bill for viewing, searching, and examining all Drugs, Medicines," etc. (1731), gives the following anecdote:—

"I hear there is three or four grocers that have erected in Old Fish Street a gew-gaw elaboratory, and fitted up a whimsical shop, without any titles to their pots, on purpose, as 'tis supposed, to elude the Physicians' inquisition; by which means they propose to serve them as some of the

* 13 George I., c. 27.

Faculty was served in a search, who when they came into an Apothecary's shop in the skirts of the city, to examine his medicines, etc., saw a shop-pot standing on the counter, entitled *Ungt. Album;* but, by accident or on purpose, I can't say which, the Apothecary had put some *Album Græcum* in it. The gentlemen got about the pot, and were viewing it ; each gave his opinion : one said it was hard, another said it did not smell enough of the camphir, a third said it ought to be softened or malax'd with some oil ; but the fourth, in a passion, was for throwing it out of doors as a medicine corrupt and decayed, and not fitted for the use of man's body. The boy all this while hearing their learned arguments, smiled, but said nothing until they were for throwing it away : then he cried, ' Pray, gentlemen, don't throw it away, 'tis a very good medicine ; I was forced to go as far as Hampstead to procure the chief ingredient of it.' ' What is it, then ? ' said one of the learned. ' Why, gentlemen,' says the boy, ' 'tis white dogs' ——; I think you call it Album Græcum.' ' And what doth he do with this Album Græcum ? ' ' Sir,' says the boy, ' he mixeth it with honey, and he gives it his patients, and cures them of their sore throats.' "

In the Pharmacopœia of 1721, many of the ridiculous remedies formerly in use were omitted ; yet this edition contains among the Materia Medica a considerable number of substances which derived their reputation from superstition or prejudice; as, for instance, bees, earthworms, millepedes, vipers, album græcum, bezoar, calculi from the human bladder and from ox-galls, spiders' webs, usnea cranii humani, cranum hominis, stercus columbarum, etc., etc.

Many of the formulæ in this work appear to be constructed on the principle of a galvanic battery, as if the intensity of the effect had depended on the number of the ingredients. One formula, although not so complicated as some others, will serve to illustrate the state of Pharmacy at that period— PULVIS AD GUTTETAM.

℞ Rad. Fraxinellæ, Visci Quercus, Contrayervæ, Serpentariæ Virginianæ, Pæoniæ maris, Seminis Pæoniæ maris, Cornu Cervis calcinati, Ungulæ Alcis, ana drachmas duas ; Rad. Valerianæ Silvestris. unciam ; Carallii rubri, Cranii humanii, ana drachma tres ; Lapidis Hyacinthi, drachmam unam; Bezoardice occidentalis, drachmam unam et semiss, orientalis scrupulum. M. fiat pulvis: cui addi possunt Moschi grana quinque, Foliorum auri N° triginta.

It was generally supposed by our ancestors that it was necessary to correct and modify the action of all medicines, by adding others of an opposite nature, and remedies were often classified as hot and cold remedies, a certain proportion of each class being combined, according to the preponderance on one side or the other, which was desired. In preparing chemical medicines, the process was frequently repeated; in some cases above twenty times, under the idea that the efficacy was thus increased or concentrated. MERCURIUS DULCIS SUBLIMATUS, was directed to be sublimed at least three times; if sublimed four or five times or oftener, it was called CALOMEL, but not otherwise.

Vessels were also sometimes used for distillation which were so constructed that the contents of the receiver might easily be thrown back into the retort, without breaking the connection, by which means the process might be continued and repeated *ad infinitum*.

A very slight inspection of the Pharmacopœia of 1746 is sufficient to show that it is, in every respect, a great improvement upon that which preceded it in 1721. This amelioration is, perhaps, in hardly any respect more evident than in the number and nature of the syrups—they are reduced from forty to twenty-one, and the formulæ are much more simple; compare, for example, the Syrupus de Althææ of the older Pharmacopœia, and the Syrupus ex Althææ of the more recent one; the former contains about twenty ingredients, while the latter is prepared simply from the root of the plant, with the requisite proportions of sugar and water. The plasters are again reduced from about twenty-six to fourteen. Among those which are omitted, are the Emplastrum de Betonicâ, containing nearly twenty ingredients; and the Emplastrum Cæsaris, of which numerous herbs form also a part, and which contain about the same number of ingredients. It must, however, detract from the praise which might otherwise be fairly bestowed on this work, that Mithridatum, with its forty ingredients, and Theriaca Andromachi, with about sixty, were suffered to remain. The ointments are, however, reduced from about forty to half that number, and their formulæ are greatly simplified and improved. Among the chemical preparations of the metals, the progress of science is, in many cases, conspicuous : for example, under the head of SAL SEU VITRIOLUM MARTIS, in the Pharmacopœia of 1721, we find the following directions for preparing sulphate of iron :—

Fit ex Spiritus Vini optimi, unciis quator.
Olei Vitrioli, unciis duabus.
Serratis simul in vase ferreo ut Chrystalli formentur.

In the Pharmacopœia of 1746, this salt, under the name of Sal Martis, is prepared by dissolving iron filings in dilute sulphuric acid, filtering the solution after having for some time kept it warm, and then allowing crystals to form.

In the preparations of Mercury, advantageous changes are also made, both in the formulæ and nomenclature.

In no part of the more recent work is the improvement greater than in the expulsion of numerous useless articles from the Materia Medica. The entire work was carefully edited, and assumes a much more scientific form than any of its predecessors.

The Corporation of Apothecaries obtained a charter * in the year 1748, empowering it to license Apothecaries to sell medicines in London, or within seven miles; and also to search the shops within that district. This occasioned a fresh altercation, and many pamphlets and books were published on both sides. One of these, entitled *Frauds Detected*, supposed to have been written at the instigation of the Apothecaries' Company, advocates the necessity of a strict adherence to the Pharmacopœia of the College, and the importance of good quality in the articles employed. It contains a summary of the various adulterations which were said to prevail at that

---

* I am informed on good authority that the increased power which the Society of Apothecaries obtained in 1748 was not conferred upon them by a new charter, but by an Act of Parliament. I have not been able to find this Act at the British Museum or elsewhere, but have reason to believe it was one of the Acts by which in the first instance the College of Physicians and afterwards the Society of Apothecaries also, obtained authority to examine the medicines in Apothecaries' shops in and around London. These Acts were renewed at intervals of a few years.

T. R.

time, and concludes with a series of arguments in favour of a
frequent and effectual visitation of shops, which, it is said,
would be an advantage to the honest and a check on the
fraudulent. Among many other abuses which are enumerated,
it is said that few foreign drugs are brought into this country
free from impurities, being generally mixed with sticks, stones,
straws, dirt, etc., and that it is a not unfrequent practice
to " beat them into the most capital compositions (such as
mithridate, Venice treacle, diascordium, etc.), with the other
ingredients unpicked, and with all their dross about them.
Nay, what is worse, sometimes to beat in nothing but the
dross left after straining, just to flavour the medicine with
the little remains of the true drug sticking to it."
It was also said, that " in the tincture of rhubarb, and in
all other compositions in which this drug has a place, it was
too frequent a practice to pick out from the heap all the bad
rhubarb and hide it in them; " that " sal prunel " was sometimes adulterated with " alom; " that in diacodium, three-
fourths of the poppy-heads were often omitted; that, in lapis
contrayervæ, the pearls were omitted, and oyster-shell powder
substituted; that in Gascon's powder, the greenish colour of
the bezoar stone was imitated by a little Spanish-juice and
ox-gall; that in elixir proprietatis, and other preparations
containing saffron, two-thirds of the quantity was omitted,
when the price of saffron was high : that in mithridate,
nearly all the expensive ingredients were left out, etc., etc.
Several answers to this publication appeared, among which
is one entitled " *An Enquiry into the designs of the late* PETITION
*presented to Parliament by the Company of Apothecaries, where-
by the Apothecaries' monstrous profits are exposed, and compared
with those of the Chemist, with respect to practice and retail, to
which is annexed a Scheme to prevent the empirical Apothecary
from practising; and the Chemist from preparing and vending
sophisticated Medicines.*" The author of this pamphlet ac-
knowledges the importance of a strict adherence to the
formulæ of the Pharmacopœia, but asserts, that even the
Apothecaries' Company do not set the example, and denies
the propriety of their being empowered to search shops. A
case is mentioned in which the inspectors appointed by the
company had been in the habit of annually visiting an
Apothecary, and extorting from him six shillings each time as

their perquisite, which he at length began to resist. On one occasion he was not at home when they called, and on examining his mithridate, they all condemned it as a medicine not fit to be used. At this moment the Apothecary returned, and on being told that his mithridate was bad, and asked for the customary fine, he said,—

"Nay, now I am convinced what a nest of villains I have to deal with, who being nettled at my refusing their usual imposition, begin to show their knavish principles, by condemning medicines of their own compounding."

He then produced the invoice from his file, and called the man as a witness who brought the mithridate from the Hall.

Having endeavoured to show, by this and other instances, that the inspectors of the company were not competent judges, the author observes,—

"And if this be true, how can you expect Apothecaries in general to compound medicines justly, when they have so bad an example ? . . .

"It is generally allowed that one half, if not three out of four of those who style themselves Apothecaries, in and about London, some too in very reputable practice, are so very illiterate, that they understand no more of compounding and preparing capital medicines than they do of the philosopher's stone. . . . Nay, there is not one in ten who perfectly understands the derivation and meaning of his technical terms, or can read the Physician's bill truly, in proper Latin, nor perhaps understands it any better abbreviated : so that these persons are under the greatest obligations to Dr. Pemberton for translating the late Dispensatory into English."

The author also observes,—

"It has been often remarked, that there are not upwards of twenty regular Chemists in London, and yet there are hundreds who style themselves so. . . . To a man who is qualified, the method of compounding *Galenical* medicines will very naturally occur, though in this there is more honesty than knowledge required; but it must be allowed, that no man knows how to mix and proportion ingredients of various qualities so well as he who is acquainted with chemical principles."

One of the objects of the Apothecaries' petition alluded to

in this pamphlet, was to obtain an Act of Parliament which would give that body the power of searching the shops of *Chemists*, as well as Apothecaries. This privilege was not granted, and the author of the pamphlet endeavours to prove that the Chemist who prepares medicine is a more competent judge of their quality than the Apothecary who procures them ready made. He admits that there are many among the Chemists, Druggists, and Apothecaries, who are unqualified and dishonest, and he proposes as a remedy, the appointment of a committee, consisting of an equal number of Physicians, Druggists and Chemists, to be annually chosen by the College of Physicians, as inspectors of shops.

In another answer to *Frauds Detected*, entitled *The Apothecary Displayed*, the several charges of adulteration are answered *seriatim*. In reference to the statement that the Druggists mix into their compositions the impure drugs as they receive them from abroad, etc., it is said,—

" It is almost impossible for men to be more diligent and careful, or to take more pains than they do ; how often may you see them with a *Seron of Bark*, first sifting away the dust, then separating the small sort, dividing the large and woody from the more delicate and curious quill; while they are thus cleansing, sorting, and dividing their drugs, one or other of the most eminent Apothecaries alights from his chariot at the door, and buys up all the raspings of the rhubarb, the siftings of the bark, and the sweepings of the shop. Does he buy it to burn, think you, or conscientiously to destroy it for the good of mankind (as they would make you believe in their petition) ? No, he says he only wants it for powder, or it will do well enough for the tincture or the syrup; or if perchance he purchases four ounces of the better sort only to keep in a glass and show his customers, has he not four pounds of the worst sort with it ? . . . If the Druggist beats in the dross with the drug, where has he the dross to beat in by itself ? You know the Apothecary bought that, and could he be supposed to beat in the dross by itself, what the DEVIL becomes of the drug ? "

This is the kind of argument which abounds in the works written at the period now under consideration, and so many ludicrous instances of ignorance and fraud are enumerated by all parties, each against the other, that a very elaborate

and amusing compilation might be made from these curious
documents. It is however sufficient for our present purpose
to introduce a few quotations as examples.

In a pamphlet, entitled "THE APOTHECARIES' MIRROR, or the
present State of Pharmacy exploded (1790)," the incompetence
of many Apothecaries who had not passed the regular examination is adverted to, and various instances are cited in
corroboration; from this it appears, that the law respecting
the licensing of Apothecaries was not generally enforced.
The author also exposes the manœuvres commonly practised
between Physicians and Apothecaries—the Physicians prescribing a vast quantity of medicines for the benefit of the
Apothecary; and the Apothecary in return only recommending
such Physicians as were in the habit of " writing well," or, in
other words, "multiplying their nauseous superfluities." Arguments are also brought forth to prove that the Apothecary
ought not to practise medicine. It is said that

" The proper business of an Apothecary is to compound
certain drugs, according to Physicians' or Surgeons' prescriptions. It may happen that some of these articles require
pulverizing; but it is presumed, that beating at a mortar
does not necessarily make a man learned. . . . All the
advantages they presume upon beyond these are only seeing
eminent practitioners' prescriptions and their patients. . . .
The compounding of medicines prescribed, and knowing why
they are prescribed, are two different things: one is an
ordinary habitual thing, the other depends upon the circumstances of the case, and cannot possibly be judged of unless
by one who understands the natural history of the human
body, and is acquainted with the mechanism and operations of
nature. These are heights of knowledge at which few
Apothecaries arrive."

The first Edinburgh Pharmacopœia was published in 1699,
and new editions appeared in 1722, 1736, and 1744. Four
years afterwards, Dr. Lewis published an English translation,
under the title of " The New Dispensatory." This work
contained much additional information, and was attended
with great success. Dr. Lewis published several editions,
and was succeeded by Dr. Webster and Dr. Duncan, and,
lastly, by Dr. Duncan, jun., who published eight editions in
the course of twelve years. Dr. James's " Pharmacopœia

Universalis, or New Universal English Dispensatory," was published in 1747.

Subsequent editions or republications of the Edinburgh Pharmacopœia appeared in 1756, 1774, 1783, 1792, 1803, 1804, 1806, 1813, 1817, 1839, 1841. It was invariably published in Latin until 1839, when the English language was adopted by the Edinburgh College.

The Apothecaries' Hall was partially destroyed at the Fire of London, and in the year 1786 it was rebuilt on a more extensive scale, and improved in every respect. This event is commemorated in an inscription on the walls of the present establishment, which is as follows:

AVLA
HIC SITA PRIVS APTATA IN VSVM
SOCIETATIS PHARMACEVTICÆ LONDINENSIS
A.D. MDCXXVIII.
RICARDO EDWARDO, MAGISTRO
EDWARDO COOKE, LEONARDO STONE CVSTODIBVS
ILLA
IN CONFLAGRATIONE LONDINENSI PENITVS CONSVMPTA
LAPSIS DECEM ANNIS ELEGANTIOR RESURREXIT
REPARATA DEMVM FVIT
MVLTVM AMPLIATA ET ORNATA
A.D. MDCCLXXXVI.
IOANNÆ FIELD, MAGISTRO
GULIELMO BALL, MATTHÆOYATMAN
CVSTODIBVS.

The Apothecaries' Hall continued to compete successfully with the Druggists and merchants in the supply of medicines to the navy, and the East India Company, as well as in other business, both wholesale and retail. This gave rise occasionally to disputes and controversies, and several pamphlets, published about this time, contain reciprocal charges made by the Druggists and Apothecaries against each other of furnishing adulterated articles.

It may be supposed that these charges were not altogether without foundation, although it appears by the result that the Apothecaries had the advantage, as they succeeded in monopolizing a large share of the export business.

The origin of the BOTANIC GARDEN AT CHELSEA, belonging to the Society of Apothecaries, is involved in some obscurity;

but it is supposed to have been founded prior to the year 1673.
The first mention of it in the records of the society is contained in a minute (dated June 21st, 1674), in which it was
resolved to build a wall round the garden, which was to be
done by subscription, provided the Court of Assistants would
agree to pay two pounds for each of the herborizings or
botanical walks. These walks were instituted in the year
1633, at which period one took place annually; but at the
time the above agreement was entered into, the number had
been increased to six. The proprietors of the laboratory stock
also gave fifty pounds towards the expense of the wall; in
consideration of which they were allowed a piece of ground
in the garden for herbs.

In the year 1679, a Committee of Management was appointed, consisting of twenty-one assistants, thirty liverymen,
and twenty of the yeomanry. In the following year a greenhouse was built, at an expense of £138. Mr. Evelyn, in his
diary, mentions a visit which he paid to the "Apothecaries'
Garden of Simples" (August 7th, 1685), where he saw
among other rare plants, "the tree bearing the Jesuit's bark,
which had done such wonders in quartan agues." He also
notices the subterraneous heat employed in the greenhouse.

The propriety of discontinuing the garden was discussed in
the year 1693, from which it would appear that it was not in
a flourishing condition. The decision, however, was in its
favour, and in 1697, Lord Cheyne granted a new lease for
sixty years. In 1708, it was found necessary to raise additional funds, and ninety persons joined in a subscription. In
1714, Sir Hans Sloane became connected with the institution,
having purchased the manor of Lord Cheyne in 1712; and in
1722 he granted a lease to the Master, Wardens, and Society
of Apothecaries, on certain conditions, of which the following
is the substance:—The garden, comprising three acres, one
rood, and thirty-five perches, together with the greenhouse
and other erections thereon, was to be held by the parties
aforesaid for ever, at a yearly rent of five pounds, payable
to Sir Hans Sloane, his heirs, and assigns, provided the
society presented annually to the President, Council, and
Fellows of the Royal Society of London, fifty specimens of
distinct plants, until the collection amounted to 2000; and
provided, also, that the garden was appropriated to the pur-

pose of cultivating plants, instructing students, and advancing science. In the event of any of these conditions being violated, or dwellings being erected on the ground, the lease was to be forfeited.

In 1743 an order was issued that no person should be allowed to gather specimens without the permission of the director or gardener; and that none but members might walk in the garden without being attended by the gardener. In 1747, Sir Hans Sloane presented £100 towards the repairs of the greenhouse, and in 1748 he gave £150 to aid in maintaining the garden. Other individuals gave liberal donations at various times, without which the garden could not have been maintained. Mr. Miller, one of the chief gardeners, was elected to that office in 1722, and retained it forty-eight years. He was buried at Chelsea, and some years afterwards a cenotaph was erected to his memory by the members of the Linnean and Horticultural Societies. Further particulars respecting Mr. Miller and other gardeners connected with the institution, may be found in a work entitled MEMOIRS, *Historical and Illustrative, of the* BOTANIC GARDEN AT CHELSEA, *belonging to the* SOCIETY OF APOTHECARIES, *London,* by those who can find the work, which is very scarce.* A statue of Sir Hans Sloane was placed in the garden in 1751. In 1771 an embankment was built to recover portions of the ground which had been washed away by the river.

The botanical walks continue to be kept up. Five of them are open to the apprentices of every member of the society; and one, which is called the general herborizing, is confined to members. As the excursions generally occupy the whole of the day, refreshments are provided for the students, who derive considerable benefit from this social and practical method of studying botany.

It was intended by the Charter of 1748,† not only to restrain Druggists from practising Pharmacy, being considered unqualified, but also to prohibit Physicians and Surgeons from selling or preparing the medicines which they prescribed. But, notwithstanding this monopoly in favour of the Apothecaries, they found it impossible to secure to themselves those

---

* A new edition, continued to the present time, has been published by R. H. SEMPLE, M.D.—1878. T. R.

† See note at page 26.

exclusive privileges provided in the Act: the law was constantly evaded, and in the year 1793 they instituted an inquiry into the defects and privations which existed among them, and which arose, as they stated, from two grand causes:— *

First—"The encroachment which Chemists and Druggists have, of late years, made on the profession of the Apothecary, by vending pharmaceutic preparations, and compounding the prescriptions of Physicians.

Secondly—"The want of a competent jurisdiction in the profession itself, to regulate its practice, and to restrain ignorant and unqualified persons from practising at all."

In the spring of this year (1793) several respectable Apothecaries formed themselves into a society for the purpose of investigating the sources of the existing evils ; and, by means of an extensive correspondence, they collected "a volume of facts demonstrative of the injury resulting to society at large, as well as to the profession in particular, from the toleration of these abuses."

On the 17th of June, 1794, a general meeting of the Apothecaries of this kingdom was held at the Crown and Anchor, in the Strand, at which about 200 attended.

The object of the meeting was stated by Mr. Chamberlaine, and it was urged in the report,

"That this unjust and innovating usurpation of the Druggists, together with the intrusion of uneducated and unskilful persons into professional practice, called loudly for some speedy and effective Act, which should at once destroy the obtrusions complained of, and restore credit and respectability to the profession.

"If we regard personal views, it was stated to be a fact, the proof of which was in the tables of calculation then present, that were the aggregate sums obtained by this infringement of the Druggists, and divided amongst the Druggists of this metropolis (a body of men unknown to the world till about the end of the last century, unauthorized by any public charter, and almost undefined by any public Act), were these sums to be divided, as they ought to be divided, amongst the Apothecaries of the metropolis, every one would have an addition of nearly £200 a year to his present income. But

* See Good's "History of Medicine."

this evil, it appeared, was not confined to the capital; it was declared to be a morbific infection—that it began at the capital as a central point, but diffused its deadly breath from thence to all the larger cities and towns throughout the kingdom. Nor stopped the contagion here. From the larger cities and towns it was beheld propagating itself to smaller cities and towns, till at length, so general was the disease, there was scarcely to be found a village or a hamlet without a village or a hamlet Druggist. If the sale of medicines and the giving of advice was not here sufficient to support the vender, he added to his own occupation the sale of mops, brooms, bacon, butter, and a thousand such articles besides."

The hardships endured by the Apothecaries having been described at some length, the report proceeds to discuss the ignorance and inefficiency of the Druggists, some of whom are said to have made fatal mistakes, and

" From want of classical education, and an incapacity of translating the directions appended to their prescriptions, have been under the necessity of disturbing Apothecaries in the night to translate for them; others who, from boldly adventuring to interpret, have given wrong directions, or who, not daring to interpret, have dispensed their medicines without any directions at all.

*   *   *   *   *   *

" The composition of prescriptions, and the vending of pharmaceutic preparations by Druggists, comprise, then, a national evil of no small magnitude. The materials they make use of must, in general, be mere offals, and the refuse of better drugs; and from want of classical knowledge, perpetual errors and negligences are discovered in their combination. The credit of the Physician is endangered, and the patient perhaps is destroyed. But if this be a source of national abuse and deceit, what infinite injury must result from the still bolder practice such men often allow themselves, of adding pretended medical advice to erroneous medical compositions? Men who have never enjoyed any other medical education than what their own counters have afforded, and who can know nothing of the powers of diseases, or of the powers of medicines to remove those diseases when present? To attempt to demonstrate this to be a public evil, and one that calls loudly for redress, is altogether to lose time : it is to light up the sun at noonday with a candle."

In order to put an end to these abuses, it was proposed to form a General Association of the Apothecaries of Great Britain, who should

" Engage to deal with such Druggists only as would immediately consent to relinquish the composition of all medical prescriptions—to retain to themselves their wholesale occupation alone—and to receive no Apprentice, and employ no Assistant, who had not had a classical education."

It was resolved also to form a general Committee, to act in the name of the whole, and to endeavour to obtain the necessary reformation by an application to Parliament.

Alluding to the chances of success, Mr. John Mason Good, whose speech is contained in the report, proceeds to state :

" As to opposition, we had no reason to expect it, but from the Druggists themselves. Nor were all the Druggists inimical to medical reform—many had already expressed their good wishes towards it, and some had even contributed pecuniary assistance to carry it into execution. But if the Druggists are to oppose us, who are to oppose the Druggists? Druggists, like all others engaged in commercial transactions, are dependent men. On whom are Druggists dependent? On Apothecaries, on ourselves. Let us then make that use of this dependence which it behoves us to make. Let us universally and individually write to every Druggist with whom we traffic, and inform him that if he values the connection between us, we insist upon it, on the continuance of that connection, that he withhold from us all personal opposition whatsoever. Let us publish to all Druggists, that if, deaf to their own interests as well as ours, they should nevertheless persist in opposing us ; should they frustrate our intentions, and wrench, if it were possible, the very statute from our hands after we had obtained it, and tear it into a thousand tatters, we have still left the former resource of associating ourselves against such opponents, we have still left the power of creating one common fund, of establishing one general magazine, of supplying ourselves from such magazine, and thus by a single act, of ruining their whole trade, and destroying their existence as a commercial community."

    *   *   *   *   *   *

It was then proposed,

" That the persons present should form themselves into a society, under the title of THE GENERAL PHARMACEUTICAL ASSOCIATION OF GREAT BRITAIN, and that all other regularly educated practitioners throughout the kingdom be invited to associate in the common cause."

A Committee of twenty members was elected; and it was resolved,

" That it have regular meetings once a month, or as much oftener as may be deemed convenient, at the BUFFALO TAVERN, BLOOMSBURY SQUARE (the first meeting to be held on the 28th day of the present month, July); that it be open to the admission of every member of the Association, and be at liberty to summon general meetings, and to report progress whenever it may seem expedient to do so."

A subscription of one guinea from each member was collected.

The Committee then undertook, by means of a systematic and universal correspondence, to communicate with every regularly educated practitioner in Pharmacy throughout the kingdom, for the purpose of urging them to join the Association, and also with a view to collect a further supply of evidence. It was found necessary to appoint special committees, and to meet regularly twice every month at the Buffalo Tavern. Mr. Good states in his report—

"The extent of their correspondence is only bounded by the extent of the kingdom; and the materials collected most voluminous and immense. The ardour evinced by practitioners, in every part of the country, to forward the common cause, is uniform and universal; and scarcely a post arrived in London for the first two months after the establishment of the Association, without new statements, from personal knowledge, of increasing evils accruing from the toleration of the abuses. There is not perhaps a single Druggist in the whole kingdom who compounds his different preparations in all respects consistently with the College Dispensatory; but the Druggists at Manchester appear to excel all others in such nefarious ingenuity, and to extend their endeavours to save trouble and expense to articles in which it could be scarcely imagined such endeavours were necessary.

"A correspondent at Croydon mentions his having been

applied to by the foreman of a Druggist for an explanation
of the words ' *cucurbita cruenta*,' which he had in vain sought
for amongst the different preparations in his dispensatory;
and at last had been happy enough to translate them ' *an
electrical shock*.'

"A Druggist of similar penetration is reported, in a letter
from Worcester, to exist in that city, who took infinite pains
to obtain, by sending to other shops, a tincture of the name
of ' *ejusdem*.' "

In order to obtain evidence of the general prevalence of
similar misdemeanours, a number of specimens of drugs and
preparations were obtained at different shops in London, and
submitted to a special Committee for examination.   The
Committee state as the result—

" That in the far greater number of instances, there were
most evidently spurious or defective drugs, and erroneous
composition.   That the most expensive medicines were all
of them, without any exception, adulterated;" "such was
the case, particularly, with Aleppo scammony, with saffron,
and Russian castor."—" Powder of gum-arabic was generally
very indifferent; and, in one instance, when formed into a
mucilage, contained no gluten * whatever, was extremely
dirty and extremely opaque."—" The preparations from extemporaneous prescriptions scarcely bore any resemblance to
what was expected, had they been compounded aright; and
no two from the same prescription were similar."—" The
directions were, in many cases, misconceived and improperly
translated; in others, not more than half translated; and in
one instance, particularly, the very reverse of what was
written."

Among other circumstances investigated by this energetic
Association, the increase in the number of Druggists claimed
particular attention;   and from the statistical information
thus obtained, it appears, that in some places the number had
increased fourfold in the space of ten or twelve years.   A
correspondent, who related the opening of three new shops
in one town within twelve months, observes,—

" But Pharmacy alone comprises too small a field for these
men of letters and ambition—they prescribe, whenever ap-

---

* " No gluten " ! !

plied to, though totally ignorant of medical science, and even pretend to reduce fractures."

The Committee, alluding to this circumstance, remark,—

" But Druggists are not the only persons who are thus adventurous. In many places the grocers of the town take upon themselves this very benevolent office, or at least a part of it. In the small town of Uckfield there are not less than three of this description, who prescribe as well as vend medicines, applying for information to the Druggists with whom they deal; who in consequence hereof send them down advice just equal to their medicines, and present them with tables of different doses."

The Committee spared no exertions in collecting from every quarter, cases of malpractice and misadventure, a few specimens of which serve to enliven their report, adding that " The secretary would satisfy the curiosity of any person who wished for farther specimens of the same destructive conduct, at any time, when properly applied to, and from proper motives."

Having collected a sufficient mass of evidence, the Committee presented addresses to the College of Physicians, the Corporation of Surgeons, and the Society of Apothecaries ; and on the sixth of February, 1795, a petition was presented to Parliament on behalf of the Association, by Sir William Dolben. It was found necessary, however, to postpone the completion of these measures until the following session, and in the meantime a full report of proceedings was circulated to all the members, calling upon them to second these efforts by means of addresses, in which the following principles were to be continually adverted to :

" *First*, That the liberty to vend pharmaceutical preparations, compound Physicians' prescriptions, etc., etc., should appertain to the Apothecary alone. *Secondly*, That no young men be taken as apprentices, who have not had an approved education. *Thirdly*, That none be assistants without having been examined as to their competency for pharmaceutical compositions, etc., etc. *Fourthly*, That none be at liberty to settle until examined; nor any person entitled to an examination until he shall have faithfully served an apprenticeship of five years at least. *Fifthly*, That to promote these purposes, a competent court be established—to consist of *a certain*

number of members, who shall have full power to make such
bye-laws and regulations as may be thought most conducive
to the welfare both of the public and the profession."

From the above brief account of the establishment of the
Pharmaceutical Association of 1794, it will be seen that, at
this period, the Chemists and Druggists were entering upon
that position which they now occupy, as dispensers of medicine.

The result of these exertions, however, was not so successful as was anticipated, and the Pharmaceutical Association
of 1794 was broken up within a short time of its formation,
without having effected the extinction, or subjugation, of
that class against which its efforts were directed. The proceedings of the Association are recorded by Mason Good,
who was a leading member, and from whose work the above
outline is taken; the absence of a similar record of particulars
on the other side forms a gap in our history. It is probable
that this violent attack, which was designed as a death-blow
to the rising class of pharmaceutists, had the opposite effect,
by obliging them in some degree to reform the system of
conducting their business, and to unite among themselves for
the protection of their interests.

In the year 1802 the Apothecaries and Chemists were
brought together and induced to coalesce for the purpose of
protecting their mutual interests against the injurious operation of the Medicine Act, passed on the 3rd of June in that
year. The Act had reference to the duties, stamps, and
licences which had formerly been confined to private nostrums
and patent "specifics," but which, by the new measure, involved, more or less, the sale of many common remedies and
articles in daily use, such, for instance, as blistering ointment,
nitre drops, lozenges, tooth powders, Indian arrowroot, salve
for ulcerations of the legs, Huxham's tincture of bark, Turkey
rhubarb, laxative pills, etc., etc. An Association having been
formed, and a Committee appointed, a petition was prepared
entitled "A Petition of Apothecaries, Chemists, and Druggists,"
which petition was addressed to the Lords Commissioners of
the Treasury, signed by Fenwick Bulmer, Strand; John
Pugh, Gracechurch Street; Edward Complin, Bishopsgate
Street; William Chamberlain, Aylesbury Street; and John
Hingeston, Cheapside. During the time that the Committee
were engaged in carrying their object into effect, they pub-

lished, in one of their reports, a caution to all parties concerned, which will serve to point out the predicament the trade was in, and the liabilities to which all venders of medicines were exposed. It is as follows:

" The Committee also think it would be the means of preventing trouble, if something like the following cautions were adopted, in all such cases where it will apply.

" *Viz.* If an informer, or any other person, should inquire for healing salve for scalds or burns, to answer that no salve is known by that name, yet they may have for that purpose white unguentum, Turner's cerate, or spermaceti ointment, etc., without a stamp. If asked for nitre drops, not to sell anything by that name, but to offer dulcified spirits of nitre. Tincture of Turkey Rhubarb, a thing not known in the shops, yet common tincture of rhubarb may be sold without restriction. If castor oil medicine should be sought for, sell simply castor oil: in this manner stamps will not be necessary.

The Committee have been informed, from high authority, that informations will not be encouraged upon articles that have been long and generally known, although they may come nearly within the letter of the Act; yet they cannot help feeling the most lively indignation, when they reflect that men so truly respectable as the Apothecaries, Druggists, and Chemists undoubtedly are, should, by any circumstances in the common practice of their profession, be under the necessity of adopting any subterfuge to avoid being plundered of their property by the innumerable host of informers which this Act will certainly engender and let loose upon them, both in town and country, after the first of September.

"EDWARD DENTON, *Secretary.*"

The final report of the Committee was published in the year 1803, and although they were not successful in obtaining a total repeal of the Act, they secured the modification of it in such a manner as to remove the chief sources of inconvenience and oppression.

The Pharmacopœia of 1809, which was translated by Dr. Powell, was prepared by a Committee of the Fellows of the College in conjunction with a Committee of the Apothecaries' Company, in whose laboratory such experiments were made on the various processes as appeared necessary. Some additions were made from the Pharmacopœias of Edinburgh and

Dublin, and a " Specimen Pharmacopœiæ " was sent by the
College of Physicians to those persons whom they thought
likely to afford assistance or information. Seventy new preparations were introduced, among which were : Acetum
colchici, confectio amygdalarum, decoctum aloës comp., and
five other decoctions; extractum aloës purificatum, belladonnæ,
hyoscyami, sarsaparillæ, and six other extracts ; infusum
anthemidis, aurantii, digitalis, and twelve other infusions;
mistura ferri comp., potassæ carbonas, sodæ carbonas, liquor
arsenicalis, etc., etc.

Notwithstanding the precautions which were taken in the
compilation of this Pharmacopœia, it was found to be defective in some particulars, and the formulæ as well as the
nomenclature were severely criticised by several commentators. Dr. Bostock published an "Essay on the Nomenclature of the New London Pharmacopœia," in which he
showed that, while the endeavour to regulate the names of
the articles in the Materia Medica by scientific principles had
failed, and led to inconsistency in many cases, it had also
involved the subject in unnecessary confusion, and added to
the intricacy naturally belonging to it.   In confirmation of
this statement he quoted the following observation of Dr.
Powell : "As by names substances are distinguished from
each other, their essential properties ought to be brevity and
dissimilarity ; and if those employed be accurately defined
and generally understood—if they be sanctioned by use and
so distinct as not to be liable to be mistaken, and, above all,
convey no false ideas of the substances they are intended to
designate, such a nomenclature may be considered as perfect."
Dr. Bostock advocated these sentiments, and pointed out a
great variety of instances in which Dr. Powell had violated
his own principle by the introduction of a nomenclature professedly " scientific," but which, from its inconsistency, did
not deserve the name.

The most severe critique which appeared on the Pharmacopœia of 1809, was a review by Mr. Richard Phillips, which
was originally published in the London Medical Review
(1810), and afterwards in a separate pamphlet (1811), entitled, *An Experimental Examination of the last edition of the
Pharmacopœia Londonensis, with Remarks on Dr. Powell's
Translations and Annotations.* Mr. Phillips observes in his

introduction that, "although individual error may be insignificant, yet when established and enforced by the authority of law, it becomes truly formidable;" and, after a few prefatory remarks, proceeds to criticise seventy-three of the preparations in the Pharmacopœia, quoting experiments in confirmation of his statements. The first sentence deserves to be quoted in italics :

"*Before I proceed to the principal object of this essay, I shall make a few observations upon the alteration of the names of measures. This was not only unnecessary, but by the mode in which it has been carried into effect, it has been productive of much ambiguity and some absurdity.*"

Mr. Phillips enumerates about twenty instances in the Pharmacopœia in which the value of the term *libra* is ambiguous.

Some of the remarks of Mr. Phillips on the preparations are rather caustic, as, for instance, the following: "According to Dr. Powell's statement, protoxide and peroxide of antimony are synonymous, and ten grains may be properly exhibited; but if we combine these assertions with those of the authorities which he recommends, it appears that, whilst ten grains of the precipitated oxide are a safe dose, 'two are a most violent and dangerous emetic,' and sixty grains 'perfectly inert;' and, consequently, that two are much more than ten, and sixty much less. Well, indeed, has Macquer observed, that some Physicians have considered this preparation as occasioning 'accidents so terrible, that instead of being called the Mercury of life, it ought to have been denominated the Mercury of death!'"

Mr. Phillips devotes thirty pages to his observations on the preparations of antimony, and confirms his statements by a detail of a variety of experiments in which he throws some light on this intricate subject.

His remarks on the liquor arsenicalis are very severe, and not without reason, as he discovered an error which ought not to have occurred, especially in a preparation containing so powerful an ingredient as arsenic. It is singular, however, that some of the "defects" pointed out by Mr. Phillips in Dr. Powell's Pharmacopœia, are to be found in a subsequent edition (1836), of which he is the authorized translator. For instance, in reference to the distilled waters, he states, "The

addition of spirit to distilled waters is altogether useless." In
Mr. Phillips' Pharmacopœia seven ounces of spirit are ordered
to two gallons of each of the distilled waters. In the extractum opii he recommends proof spirit to be employed instead
of water. In the Pharmacopœia of 1836, distilled water is
ordered as the menstruum without any animadversion. In the
hydrargyri oxidum cinereum, he recommends potash in preference to lime; yet in his own Pharmacopœia lime is ordered.
A few other cases might be mentioned.

Although Mr. Phillips criticised without mercy the imperfections of the Pharmacopœia, he found some merits in the
work, to which he gave their share of commendation; and
his review was found to be so far entitled to attention, being
based upon practical experience, that some of his suggestions
(as well as those of some other commentators) were adopted
in the next edition, which appeared in 1815. In this edition
several new articles were introduced, others which had been
expunged in 1809 were restored, and some of the names were
changed. The work was on the whole a decided improvement on its predecessor ; but it did not yet come up to Mr.
Phillips's ideas of perfection, and accordingly, in the year
1816, he published some " REMARKS on the EDITIO ALTERA of
the PHARMACOPŒIA LONDINENSIS."

It happened, unfortunately for Dr. Powell, that he had
omitted to give Mr. Phillips credit for those improvements
which, at his suggestion, he introduced into the Pharmacopœia,
and that he stated nevertheless in the preface, "I am not conscious that in any instance I have purloined the observations
of others or used them without due acknowledgment." This
gave Mr. Phillips a pretext for recapitulating some of his former
statements, pointing out the instances in which his directions
had been followed, but not acknowledged, and making a
fresh attack on those errors which had not been rectified.

While it cannot be denied that there was some foundation
for these criticisms, it must be admitted that Dr. Powell's
Pharmacopœia met with a most unmerciful reception, and
that he did not enjoy a fair share of indulgence. Dr. Powell,
as a Physician, could not be expected to compete in practical
experience with the manufacturing Chemists, many of whom
devoted their whole lives to a small section merely of the art
of pharmacy, and who were not likely to reveal the secrets by

which they sustained their reputation, for the benefit of a work in which they were not interested and for which they would gain no credit. Many processes might appear to answer the purpose when conducted on a small scale, by way of experiment, and yet they might not be adapted to the manufacture of the articles in quantity, and this, in fact, was found to be the case in several instances. On the whole, the work appeared in its most unfavourable aspect, when seen through the medium of the searching and practical satire of Mr. Phillips.

The improvement which was taking place among the Apothecaries, in consequence of the increased attention which they devoted to medical and surgical practice, tended materially to strengthen the position of the Druggists as dispensers of prescriptions : this office, being *comparatively* neglected by the one class, naturally fell more and more into the hands of the other. But the Apothecaries, while they were losing ground in the "trading" department of their profession, possessed no other legitimate means of obtaining remuneration, the amount of their receipts being chiefly regulated by the quantity of medicine they supplied to their patients. To use the words of Dr. Burrows, " The practising Apothecaries justly complained that the dispensing Chemists and Druggists had greatly deteriorated the profits of their business ; but the practice had existed so long, that *it had acquired from custom the force of law*, and it was impossible by sudden or violent means to suppress it. It had indeed become difficult to define who was, or who was not, an Apothecary. . . ."

In addition to the falling off in their dispensing business, and the inroads made upon the profession by irregular and uneducated practitioners of every description, the Apothecaries sustained another grievance, namely, an increase in the taxes on drugs and other necessary commodities, which pressed with peculiar severity upon them. The exorbitant duty on glass, which was imposed by Government in the year 1812, brought their misfortunes to a climax, and occasioned a public meeting of their body, which was convened on the 3rd of July of that year, at the Crown and Anchor Tavern, by Mr. Burrows,* Mr. Cates, and Mr. Wells.

---

* Afterwards Dr. George Mann Burrows.

Several meetings had been held on the subject of the duty on glass, to very little purpose, when Mr. A. T. Thomson having accidentally attended one of them, diverted the attention of the meeting from the subject of glass, which he considered derogatory to the profession, to the more important matter of improving the condition of that branch of it, in a professional point of view.

An Association was formed, of which Mr. Burrows was appointed chairman, and Mr. Ward secretary. Mr. Kerrison,* who had declined taking a share in the proceedings respecting the duty on glass, became an active member of the Committee, when a more enlarged scheme was undertaken, and Mr. Thomson,† Mr. Good,‡ and Mr. Upton, as well as other influential practitioners, joined with great spirit in the enterprise.

The exertions of the Association were directed to the framing of a bill to be brought into Parliament, the objects of which were :—

To constitute a fourth Medical body which should be empowered to examine Apothecaries, Surgeon Apothecaries, Accoucheurs, Midwives, Dispensing Chemists, and Assistants; to prohibit the practice of Medicine, Surgery, Midwifery, or Pharmacy, by uneducated persons ; and to vest in the new body the prerogative of granting licences to such persons as they should find on examination to be competent, which licences should be annually renewed on payment of a fee, the examiners possessing the powers of withholding them from persons whose conduct had been immoral or discreditable.

To introduce certain regulations respecting apprentices, and to found a school § for the education of pupils in medicine, surgery, pharmacy, etc.

---

* Afterwards Dr. Kerrison.
† Afterwards Dr. A. T. Thomson.
‡ Afterwards Dr. Good.
§ In the London Repository, vol. iv., pp. 487-8, the following remarks, from the pen of Dr. Burrows, in reference to the subject of education, are worthy of notice : "There is in London another defect, which we will cursorily mention, and that is the want of a regular School of Pharmacy. The Apothecaries' shops in England do not furnish those means of instruction in this important science which are necessary to form a good Pharmaceutist. Young men cannot acquire in such situations a practical

It was the original intention of the Association to apply to Parliament through the medium, or with the concurrence, of the Colleges of Physicians and Surgeons, and the Society of Apothecaries, and letters were written to these bodies, representing the urgent necessity for some measure of reform, and respectfully requesting their co-operation and support.

The COLLEGE OF PHYSICIANS declined taking any share in the matter, stating, that they " could not give any advice or assistance on the occasion." The COLLEGE OF SURGEONS concluded their reply with these words, " The Court of Assistants does not intend to interfere with the subject of such letter." The SOCIETY OF APOTHECARIES, after having consulted the College of Physicians, stated, that "They could not, *as a body*,* concur with the Committee in the intended application to Parliament." The *Associated Apothecaries*, therefore, being left to their own resources, prepared a bill, which was introduced to the House by Messrs. Wilberforce, Calcraft, Whitbread, and Rose, in the month of March, 1813. The Colleges of Physicians and Surgeons, laying aside the apathy which they had originally evinced on the subject, when they perceived that active steps were in progress, openly opposed the bill and presented petitions against it. The Society of Apothecaries maintained a certain degree of neutrality, as they could not offer direct opposition to a measure in which a majority of their body was prominently engaged.

The Chemists and Druggists, against whom some of the most important provisions in the bill were levelled, and to whom no application had been made for advice or assistance, spontaneously took the alarm, and the standing Committee of the Society, which they had formed for the protection of

---

knowledge of Chemistry, of Materia Medica, or of Botany; and when in London, if they are laudably desirous of prosecuting such studies, there are no institutions affording all the requisities for pursuing them with full advantage. A school, therefore, should certainly be established in this metropolis, where all these sciences and arts would be practically taught and illustrated, especially Pharmacy, even to the very manipulations of the art. These projects are not chimeras: they are obvious, simple in principle, and facile of adoption, and such as we hope ere long to see carried into effect."

* Although three-fourths of .the body were actually among the petitioners! See "An Inquiry," etc., by Robert Masters Kerrison, p. 76.

their interests in the year 1802, convened a general meeting
for the purpose of opposing the new bill.

The following account of their proceedings is copied from
the minute-book:

> At a general meeting of the Chemists and Druggists in
> the metropolis, held, in pursuance of public advertise-
> ment, at the Freemasons' Tavern, Queen Street, Lin-
> coln's Inn Fields, on Thursday, March 4th, 1813, to
> take into consideration "An Abstract of a Bill for
> regulating the Practice of Apothecaries, Surgeon
> Apothecaries, Practitioners in Midwifery, and Com-
> pounders and Dispensers of Medicines throughout
> England and Wales," published by order of the
> general Committee,

MR. HUDSON in the chair,

The following Resolutions were passed:

"*First—Resolved*, That the abstract of a bill, published and
proposed to be brought into Parliament by certain Apothecaries, contains many clauses deeply injurious to the Chemists
and Druggists who compound and dispense medicines, and
to the public at large, inasmuch as the operation of these
clauses will be to put all compounders and dispensers of
medicines under the control of a Committee of Apothecaries
(distinct from the corporate body of Apothecaries), and to
give that Committee a power, by the making of bye-laws, and
the issuing of annual licences, to use means of the greatest
oppression and injustice, and eventually to place a monopoly
of compounding and dispensing medicines in the hands of
the Apothecaries, which will increase the price of medicines,
and consequently diminish the means of a large body of the
community to procure necessary medical assistance.

" *Second*—That the Chemists and Druggists having, for a
great number of years, exercised the trade of compounding
and dispensing medicines (by which they mean making up
the prescriptions of Physicians and Surgeons) to the satisfaction and advantage of the public, consider it highly important
to oppose this bill in all its stages, so far as it interferes with
their established and universally acknowledged business.

" *Third*—That a Committee be chosen, five of whom shall

be a quorum, to take the necessary steps for opposing the bill; and that the Committee do consist of the following persons, with power to increase their number :—

> Messrs. ALLEN, Plough Court.
> BELL, Oxford Street.
> COOKE, Southampton Street.
> COLE, Newgate Street.
> COMPLIN, Bishopsgate Street.
> CURTIS, Old Fish Street.
> HASTINGS, Haymarket.
> HUME, Long Acre.
> HUDSON, Haymarket.
> PHILLIPS, Poultry.
> SAVORY, Bond Street.
> SMITH, Haymarket.
> TEBBS, Bond Street.

" *Fourth*—That a subscription be entered into for defraying the expenses attendant on prosecuting the opposition to the bill; that Mr. Complin be treasurer; and that no moneys be paid but on an application, in writing, signed by at least three members of Committee, in Committee; and that subscriptions be received by all the members of the Committee.

(Signed)　　　W. B. HUDSON, *Chairman.*"

The Committee met on the 5th of March, at the house of Mr. William Allen. Mr. Hudson, the chairman, stated, that he had had an interview with Mr. Wilberforce, who recommended a meeting, by deputation, between the Apothecaries and Chemists; but on a full consideration of circumstances, the Committee thought this measure inexpedient. The chairman was, therefore, requested to inform Mr. Wilberforce of this determination.

It was also resolved to publish an address to the country Chemists and Druggists in the following papers : *Times, Morning Herald, Chronicle, Ledger, Star, Courier,* and *Statesman.*

It was resolved to retain Mr. Brougham as counsel.

A Sub-Committee was appointed to prepare the address, the Secretary was requested to draw up the form of a petition, and the Committee adjourned to the 8th, on which day they

met at the Globe Tavern. They also met on the 12th, 15th,
17th, and 18th. Mr. Brougham being out of town, Mr. Adam
was retained as counsel, and Mr. Harrison to assist at consultation. The result of the labours of the Committee during
the above space of time is detailed in the following report:

At a general meeting of the Chemists and Druggists in
the metropolis, held, in pursuance of public advertisement, at the Freemasons' Tavern, Great Queen Street,
Lincoln's Inn Fields, on Monday, 22nd March, 1813,

Mr. HUDSON in the chair,

The following report was presented by the Committee :

"Your Committee, in reporting their progress since the last
general meeting, have to observe, that, after advertising the
resolutions of that day in the most widely-circulated London
newspapers, they directed their attention to the best means
of informing their fellow-tradesmen individually throughout
the kingdom of the steps already taken to oppose the Apothecaries' Bill, and to request their communications and subscriptions in support of that object. This was done by a
circular letter, addressed to all whose names could be collected
in town and country. They have now the gratification to
state, that their exertions in this respect have been highly
successful. From most parts of the kingdom they have
received the most hearty concurrence in their views; many
towns have formed associations, and transmitted liberal subscriptions—some have published and adopted the substance
of the resolutions of the general meeting as their own.
Numerous subscriptions have also been received from individuals where associations could not be formed; and communications have been received from associations promising
an early remittance of their funds—almost *all* offering more
assistance, if necessary.

"Your Committee, in acknowledging communications or
remittances, have not failed to urge upon their correspondents
the importance of soliciting their town and country members
to oppose the bill.

"The expected reading of the bill a second time on an
early day after the first reading, necessarily presented great

difficulty and inconvenience to your Committee in preparing their opposition to it; but in consequence of an interview between the mover of the bill (Mr. Calcraft) and one of their body, Mr. Calcraft very handsomely deferred the second reading till Friday, the 26th instant, an indulgence which your Committee acknowledged with due respect.

"Many Members of Parliament have been waited upon, and their opposition to the bill solicited. Your Committee are happy to state, that several of them were fully sensible of its obnoxious tendency; and others, who were before unacquainted with it, have promised to give it their attention and consideration.

"In the course of their exertions and inquiries, your Committee have found that many Apothecaries, both in town and country, were not only unacquainted with the bill brought into Parliament, but that they were averse to many of its provisions.

"A petition, prepared under the direction of your Committee, is now to be brought forward for your approbation and signature. A circular letter for Members of Parliament is in the press."

The following is a copy of the circular:

"SIR,—The Committee of Chemists and Druggists respectfully solicit your attention to the following provisions of a bill, now pending in Parliament, 'for regulating the Practice of Apothecaries, Surgeon Apothecaries,' etc., etc.

" Section. Page.
" 1.   2. Provides a Committee of twenty-seven Apothecaries and eight Physicians and Surgeons, 'for ever,' to regulate not only the practice of Apothecaries, but all the Chemists and Druggists in England and Wales.
" 2.   3. Excludes all Chemists and Druggists from any vote or influence in directing the operation of the bill.
" 7.   5. Enables the Committee to employ informers, under the description of 'such other officers as the Committee shall adjudge to be necessary.'

52   FURTHER OBJECTIONABLE PROVISIONS.

"Section. Page.

" 9. 6. Enables the Committee to make bye-laws for its
own regulation, advantage, and 'interest,' and
to alter them at pleasure.
" 11. 7. Appoints medical provincial districts, subject
to the absolute control of the London Committee.
" 20. 11. Empowers the Committee to determine the necessary qualifications of compounders and dispensers of medicines, and their assistants.
" 25. 13. Requires a sum to be paid for certificate of examination.
" 30. 15. Requires an annual licence to be taken out by
every Chemist and Druggist, on pain of
penalty.
" 34. 16. Licences may be refused on a charge of im-
morality of character, to be judged of by the
Committee.
" 35. 17. Appeals from all parts of England and Wales to
be determined by the London Committee.
" 43. 20. Gives great encouragement to informers, and
provides a permanent fund for prosecutions.
" 47. 21. Gives the magistrate authority to imprison for
small penalties.
" 48. 22. Protects the prosecutor under any informality,
and affords no redress but by an action at law.

"It will be observed, that in the constitution of the Committee, the Apothecaries are to possess a majority so over-
bearing, as virtually to reduce the Physicians and Surgeons
to nothing; and the obvious tendency of the bill is to depress
and ruin, and eventually to extirpate, the compounding
Chemists and Druggists; for though their existence is to be
suffered, yet they are to be entirely excluded from any share
or voice in directing the operation of the bill; and the
inquisitorial power it will establish over them and their
assistants, must produce infinite confusion, embarrassment,
and injury.

"By the great encouragement held out to informers, any
medical advice or interference on the most urgent or most
trivial occasion, whether real or pretended, may subject the

Chemists and Druggists to frivolous and vexatious proceedings and penalties.

"The clause enabling the Committee to make bye-laws of an indefinite nature, may be the instrument of grievous oppression and injustice.

"The Chemists and Druggists conceive that their long experience in making up prescriptions, and their extensive employment in preparing the various articles of the Pharmacopœia, for the use of medical practitioners, must necessarily render them more competent than Apothecaries to compound medicines, and to judge of the qualifications of the assistants they employ for that purpose, and it is scarcely necessary to add, that their interest and reputation are deeply concerned in the selection of proper persons.

"The annual licence will not only operate as a tax upon persons not represented in the legislating body, but may be withheld upon vague charges against their characters—Apothecaries being the judges.

"Great hardship and injustice may arise in the country districts, where it will be very easy for Apothecaries to combine against a Chemist and Druggist, or to harass his assistants; and much expense as well as loss of time must be incurred by travelling up to London, from all parts of the kingdom, for redress from the superintending Committee.

"Persons convicted in small penalties, on the evidence of a single witness, may be distressed and imprisoned on the authority of a magistrate's warrant, and the distressing party is to be protected under any informality, while the aggrieved person can obtain no redress but by an action at law: a single individual, perhaps already ruined, against an organized body with a permanent fund!

"The middle and lower classes of the community will suffer material inconvenience and injury from the operation of the bill. In large towns it is usual for Physicians to prescribe *gratis* for the poor, and to send them to a Chemist and Druggist for the medicines; and in populous districts, ineligible for the residence of a Physician, and unfavourable for the formation of local charitable institutions, simple remedies are often procured from the Chemist and Druggist at a cheap rate; but if these classes are obliged on every slight ailment to employ a professional man, who can legally charge for attendance and medicine, they must encounter the greatest pecuniary inconvenience, or the distressing con. sequences of protracted sickness.

"*March* 22*nd*, 1813.

"*First*—It was *resolved unanimously*, that the above report be received.

"*Second*—*Resolved*, That a petition * be presented to the House of Commons from this meeting; and that the petition, as prepared, be now read.

"*Third*—*Resolved*, That the petition just read be approved and signed by the Chemists and Druggists of the metropolis.

"*Fourth*—*Resolved*, That the Committee be empowered to put the petition into the hands of such Members of Parliament as they shall think most favourable to their cause, to have it presented to the House of Commons.

"W. B. HUDSON, *Chairman*."

In consequence of the determined opposition which was made in all quarters to the bill at its first reading, the Committee of the Associated Apothecaries modified it considerably, and on the 25th of March, 1813, sent the following notice to the members of the House of Commons :—

The general Committee of Apothecaries and Surgeon Apothecaries, think it requisite to inform the members of the House of Commons, previously to the second reading of their Bill, of the following circumstances :

" 1. That in the event of the bill passing into a Committee, they mean to expunge from it everything affecting the compounding Chemist and Druggist.

" 2. That the idea of erecting a medical school has been abandoned, and that instead of interfering with the rights of the Royal College of Surgeons, they wish to make it imperative on every Surgeon Apothecary to have a diploma from the College of Surgeons.

" 3. That the idea of uniting the different heads of the already-constituted medical bodies with Apothecaries and Surgeon Apothecaries in the superintending body, may be abandoned.

---

* It is not considered necessary to quote the form of petition.

"4. That the views of the bill will be altogether confined to rendering the Apothecary and Surgeon Apothecary competent practitioners, by examinations, and obtaining for them a different mode of recompense for their visits and professional skill."

The Committee of the Chemists and Druggists met at the Globe, on the 29th of March, and also on the 1st and 7th of April. On the 8th of April a general meeting took place, of which the following is a report:—

> At a general meeting of the Chemists and Druggists in the metropolis, held in pursuance of public advertisement, at the Freemasons' Tavern, Great Queen Street, Lincoln's Inn Fields, on Thursday, the 8th day of April, 1813,
>
> MR. HUDSON in the chair,

The following report was presented by the Committee:—

"Your Committee have now the satisfaction formally to announce to you, that the measure which first occasioned our meeting together is abandoned for the present session—the Apothecaries' Bill was withdrawn by the mover, on Friday, the 26th of last month, the day appointed for the second reading. The motives for this procedure are thus stated in the public advertisement of the Committee of Apothecaries, inserted in the newspapers of the succeeding day, as follows:— 'The great importance of the objects embraced by the bill lately introduced before Parliament for regulating the concerns of the profession, the complexity of its interest, and the very extensive communications from the country, many of them entitled to more attention than the shortness of the period allowed by the present session will permit, have induced the Committee to withdraw the bill from the House, in order that it may be submitted, in the course of the next session, under a more perfect form.'

"The petition submitted to you at the last general meeting was signed by a very large majority of the Chemists and Druggists in the metropolis. It was presented to the House of Commons on the 24th ult., by the Right Hon. Geo. Canning, who previously honoured a deputation of your Committee with an interview, to enable them to explain to him the particular grounds of their opposition to the Apothecaries' Bill.

"A circular letter was also distributed amongst the members of the House of Commons; and in the interviews which individuals or deputations of your Committee had with various members, they had the satisfaction to find a general concurrence in the views, as to the oppressive and injurious operation of the proposed bill upon the Chemists and Druggists.

"The avowed intention of the Apothecaries to introduce another bill into Parliament next session, and the recollection of the previous harassings the trade has experienced, cannot fail to convince you of the necessity of a continued watchfulness to protect and preserve the interests of all concerned in t. Your Committee, therefore, feel it to be their duty to recommend to the consideration of this meeting the adoption of some measure for this purpose, and at the same time to submit to you the importance of providing a fund, to be ready on any emergency, to enable them to adopt the most speedy and most effectual measures without incurring the great labour, inconvenience, and delay attendant on an extensive correspondence with the country.

"The amount of subscriptions already received is a little more than £500, and the expenses are now short of £100, when the whole of the business is concluded, they will be within £120.

"*Resolved*, That the report now read be received.

"*Resolved*, That the present Committee do remain a permanent Committee, for the protection of the interests of the Chemists and Druggists.

"*Resolved*, That the surplus of the subscriptions, after the expenses are paid, be funded in the names of Trustees.

"*Resolved*, That the Trustees be the Chairman, Mr. Allen, and Mr. Horner, subject to the direction and control of the Committee.

"*Resolved*, That these resolutions be printed on the same sheet with the circular letter to Members of Parliament, and sent to all the Chemists and Druggists in town and country, in order that they may be accurately informed of the particular grounds taken by the Committee, in their opposition to the Apothecaries' Bill.

"At the same time urging those who have not yet sent their subscriptions to remit them immediately, that they may be added to the permanent fund.

" The Chairman having left the chair,

" *Resolved*, That the thanks of this meeting be given to the Committee for their prompt and persevering exertions in this business.

" W. B. HUDSON, *Chairman.*

" Mr. Savory having been voted into the chair, it was

" *Resolved*, That the thanks of this general meeting of Chemists and Druggists are due, and are hereby presented, to W. B. Hudson, Esq. (Chairman), accompanied with a piece of plate, of the value of thirty guineas, as an acknowledgment of his services rendered the trade by his prompt, zealous, and unremitted attention to their interests, in the opposition to the late injurious bill introduced into Parliament by certain Apothecaries."

Notwithstanding the modifications in the bill, and the persevering efforts of the Committee of Associated Apothecaries to conciliate the three constituted medical bodies, these advances met with no encouragement, and the Committee, on the 19th of November, 1813, passed the following resolution:—

" *Resolved*, That this Committee determine not to apply for the formation of a fourth Medical body for the purpose of examinations, if the powers of the present Chartered Bodies can be so extended as to accomplish the objects which the printed resolutions of the 4th of September embrace."*

This resolution was sent, with an appropriate memorial, to each of the three bodies, and the following replies were received :—

" *Apothecaries' Hall, October* 29, 1813.

" *Resolved*, That this Court, after taking into consideration the memorial addressed to them from the Committee of the Society of Apothecaries and Surgeon Apothecaries of England and Wales, together with the reply of the Royal College of Physicians, enclosed to their memorial, are of opinion that this Court cannot enter into measures for any improvement in Pharmacy, but in conjunction with that learned body.

" S. BACKLER, *Clerk.*"

Dr. Latham, on behalf of the ROYAL COLLEGE OF PHYSICIANS, transmitted a copy of a resolution as laid before the

---

* The substance of these resolutions has already been stated.

College at the last *comitia*, enclosed in a short note dated January 27, 1814, in which he stated that he was "sincerely happy in the prospect afforded of matters being, at last, satisfactorily adjusted."

"*Resolved*, That the President be empowered to inform the Right Hon. George Rose, that the Royal College of Physicians have no objection to the formation of a bill to be brought into Parliament by the London Committee of Apothecaries, upon the basis of certain resolutions passed by the said Committee, and dated 4th of September, 1813, provided the powers therein contained be vested in the Society of Apothecaries as established by the charter of King James, and provided the bill, before it shall be brought into the House of Commons, be submitted to the consideration of the College of Physicians for their approval."

This report, which had been drawn up by a Committee, was approved by the College, with a slight exception, relating to Army and Navy Surgeons, which it is unnecessary here to particularize.*

The following is the laconic answer of the COLLEGE OF SURGEONS':—

"*Royal College of Surgeons, February* 12, 1814.

"SIR,—I am directed by the Master of the College to acknowledge the receipt of your letter and enclosures of the 8th instant, and to return you his thanks for the same.

"I am, Sir, your most obedient Servant,

"EDW. BALFOUR, *Sec.*"

"Wm. T. Ward, Esq."

A general meeting of the Associated Apothecaries was held on the 12th of May, 1814, Mr. Burrows in the chair. The report of the Committee contained a detailed account of their reasons for abandoning their original design, and of the progress the Society of Apothecaries had made in framing a new bill, which they proposed to bring into Parliament at their own expense, under the sanction of the College of Physicians.

The report having been read, Mr. A. T. Thomson ex-

---

* See "The London Medical Repository," vol. i., page 266.

pressed at some length his conviction, that although the proposed bill was in many respects defective, and by no means so
satisfactory and complete as the one which the Committee had
been compelled to withdraw, yet the circumstances of the
case rendered it advisable to unite with the Society of Apothecaries in the work which they had undertaken, and thus to
secure a portion at least of those advantages which it appeared impossible to obtain to the full extent.

Mr. Good, who had been absent from some of the late
meetings of the Committee, dissented from the report, and
denounced the proposed bill " as a measure which had been
raked from the musty records in which it had mouldered for
two hundred years, to disgrace the enlightened period of the
nineteenth century." He objected to the omission of what he
considered one of the most important features in the original
bill—examinations in Anatomy, Surgery, and Midwifery. He
objected to the inquisitorial power being vested in any body
of men, of entering premises under pretence of " searching for
drugs, unlawful, deceitful, corrupt," etc. ; and severely handled
the clause which subjects an Apothecary to a penalty " if he
shall at any time knowingly, wilfully, and contumaciously
refuse to compound," or shall " falsely, unfaithfully, fraudulently," compound any medicines, etc., as directed in any prescription signed with the initials of a Physician.   .   .

The Chairman explained that a separate bill was contemplated for the regulation of Surgery and Midwifery—that the
clause respecting the visitation of shops would be modified in
committee, and that the penalty for refusal to compound prescriptions was designed merely to give the Physician authority
over the patient and the treatment adopted, and not to oblige
Apothecaries to compound prescriptions whether it suited
their convenience or not.

Mr. Good was not at all satisfied with this explanation, and
concluded his speech by insisting, that the bill was "a measure made up of restrictions, penalties, and imprisonments;
founded in tyranny and oppression," which he felt confident
the meeting would reject. After several members had briefly
expressed their opinions, Mr. A. T. Thomson replied to Mr.
Good in an elaborate speech, in which he answered the
various objections *seriatim*, contending that it would be unwise, because the whole of what was desired could not be

obtained, to refuse a part; and stating that the Committee were still on the alert, and would, he trusted, continue their exertions until, sooner or later, they had succeeded in accomplishing all that they had undertaken.

The motion in favour of supporting the bill was carried by a large majority.

The Committee of the Associated Apothecaries met at the Crown and Anchor, May 26th, and drew up an amended clause, which they desired to substitute for that which makes it penal for an Apothecary to *refuse* to compound a prescription, which, with a few other suggestions, they forwarded to the College of Physicians.

The clause, however, remains as it originally stood.

When this unfortunate bill was brought into the House, on the 23rd of February, the College of Physicians signified their determination to oppose it, without stating the ground of their objection. When the several portions of the bill came under discussion, it was found necessary to make considerable alterations in order to meet the wishes of the College. The House of Lords also introduced amendments, in consequence of which it was rejected by the Commons, and it was necessary *pro formâ* to bring in a new bill. These proceedings occasioned so much delay that the close of the session had almost arrived before the bill was completed, and it was ultimately hurried through Parliament in a state which was not altogether satisfactory to the promoters of the measure, although they chose the alternative of securing it in that condition, hoping to obtain an amended Act during the ensuing session, and fearing that by further procrastination they might be defeated altogether.

But we must not omit to notice the proceedings of the Chemists and Druggists, who met this bill with the same determined opposition with which they encountered its predecessor.

At a general meeting of the Chemists and Druggists in the metropolis, held, in pursuance of public advertisement, at the Freemasons' Tavern, Great Queen Street, Lincoln's Inn Fields, on Monday, the 6th day of March, 1815,

Mr. HUDSON in the chair.

The following are the principal clauses of the report which was presented by the Committee:— *

"Your Committee, in reporting their progress since the last general meeting, have to acquaint you, that the Society of Apothecaries have procured a bill to be brought into the House of Commons, entitled, 'A Bill for enlarging the Charter of the Society of Apothecaries in the City of London, granted by His Majesty King James the First, and for better regulating the Practice of Apothecaries throughout England and Wales;' and such bill appears to your Committee to be equally objectionable as the former bill presented by the Associated Apothecaries, and as injurious to the Chemists, Druggists, and to the public at large.

"*On Monday, the* 16*th May,* 1814, a Sub-Committee was appointed to confer with a Sub-Committee of the Associated Apothecaries, on the bill proposed to be brought into Parliament, 'For enlarging the Charter of the Society of Apothecaries,' etc., and to report to the Committee the result of such conference. In answer to the letter proposing a conference, the following was received:—

"*Bloomsbury Square, May* 18*th,* 1814.

"Sir,—In answer to your favour of yesterday, permit me to remark, that I apprehend your application is made to me under the impression that the bill about to be introduced to Parliament is a bill formed by the Committee of Associated Apothecaries, and that they carry it into the House.

"For the information of yourself and the gentlemen acting with you, permit me also to say, that it is arranged by the Society of Apothecaries, in conjunction with the College of Physicians, that it has been submitted for the remarks of the Committee to which I belong, and received, after some amendments are made which were proposed, the approbation of a general meeting of Apothecaries, held last Thursday, to take the bill into consideration.

"I have the honour to be, Sir,
"Your obedient humble Servant,
"W. B. Hudson, Esq."   "G. M. Burrows.

---

* At a meeting of the Committee, held at the Globe, on the 2nd of March, 1814, Mr. Westwood, of Newgate Street, and Mr. Butterfield, of the Strand, were added to the Committee.

" *On Thursday, November* 24th, 1814, the accounts of subscriptions and disbursements were audited and approved, whereby it appeared that £550 five per cent. annuities were standing in the names of the Trustees, which cost the sum of £502 1s. 6d., and that a balance of £36 4s. remained in the hands of the Treasurer; and it was resolved, that a circular letter should be sent to all the Chemists and Druggists in town and country, informing them of the proceedings of the Committee since the last general meeting.

"*Resolved unanimously,* That the report now read be received and approved.

"The Chairman then informed the meeting that the Apothecaries' Bill was now to be submitted to the meeting. The bill having been read and discussed, it was

"*Resolved,* That it is the opinion of the meeting that the bill now read contains much matter highly injurious to the Chemists and Druggists and the public at large, and that therefore it ought to be opposed.

"*Resolved,* That a petition be presented to the House of Commons against the aforesaid bill, and that a petition for this purpose be now read.

"*Resolved,* That the petition now read be approved, and be signed by the Chemists and Druggists of the metropolis.

"*Resolved,* That the Committee be empowered to take measures to have the petition presented to Parliament, and to employ such other means as they shall think fit, and may be necessary for opposing the said bill.

"*Resolved,* That the resolutions be advertised in the *Times, Morning Chronicle,* and *Courier.*

"W. B. HUDSON."

On the 17th of April, Mr. Gifford was added to the Committee.

At a general meeting of the Chemists and Druggists in the metropolis, held at the Globe Tavern, Fleet Street, London, on Friday, the 21st day of April, 1815, in pursuance of advertisements,

Mr. HUDSON in the chair.

REPORT OF THE COMMITTEE.

"Your Committee, in reporting their progress since the last general meeting, have to acquaint you that, in order to carry into execution the resolutions of the general meeting of the 6th day of March last, relative to the bill brought into Parliament by the Society of Apothecaries, they met together the next day, when a Sub-Committee, consisting of the Chairman, Mr. Smith, Mr. Allen, Mr. Cole, and Mr. Savory, was appointed to confer with the Committee of the Society of Apothecaries on the subject of the said bill, and that any two of them should be competent to hold such conference, and report the result thereof.

"*Monday, the* 13*th of March.*—The Chairman reported from the Sub-Committee, that he had written to the Master of the Society of the Apothecaries' Company, requesting a conference with the Committee of the said Society, on the subject of the said Bill; and that he had received a letter from their Secretary appointing Wednesday next, at one o'clock, to receive the deputation.

"*Wednesday, the* 15*th of March.*—The Chairman reported that Mr. Smith, Mr. Savory, and himself had waited upon the Society of Apothecaries that day, according to their appointment, and that the Society declared it to be their intention not to interfere at all with the Chemists and Druggists by their bill now in Parliament, and they offered to prepare a clause to that effect, to be added to the bill, for the satisfaction of the Chemists and Druggists.

"*Monday, the* 20*th of March.*—The Chairman reported that he had received the following letter from the Solicitors to the Society of Apothecaries, inclosing a clause proposed to be added to their bill, now pending in Parliament, for exempting the Chemists and Druggists from the provisions and effect of the said bill.

"*SIR,—We are instructed by the Committee of the Society of Apothecaries to forward to you the clause which they propose, at the requisition of the Committee of your body, to introduce into the Act now before the House of Commons, and which, we trust, will meet the wishes of the parties whom you represent.*

"*The Committee of the Society of Apothecaries see with concern that misrepresentations have been made of their object, which is the improvement of their branch of the profession in medical knowledge. To this their views are so entirely directed, that they have no disposition to insist on any clause which is not essentially connected with it. If the power enabling them to purchase land (a power which was asked for only because the opportunity of obtaining it without expense presented itself) be a clause which excites any jealousy, and of which the omission would conciliate the Chemists and Druggists, they have no hesitation in stating, that they shall recommend it to the Court o Assistants not to press its insertion.*

"*We are,* SIR, *your obedient Servants,*
"FLADGATE AND NEELD.
"*Essex Street,* 17*th of March,* 1815."

The clause proposed :
"*Provided always, and be it further enacted, That nothing in this Act contained shall extend, or be construed to extend, to prejudice, or in any way to affect the trade and business of a Chemist and Druggist; but all persons using or exercising the said trade, or who shall or may hereafter use or exercise the same, shall and may use, exercise, and carry on the same trade in such manner and as fully and amply to all intents and purposes as they might have done in case this Act had not been made.*"

"Your Committee directed that the charter of the Apothecaries, the new bill in Parliament, with the proviso above proposed, and the letter of the solicitors of the Apothecaries' Company, should be submitted to the consideration of counsel as to the effect the same might have on the Chemists and Druggists, and that the Secretaries should lay the same before counsel with proper instructions accordingly.

"*Monday,* 17*th April.*—The Secretaries laid before the Committee the case submitted to counsel on behalf of the Chemists and Druggists, with the charter and bill in Parliament, and counsel's opinion thereon ; also the proviso proposed by the Solicitors of the Society of Apothecaries, as settled by counsel. And it was resolved, that the following clause should be recommended to the general meeting, to be added to the bill now pending in Parliament; and that it be also recommended to the general meeting to request the Society of Apothecaries to withdraw the clause introduced into their bill for enlarging their powers of purchasing lands."

Amended clause :—
"*Provided always, and be it further enacted, That nothing in this Act contained shall extend or be construed to extend to prejudice, or in any way to affect the trade or business of a Chemist*

and Druggist, in the buying, preparing, compounding, dispensing, and vending drugs and medicinal compounds, wholesale and retail; but all persons using or exercising the said trade or business, or who shall or may hereafter use or exercise the same, shall and may use, exercise, and carry on the same trade or business, in such manner and as fully and amply to all intents and purposes as the same trade or business was used, exercised, or carried on by Chemists and Druggists before the passing of this Act."

" *Resolved unanimously*, That the report now read be received.

" *Resolved unanimously*, That on the insertion of the last stated clause in the bill of the Society of Apothecaries now pending in Parliament, and on the withdrawment of the clause in the said bill for the enlargement of the power of the Society to purchase lands, the Chemists and Druggists do withdraw their opposition to the bill.

" *Resolved unanimously*, That the last resolution be sent, with a copy of the amended clause, to the Society of Apothecaries."

At a general meeting of the Chemists and Druggists in the metropolis, held in pursuance of public advertisements, at the Globe Tavern, Fleet Street, London, on Friday, the 11th day of August, 1815,

Mr. HUDSON, in the chair,

The following report of the Committee was read :

" Your Committee have now the pleasure to report to you the termination of their labours on the Apothecaries' Bill. The clause to protect the Chemists and Druggists from the operation of the bill, which received the sanction of the last general meeting, was agreed to without alteration by the Society of Apothecaries, and subsequently approved by the Committee of the House of Commons on the bill; the Chairman attended the Committee with the Counsel and Secretary, and they had the satisfaction to find that the Counsel for the College of Physicians was also well satisfied with the clause.

" The earnest desire your Committee had to make some decision on the subject, that the trade might be relieved of the great expense and trouble heretofore experienced, led them to adopt every possible means to obtain a perfect under-

F

standing of the charter of the Society of Apothecaries, in order to form a clear idea of their own duty. This, and the necessary attendance of the bill before the Committee of the House of Commons, has necessarily brought on a considerable expense of Counsel not before incurred; the result, however, has fully equalled their expectations, and they trust will be satisfactory to those whose interests they have been endeavouring to protect and support.

"The state of the funds since the last audit is as follows :—

1815.	£	s.	d.	1815.	£	s.	d.
Balance then in hand	36	4	0	Paid Postages, 1814	7	17	11
April Dividends	12	7	6	Advertisements and Room	16	18	8
Subscriptions	18	12	0	Printing	3	4	6
August Dividends	12	7	6	Now due, Expenses of Counsel	57	18	0
				Agents of both Houses of Parliament	23	3	6
				Secretary's Bill, including Printing, Advertisements, Postages, and Attendances	95	4	2
					£204	6	9

	£	s.	d.
Balance now in hand	51	9	11
Navy 5 per Cents. in hand £550, worth about	500	0	0 Sterling.

"Some further expenses of printing, postages, &c., will be necessary to convey a circular letter of information to the subscribers.

"The Committee have only to observe in conclusion, that they beg to recommend to the consideration of this general meeting, that the surplus of the fund should remain in the Navy 5 per cents., in the names of the present Trustees, to be appropriated to any purpose of trade for the benefit of the subscribers which shall be sanctioned by a general meeting, and that *future subscriptions shall not be less than Two Guineas each.*"

"*Resolved unanimously*, That the report now read be received and approved.

"*Resolved unanimously*, That the surplus of the fund, after defraying the expenses, do remain in the Navy 5 per cents., in the names of the present Trustees, to be appropriated to any purpose of trade for the benefit of the subscribers which shall receive the sanction of a general meeting, and that future subscriptions shall not be less than Two Guineas each.

"*Resolved unanimously*, That the thanks of this meeting be presented to the Right Honourable Lord Lascelles, for presenting the Petition of the Chemists and Druggists to the House of Commons, and for his constant attention to their interest.

"*Second Resolution*, Reconsidered and amended, and carried unanimously.

"*Resolved unanimously*, That the substance of the resolutions of the general meetings be printed under the direction of the Committee, and sent to all subscribers to the fund, in town and country.

"*Resolved unanimously*, That the cordial thanks of this meeting be presented to the Committee for their unwearied and successful services in securing to the Chemists and Druggists the free and undisturbed exercise of their trade and business.

The Chairman having left the chair,

Mr. Hume was voted to it.

"*Resolved unanimously*, That the thanks of the meeting be given to the Chairman for his attention to the business of the day."

An account of the proceedings of the Associated Apothecaries, in reference to the Act of 1815, is contained in the Transactions of that body, a volume published in the year

1823, and also in the London Medical Repository of 1814 and 1815.

The above brief outline is introduced for the purpose of connecting into one concise history the principal circumstances of the controversy, and the policy adopted by the various parties concerned, in order that we may benefit by the experience of our predecessors.

The avowed object of the Act was to protect the public from the dangers resulting from the ignorance of unqualified practitioners, to improve the character and respectability of the educated Surgeon Apothecary, to establish a school of Medicine and Pharmacy, and to secure to qualified persons a fair remuneration for professional skill. The result is emphatically described in the Transactions of the Associated Apothecaries (Introductory Essay, page lviii.).

"That it was very unsatisfactory may be seen, by comparing the Apothecaries' Act as it is with the bill as first projected by the Association. Shorn, indeed, is the latter of its fair proportions! The practice of medicine is doubtless placed under certain but very inadequate restrictions; but, whilst that of Surgery and Midwifery is still open to every unprincipled pretender, the Druggists are neither prevented from making up Physicians' prescriptions, nor even from practising medicine; no provision is made for securing a supply of qualified assistants; and lastly, while the public are thus denied so many and such great advantages, not only is the general practitioner not relieved from his burdens, but he is subjected to new and vexatious restrictions."

Gray, in his supplement to the Pharmacopœia, makes the following observations on the subject :—

"This Act has had the singular fortune of being violently opposed, as insufficient, by those who were its original promoters; of being esteemed a burden by many of those whom it was meant to benefit; and of being looked upon with indifference by those against whom it was intended to act; since the Act was altered and restricted to those who *practise as Apothecaries*, with an express declaration that it did not extend to the Chemists and Druggists, whose shops are in general confounded with those of the Apothecaries, and whose business differs no otherwise than that with the dispensing Physician or modern Apothecary medical practice is the principal object, retail and dispensing the secondary: while, with the Chemist and Druggist, or old Apothecary, retail and dispensing are principal, and medical practice mostly confined to the counter, or to a few personal acquaintance; *à fortiori*, the midwives, herbalists, cuppers, barbers, electricians, galvanizers, dentists, farriers, veterinary surgeons, village wisemen, and cow-leeches, are left in full possession of their ancient practice, and may be consulted by those who place confidence in them, as they cannot be confounded with Apothecaries, though the Chemist and Druggist may."

Dr. George Mann Burrows continued his exertions as Chairman of the Committee of Associated Apothecaries until August, 1817, and pointed out a variety of defects in the bill, which the Committee submitted to the notice of the Court of Assistants of the Society of Apothecaries. But it was found impossible to induce that body to take the needful steps for rectifying these defects, and although proposals were entertained for applying to Parliament for an amendment of the Act, no decisive result ensued.

The Association continued to meet periodically for some years, their chief attention being directed to the suppression of irregular and unqualified practitioners, but their efforts were not seconded by the medical bodies, and although the Association comprised upwards of 3,000 members, their labours in this particular ended where they began.

The formation of so large an association of Apothecaries, distinct from the chartered Society of Apothecaries, especially as many of the members belonged to both bodies, is an anomaly the object of which it is not easy to comprehend; it appears that this Association was, in fact, a revival of that which was formed in the year 1794, and which was also unconnected with the three constituted medical bodies; but as its attention was directed to a new object, namely, that of ensuring the competence of Medical and Pharmaceutical practitioners of all ranks, and establishing a fair system of remuneration, the result ought to have been more successful than it was. But the want of unity in the profession itself, and the party spirit which prevailed throughout the controversy, diverted the influence into so many channels that a partial failure was the natural consequence. The Chemists and Druggists, on the contrary, who had already acquired a

standing as dispensers of medicine, by uniting their strength
on the occasion, secured to themselves a continuance of all
their former privileges, although they did not at that time
aspire to the scientific improvement which they have now
undertaken to bring about. Their Committee retained the
powers which had been confided in them, and kept a watchful
eye on any proceedings or events which appeared likely to
influence the welfare of their body, or in which their credit as
Pharmaceutists was concerned. In the year 1819 they called
a public meeting, of which the following is the report:—

> At a general meeting of Chemists and Druggists, in
> the metropolis and its neighbourhood, held in pur-
> suance of public advertisement, at the Globe
> Tavern, Fleet Street, on Thursday, the 24th day of
> June, 1819,
>
> Mr. HUDSON in the chair,

The following report was presented by the Committee:

"Your Committee have called you together on the present
occasion to lay before you some information respecting a bill
which was brought into Parliament during the present session, entitled 'A Bill for establishing Regulations for the
Sale of Poisonous Drugs, and for better preventing the mis-
chiefs arising from inattention or neglect of persons vending
the same.'

"Your Committee procured copies of the bill as soon as it
was printed, and met to consider its provisions, some of which
appearing to them 'likely to embarrass the dispensing of
medicines, and not calculated to effect the object intended,'
they prepared a petition to that effect, which was presented
to the House of Commons. They were subsequently favoured
with a hearing before the Committee of the House, to whom
the bill was referred, and the bill was shortly after withdrawn.

"Your Committee, however, being deeply sensible of the
importance of the subject, and anxious to employ every possible means to attain the object intended by the bill, beg to
recommend to the Chemists and Druggists, and all others
who vend poisons or poisonous substances, the adoption of the
following regulations in their shops:

"*First*—That no arsenic, oxalic acid, or corrosive sublimate, be issued by any vendor, without a printed label of the name of the article, and the word 'POISON' being affixed to every wrapper, box, bottle, or other vessel containing the same.

" *Secondly*—That on every wrapper or vessel containing any drug or preparation likely to produce serious mischief, if improperly used, the name of the article be affixed in a legible form; and as many persons can read print who cannot read writing, they would recommend that printed labels be used where possible, in preference to written ones.

" *Thirdly*—That no person be allowed to serve poisons, who is not of sufficient age and experience to judge of the importance of the great caution necessary in avoiding the sale of them to improper or ignorant persons.

" *Resolved unanimously*, That the report now read be received and approved, and that the same be printed and circulated as widely as possible among the Chemists and Druggists and all other persons who vend poisons or poisonous drugs throughout the United Kingdom."

In the year 1824 another edition of the London Pharmacopœia was published, and Sir George Tuthill produced the English translation. On this occasion Mr. Phillips, instead of repeating his strictures on the work of the College, gave a specimen of his own performance in " A Translation, with Notes and Illustrations," which he published shortly after that of Sir George Tuthill. The merit of this work was appreciated by the College, as would appear from the subsequent appointment of Mr. Phillips as the official translator of the Pharmacopœia of 1836.

Dr. A. T. Thomson's " London Dispensatory " appeared in the year 1814, and has undergone a succession of improvements and amplifications up to the present time. The fame and merits of the work are too well known to require any particular notice ; it comprehends in one volume a sufficiently ample account of all the substances comprised in the Materia Medica, a very useful explanation of the science of Chemistry, as applied to Pharmacy, a compendium of the three Pharmacopœias, with copious notes, and a list of substances incompatible with others in extemporaneous prescriptions. The tenth edition has lately been announced.

The Committee of the Druggists' Association of 1802 met in the year 1829, in consequence of the vexatious proceedings of the Commissioners of Stamps, aided by common informers, in reference to the Medicine Act. Numerous penalties were inflicted on individuals in various parts of the country for selling lozenges and other articles, by weight, without a stamp, which had hitherto been considered legal, provided printed directions for their use were not affixed. The injustice of these proceedings became so glaring, that it was considered necessary to take some steps for protecting the trade. Accordingly a meeting was called on the 31st of December, 1829. The following resolutions are inserted, as they show the disposition which prevailed at that time to form a permanent society :

" That the individuals composing this Society disclaim all motive of opposition to any act of the legislature. They declare their sole object in associating to be the concerting, in unison, the fair means of protecting themselves and the trade from the losses and annoyance in business to which they are subjected, on the part of the stamp-office, by prosecutions for penalties, under what they honestly conceived to be, and are legally advised, is a misconstruction of the Medicine Stamp Act.

" That a Society be formed, to be intituled ' The General Association of Chemists and Druggists of Great Britain,' for the purpose of obtaining a *judicial* construction of the Medicine Stamp and Licence Acts, by assisting those who have been improperly prosecuted to bring their cases before a court of justice, and, if the Acts should be there held to have been rightly construed, for the further purpose of obtaining a revision of them by the legislature.

" That a Committee of twelve, with liberty to add to their number, be chosen annually—five to form a quorum : the Committee to meet once in every month.

" That a general meeting of the Association to be called by advertisement, and by circulars to all the members, be held twice in each year (viz. May and November), at which meetings the Committee shall report its proceedings.

" That the Committee be empowered to convene special general meetings, when any circumstances shall arise to render such meetings desirable.

" That every member shall pay a yearly subscription of twenty shillings, and in default of payment, after two months' notice from the Secretary, he shall be excluded the Society, and debarred from all privileges and advantages.

"That every member claiming protection from the Society, shall lay before the Committee a full and fair statement, in writing, of all the circumstances of the case upon which he grounds such claim.

"That the Committee shall have power to receive, examine, and consider any claim for protection, and decide thereon ; and if the case be defensible at law, the expenses of such defence shall be defrayed out of the funds of the Society.

"That the Committee be authorized to obtain such legal advice as they may deem necessary.

"That no money be paid by the Treasurer without an order, in writing, from the Committee.

"That at any general meeting bye-laws may be enacted, which shall be as binding as the original rules; but that no bye-law to alter or rescind any of the original rules shall be passed, unless notice be given in the circular calling such general meeting.

"That Auditors (not being members of the Committee) be elected annually, to examine and pass the Treasurer's accounts, which accounts are to be exhibited at the two named general meetings.

"That all the offices, except the Secretary of the Society, be honorary: That the officers be elected annually, by the members of the Society, at one of the general meetings, and that they be eligible to re-election."

This Association flourished for several months; Dr. Reece, Messrs. Midgley, Ancell, Gifford, Gray, Waugh, Watts, Binge, and Winstanley, were among the most active members. Petitions were drawn up and ready for presentation to Parliament, when an alteration took place in the law, the evil was at an end, and the Association was broken up. Mr. Hudson, the treasurer of the Association of 1812, declined to hand over the balance of subscriptions, as it appeared, on maturely considering the subject, that the objects of the two Associations being different, he was not justified in amalgamating the funds.

About the year 1830 another attempt was made to introduce a reformation in the practice of Pharmacy in this country, and for this purpose it was proposed to address the government on the subject, petitioning for an ACT which should regulate those who follow this department. Mr. John Savory took the lead on this occasion, and his efforts were seconded by the late Mr. Hudson and Mr. Butler. The memorial which was prepared contained a brief and appropriate exposition of the importance of Pharmacy to the health and life of his Majesty's subjects; the necessity of education and integrity in those whose duty it is to carry into effect the instructions of medical men; the prevalence of ignorant and incompetent persons calling themselves Chemists and Druggists, and the frequency of injury to the public from this source; the difficulty of detecting adulterations and the necessity of proper qualification in Pharmaceutists, in order to enable them to perform their duty in this respect; the advantages resulting from Pharmaceutical education in foreign countries; the danger arising from the uncontrolled sale of poisons by ignorant persons; and, finally, the absolute necessity of some sanitary regulations for the elevation of this department in the profession, and the protection of the public.

Mr. Savory waited on a considerable number of the Chemists and Druggists in London, soliciting signatures to this memorial; but so little encouragement was given to the proposed measure of reform that the project fell to the ground. A notion appeared to prevail, that the trade had been so often attacked, that it was hazardous to court a repetition of former annoyances by introducing so delicate a subject, and thus giving the cue to parties who might be interested in bringing about a destructive revolution. It was also considered by many to be a chimerical scheme on account of the want of unanimity in the trade, and it seemed to be the opinion of the majority that it was

" Better to bear the ills we have,
Than fly to others that we know not of."

Accordingly the memorial proved abortive, not from any doubt of its propriety or justice, but because the parties concerned, who might have promoted its object, were not disposed, in the absence of an exciting cause, to coalesce, and embark in an undertaking which would have involved a departure from the strictly *defensive* policy hitherto adopted by the trade.

The rapid progress of the science of Chemistry, and the recent introduction of various substances and preparations into medicinal use, had by this time thrown the Pharmacopœia of 1824 into the shade, and a new edition was anxiously anticipated. Some delay arose from the endeavour to compile, "not as before, a London Pharmacopœia, but one which should include Scotland and Ireland with England," for which purpose "it was requisite to consult with the Fellows of both colleges; and as, on account of the great distance, this was with difficulty accomplished," the college was "constrained to abandon the negotiation, which had been commenced." *   There was, however, another obstacle to this project, namely, there was a considerable stock on hand of the Dublin Pharmacopœia, which must have been sacrificed at a heavy loss to the publisher (or the college), if the amalgamation had been carried into effect. It must also be recollected, that at the time the "great distance" was considered an insurmountable bar to the union, the railroads and the penny postage had not come into operation.

In the year 1836 the London Pharmacopœia was completed, and Mr. Phillips, who had been engaged in the practical details of its compilation, was officially authorized to publish the translation. Among the most important additions, we may mention the alkaloids—morphia, aconitina, strychnia, and veratria; several preparations of iodine; hydrocyanic and phosphoric acids, and a few conventional formulæ, such as pilula rhei composita, mistura spiritus vini Gallici, etc., etc.

In this Pharmacopœia an alphabetical arrangement is adopted, from which however a few substances are excepted, forming separate sections. Mr. Phillips, in his translation, gives explicit instructions for testing the strength of preparations, and for detecting impurities. The known (or supposed) constitution of the various compounds is explained by diagrams and symbols, a list of synonyms is affixed to each preparation, tables of equivalents and symbols are given in addition to the other tables, and many valuable remarks and directions are added, which make the work very complete and voluminous.

---

* Pharmacopœia Londinensis, 1836, Phillips' translation, preface, p. 7.

The alterations in the nomenclature have been so much commented upon, that it is unnecessary to notice them in detail. Our only cause for regret is, that the multiplication of terms and synonyms has occasioned considerable ambiguity, which is not unfrequently productive of inconvenience as well as mistakes. Some of the alterations in names have little or no reference to scientific considerations; as, for instance, pilula saponis composita for pilula saponis cum opio, tinctura camphoræ for spiritus camphoræ, mistura acaciæ for mucilago acaciæ, syrupus for syrupus simplex, etc. These changes are of no importance, except in a few instances, in which they occasion a little want of perspicuity.

The adoption of the imperial measure, in conformity with the Act of Parliament by which measures in general are regulated, has given rise to some discussion. As the College of Physicians is authorized by law to publish a Pharmacopœia, and to enforce its observance by those who compound and prepare medicines, it may fairly be doubted whether that body comes within the pale of the Act by which publicans and wine-merchants are governed; and as the medical profession has adopted, and continues to use "Apothecaries' Weights," it cannot be denied that "Apothecaries' Measure" might with equal propriety be allowed. In adverting to the disadvantage of unnecessary changes of this description, we may recur to Mr. Phillips' remarks on the *libra*, quoted page 43, which with a slight variation would apply to the recent change in the value of the term *octarium*. In the present instance, however, it may also be observed, that the old pint is more convenient than the new, as it admits of subdivision to a greater extent without fractions, and is therefore better adapted to the calculations of the Pharmaceutical Chemist. Some medical men, in order to avoid the ambiguity which now exists respecting the octarium, use the term *libra* (meaning 16 oz.); but this is no less ambiguous, as the Apothecaries' pound is 12 oz. and the fluid pound is obsolete. Others avoid the use of the terms *pound* and *pint* altogether, which indeed is the only effectual method of avoiding confusion.

In the year 1837, Dr. Collier published a caustic and acrid pamphlet, in which he disputed the title of the College to secure the copyright of the Pharmacopœia to Mr. Phillips, enumerating a number of instances in which translations of former Pharmacopœias had been published without authority, among others a translation by himself, in the year 1820, and the one by Phillips in 1824.   In this pamphlet he announced his intention of again appearing in the field, and shortly afterwards produced his translation of the Pharmacopœia of 1836, with copious notes and comments.

The next event which we have to notice in the annals of Pharmacy is the Parliamentary inquiry, instituted by a Committee of the House of Commons, in 1839, of which Mr. Warburton was chairman.   The object of this Committee was to revise all the laws relating to the medical profession, to obtain authentic and satisfactory evidence in every department of the subject, and to reform any abuses which might be found to exist.   Every person who was supposed to be likely to possess information of any importance was examined, and the mass of evidence thus collected was, as might have been expected, very voluminous.   The fire which took place at the House of Commons was an obstacle to the completion of the work, as a portion of the evidence, including that which related to Pharmacy, was burnt when on the eve of publication.   Sufficient materials, however, were collected and preserved to enable Mr. Warburton, assisted by Mr. Wakley and Mr. Hawes, to prepare a bill, entitled " A Bill for the Registration of Medical Practitioners, and for establishing a College of Medicine, and for enabling the Fellows of that College to practise Medicine in all or any of its branches, and hold any Medical Appointments whatsoever, in any part whatsoever of the United Kingdom."   This bill contained no provision for the prosecution or punishment of unqualified practitioners, but it provided for the registration of those who had passed the requisite examinations, and who were to pay an annual tax towards the expenses of the establishment, in return for which they were to enjoy the privileges of registration, and holding offices of emolument in the profession.   According to the principles advocated by Mr. Warburton, the public were to be furnished with qualified practitioners in every department, and ample means provided for distinguishing between those who possessed the requisite proficiency and others ; but no penalties were to be inflicted on persons who presumed to practise without a qualification, it being considered that the public are responsible for the results of patronizing such persons.

The machinery of the plan proposed by Mr. Warburton for registering medical and pharmaceutical practitioners was so complicated, and the provisions of the bill so unsatisfactory to those who advocated the restraint of unqualified practitioners, and who constituted the bulk of the "Medical Reformers," that the bill was withdrawn at an early stage; those who had been engaged in the work divided themselves into two or three parties, and other bills were prepared which were destined to share a similar fate. •But before entering on the notice of these bills, it may be as well to advert to the operation of the Apothecaries' Act, in reference to Chemists and Druggists. In the evidence of Mr. Nussey, in the Parliamentary Committee, June 9, 1836, the following statements were elicited :—

34. The Act of 1815 reserves to Chemists and Druggists whatsoever privileges they possessed at the time the bill passed; among which they reckon the privilege of prescribing and dispensing in their own shops : does not this privilege occasion medicine to be practised by a number of persons who have not received any regular medical education ?—Most undoubtedly.

35. Why would you put down unqualified practitioners of one description, when you maintain in possession of a right to practise an unlimited number of persons of another description, who, for the most part, have received no medical instruction whatever ?—I do not admit that the Chemists and Druggists have the power of prescribing.

36. Do they not contend that they have the right to prescribe in their own shops, and do they not exercise that right ?—That may be, but the law is decidedly against them.

37. Has any prosecution been instituted by your society against a Chemist and Druggist ?—No.

38. Surely the Chemists and Druggists have exercised that right since 1815 ?—Yes; but it is in private. We have no means of getting information upon that point.

From this it appears, that during twenty-one years after the passing of the Apothecaries' Act, no attempt was made to restrain the Chemists and Druggists from prescribing in their own shops, as they had previously been in the habit of doing.

If the Apothecaries had the power of prosecuting in such cases, it is remarkable that they *enjoyed* (?) it so long without *exercising* it.

At the time the Act passed, it was fresh in the recollection of those who framed it, that "it was their intention not to interfere at all with Chemists and Druggists;" * but after a lapse of twenty-five years, it was found expedient to recon-sider the words of the Act, in order to discover how far they could be construed to meet certain cases in which its spirit was said to have been violated. It had by this time become notorious that persons who desired to establish a medical and surgical practice, without incurring the expense of a proper education, assumed the name of Chemist and Druggist in order to come within the pale of the protective clause, while they professed to act in every respect and to all intents and purposes as medical practitioners. Some of these equivocal "Chemists and Druggists" undertook to cure every disorder, and performed surgical operations of all kinds, both minor and capital, attracting a large number of patients by advertis-ing the wonderful cures which they had performed. The Apothecaries, in order to put a construction on their Act favourable to themselves, and which had not been contem-plated at the time it was passed, consulted the most eminent lawyers, and all their ingenuity was directed to the task of demolishing the privilege which had been abused. The words were twisted in every variety of form, and conflicting opinions were given. On one side it was urged, that the trade or busi-ness of a Chemist was restricted in that clause to "the buying, preparing, compounding, dispensing, and vending drugs and medicinal compounds, wholesale and retail;" and that the words "recommending" or "prescribing" not being intro-duced, the clause did not afford protection to them in exercis-ing these functions. On the other side it was contended, that the clause empowered all Chemists and Druggists "to use, exercise, and carry on the same trade or business in such a manner, as fully and amply, to all intents and purposes, as the same trade or business was used, exercised, or carried on by Chemists and Druggists before the passing of this Act." It was well known that Chemists and Druggists were in the

---

* See page 64.

habit of prescribing prior to 1815 ; * but so many years having elapsed, it was not so easy as might at first have been
imagined, to obtain such evidence on this point as would be
received in a court of justice. On this, therefore, hinged the
chief difficulty of the question, and the first case which was
brought into court was decided in favour of the Chemist and
Druggist ; Mr. Justice Maule having considered that the protective clause entitled him to give advice as well as medicine.
But this decision was afterwards reversed by the Court of
Queen's Bench, a new trial having been granted. In allusion
to this case the Editor of *The Lancet* observes (Oct. 30,
1841) :

"The Act of 1815 has assumed a new form. Hitherto it
has been viewed by many as an useless document, or even as
an instrument of mischief. By several it has been felt to be a
law of oppression and injustice, and *the earlier decisions of the
judges* against Surgeons and Physicians, while the unqualified Druggist was allowed to practise with impunity, were
regarded as *offences against common sense and justice*, which
few honest hearts could tolerate. Men of rank and medical
education were prosecuted by the Company, while the uneducated pretender revelled in success and luxury."

This then was the construction put upon the Act, which
had never been deviated from during the space of twenty-six
years, at the end of which period the Court of Queen's Bench
set the old words to a new tune. It must be clear to every
reflecting mind that the lawyers who framed the words performed the task with consummate skill, since they obtained
credit from both parties at the time, and paved the way for a
rich harvest for the members of the legal profession. The
intention of the legislature was so well understood when the
law was passed, that the words were interpreted by all parties
in their true and literal sense, but it was policy in the lawyers
to have a double meaning in reserve for their own future
benefit.

On the 23rd of February, 1841, a meeting, convened by Mr.
Warington, for the purpose of taking into consideration the
formation of a CHEMICAL SOCIETY, was held in the rooms of
the Society of Arts.

---

* See pages 39, 45, etc.

The meeting was attended by several professors and other scientific men, and a society was established "for the advancement of Chemistry, and those branches of science immediately connected with it; for the communication and discussion of discoveries and observations relating to such subjects; the formation of a library of scientific works, and a museum of chemical preparations and standard instruments."

On the 30th of March, Professor Graham was appointed president; Professor Brande, J. F. Cooper, Esq., Professor Daniell, and R. Phillips, Esq., vice-presidents; Arthur Aikin, Esq., treasurer; E. F. Teschemacher and Robert Warington, secretaries. The council consisted of Dr. T. Clark, Professor J. Cumming, Dr. C. Daubeny, T. Everitt, Esq., T. Griffiths, Esq., W. R. Grove, Esq., H. Hennell, Esq., G. Lowe, Esq., Professor W. H. Miller, W. H. Pepys, Esq., R. Porrett, Esq., and Dr. G. O. Rees.

At that time the members amounted to seventy-seven, and the society has continued to increase and flourish. Its object being purely scientific, it numbers among its members men in various professions, who are devoted to the study of Chemistry, and embraces within its sphere every department of that science.

The origin and progress of Apothecaries' Hall having been noticed in general terms, it appears requisite to give a brief description of the establishment in its mature condition. In the 16th volume of the Quarterly Journal of the Royal Institution, the desired information is contained, in an article by Professor Brande, who has described the laboratories and apparatus in terms so concise and perspicuous that the substance of it is annexed as a quotation. A few improvements have subsequently taken place in some of the details, but the following account will serve to give a sufficiently correct idea of the extent and capabilities of the institution :—

" The principal laboratory is a brick building about fifty feet square and thirty high, lighted from above and subdivided by a brick wall into two compartments, the dimensions of the larger one being fifty feet by thirty; and of the smaller fifty feet by twenty. The former may properly be termed the *chemical laboratory*, all the open fires and furnaces being situated in it, and all operations requiring intense heat being there conducted. The latter is usually termed the *still-house*, all distillations and evaporations being performed there, exclusively by steam, which is furnished in a manner afterwards to be described. Immediately connected with the above mentioned building is a *chemical warehouse* for such articles as are in immediate consumption in the laboratory, above which is a small house for a clerk, the whole being shut off from the laboratory by iron doors. The principal entrance to the chemical laboratory is through the *mortar-room*, which is forty feet long and twenty-two broad, and appropriated to mortars, presses, and generally speaking to all mechanical operations performed by manual labour. At its eastern extremity is a large drying-stove, heated by flues, for the desiccation of those articles which cannot be dried conveniently at a temperature easily obtained by steam. At the west end of this apartment a room twenty-two feet by fifteen is divided off, in which is an apparatus for the production of gas from oil, with which the hall and its various departments both externally and internally are lighted.* Above the mortar-room is a gallery fitted with shelves for various utensils and apparatus, opening at one end into a room appropriated to the use of the labourers, and at the other into the *test-room*, a small laboratory fitted up with the requisite apparatus for minute and delicate investigations, and in which chemical tests and other articles requiring peculiar attention and cleanliness are prepared. Annexed to the *gas-room* is a counting-house, behind which a room, twenty-two feet square, commonly called the *magnesia-room*, is appropriated to the preparation of that article, and also to the manufacture of the most common saline preparations.

" In a detached building there is a steam-engine of eight-horse power, which is employed, with proper machinery, for grinding, sifting, triturating, pounding, and a variety of other operations. There are also connected with the establishment suitable warehouses, shops, and all other requisite conveniences for carrying on an extensive trade.

" In the construction of the new laboratory safety is

---

* In 1816, coal-gas was made on the premises for illumination ; in 1819, this was replaced by the oil-gas apparatus, which was discontinued in 1838, the gas being laid on from without. In the same year, a well (300 feet deep) was sunk, which supplies the establishment with water.

insured by the whole being fire-proof, and it is ventilated by a series of apertures in the roof, which may be opened or closed at pleasure. The main chimney is erected in the centre, and has opening into it below the pavement of the laboratory four large flues, one of which enters upon each side of its square base. The shaft is one hundred feet high from the foundation, and is accessible in its interior from one of the underground flues. The flues of the furnaces, which are placed against the walls of the laboratory, are each supplied with registers, and open into a common channel, which surrounds the building, terminating in the chimney as already described. Each of the four large flues has also a separate register, which may be more or less closed or opened, according to the operations which are going on in the various furnaces connected with it. The furnaces thus arranged are— a subliming apparatus for benzoic acid; a furnace for the preparation of sulphate of mercury; a high pressure steam boiler; a reverberatory furnace; a sand-bath; an apparatus for muriatic acid; ditto for nitric acid; ditto for the distillation of hartshorn, and a calcining furnace. There are also a series of furnaces built against the sides of the main chimney, and communicating directly with it by flues of their own, which, as well as the common openings by which they enter the chimney, are supplied with effectual registers, so that when not in use they may be perfectly closed. Of these furnaces four are chiefly employed for various sublimations and fusions; four more retort-pots. The third side of the chimney is occupied by a powerful wind furnace, and the fourth by a furnace for the sublimation of calomel. In this laboratory there is, moreover, a very plentiful supply of water both hot and cold; and an engine hose and pipe is always attached to the water-main in case of accident by fire, as well as for the purpose of cleansing the pavement. Beneath the building are extensive vaults for fuel, with which there is a direct communication by steps descending in one of the angles of the laboratory.

"The *still-house* contains six stills of various dimensions and constructions, twelve pans or boilers, and a drying stove, all of which are exclusively heated by steam supplied from an eight hundred gallon copper-boiler placed in an annexed building below the level of the still-house; and the flue of which, passing under the pavement of the laboratories, enters the main chimney already described. The boiler is calculated to supply steam under a pressure of an atmosphere and a-half, and is fed with hot water by a forcing pump kept in constant operation by the steam-engine.

" The main steam pipes, after ascending from the boiler, send off descending branches which ramify under the pavement of the still-house in channels of brick-work, covered by cast-iron plates. These send off a steam pipe, fitted with a register cock, to each still and boiler, from which there passes off an eduction or condensed water-pipe entering the condensed water main, the ramifications of which accompany the steam main and deliver their contents into a cistern, whence the boiler is supplied with hot water. A large branch of the steam-pipe circulates in five convolutions at the bottom of the drying stove, so as to heat a current of air which is made to pass through it; and another branch arising perpendicularly through the pavement is properly fitted with cocks and screws for the occasional attachment of leaden or other pipes, for boiling down liquids in moveable pans and vessels.

" In this building one of the stills is of a distinct construction and heated by high pressure steam, supplied from the boiler already mentioned in the description of the laboratory. Another still together with its condensing pipe is composed entirely of earthenware. The former is chiefly used for the first distillation of sulphuric ether, and the latter for that of spirit of nitric ether. The stills and vessels are generally heated by the circulation of steam upon their exterior, but sometimes serpentine pipes traversing the liquor are employed. In the still-house all spirits and waters are distilled; extracts and plaisters are prepared, and all operations are carried on which involve risk by fire or in which damage is likely to occur from excess of heat. The magnesia-room contains proper vats and boilers for the production and evaporation of saline solutions; the apparatus for the precipitation of carbonate of magnesia, and a series of vessels for saturating alkalies with carbonic acid."

In the commencement of the year 1839, a commotion arose among the Assistants of the Druggists and Apothecaries of London, who held several meetings for the purpose of taking into consideration the hardships they suffered on account of their close confinement during every day in the week, Sundays included, and the want of that recreation which their bodily health and mental improvement required. It was urged as an anomaly which demanded an effectual remedy, that while the Pharmaceutical Assistants were labouring to provide for the health of the public, they were sacrificing their own; and that while they were engaged in an occupation in which the cultivation of their minds in the study of Chemistry and other sciences was essential, their whole time was occupied in the mechanical drudgery of the shop, which precluded the possibility of acquiring the needful education. A Committee was appointed, and after several discussions had taken place, a memorial was sent round to the Principals, respectfully representing the grievances complained of, and requesting them to call a meeting of the trade for the purpose of providing a remedy.

Accordingly, a meeting was held on the 18th of February, 1839, at which the opinions on both sides of the question were fully and fairly stated. Many of the masters advocated warmly the expediency of adopting to a certain extent the measures proposed by the Committee of Assistants, closing the shops at an earlier hour every evening (except Saturday) and keeping them entirely closed on Sundays. Others considered that, however expedient this regulation might appear, it was nevertheless impracticable, on account of the impossibility of compelling all parties to adhere to it, and also from the difficulty of making any law in a case of this kind which would be applicable to all parts of London, it being well known that, in some localities, business in general is in the height of activity at the time in the evening at which, in other localities, almost every shop is closed. The hardships detailed by the Assistants were admitted to be great and pressing, and the desire to provide a remedy was only equalled by the difficulty of finding one.

After a long debate it was decided, that the meeting had not the power of enforcing the cessation of business at an earlier hour in the evening; but a general opinion prevailed that this would be very desirable wherever it could be effected. A resolution was unanimously passed, recommending the entire closing of shops and the discouragement of all business, except in cases of absolute necessity, on Sunday. A Committee was appointed to carry out this resolution, and bills were printed and circulated extensively among the trade, containing a copy of the resolution, and a brief statement of the facts which had led to it, which bills were designed to obtain the concurrence of the public in the measure. A considerable number of Chemists acted upon this resolution, which came into operation on the first Sunday in March.

In some instances, however, the adherence to the regulation was but ephemeral; the Assistants, in several establishments, complained of the darkness of the shop, and said that their labour was considerably increased by the trouble of opening the door for every customer. They therefore requested that the door-shutters might be removed, and the new regulation was laid aside. In other cases the regulation was violated without any reason being assigned, which gave offence to many of those who had adhered to their resolution, some of whom followed the example. The result was generally considered an illustration of the difficulty of legislating for a large body of men, in a matter in which individual interests and local circumstances are likely to interfere. A considerable number have continued, up to the present time, to close their shops on Sundays, and have had no reason to regret so doing. The credit of drawing the attention of the Assistants to the subject belongs to Mr. Hewett, the secretary of the Committee, and Mr. Fuller, who acted as chairman. Mr. Payne, Mr. Hallows, and the late Mr. Hudson, took an active part in the proceedings.

In the year 1841, Mr. Hawes, Mr. Ewart, and Mr. Hutton endeavoured to reform the profession by introducing a bill which was printed in the beginning of February. It having been generally understood that no material change would take place in the Pharmaceutical department, the Chemists took little or no interest in the measures in progress.

The Patent Medicine Venders had, however, already exerted their influence in obtaining the insertion of a clause which secured to them all their former privileges, and an exemption from any interference; but the Chemists and Druggists remained inactive, until the bill had been published and circulated. It was then discovered that the contemplated measures were very different from those which had been advocated by the Chairman of the Parliamentary Committee. Before re-cording the proceedings of the Chemists and Druggists, it may be as well to state briefly the grounds of their opposition to the bill.

In the interpretation clause, it is stated, that

The words "Practising Medicine," shall be construed to include within their meaning the recommending, prescribing, or ordering, either directly or indirectly, any medicine, remedy, or application whatsoever, for the relief or cure of any disorder, ailment, or illness of the body or mind, or any part thereof, or performing any surgical operation, minor or capital, or practising midwifery: and the words "Medical Practitioner," shall mean a person qualified under this Act to practise medicine: and that the words "Chemist and Druggist," shall mean a person who shall sell, deal in, mix, or dispense for sale, any drug or medicine for the cure or relief of any bodily disorder, ailment or illness, save and except such person as shall have obtained a certificate to practise medicine.

It was provided (sec. 33),

That no male person whatsoever, on or after the 1st day of February, 1842, be permitted to practise medicine for remuneration or gain, either directly or indirectly in any part of the kingdom of Great Britain and Ireland, unless such person shall have obtained a certificate to practise the same according to the provisions of this Act; nor shall any person whatsoever, on or after the first day of December, 1842, be entitled or permitted to carry on the trade or business of a Chemist and Druggist in any part of the United Kingdom of Great Britain and Ireland, unless such person shall have obtained a licence to carry on the said trade and business according to the provisions of this Act.

The licence to be renewed annually on payment of a fee.

Sec. 48. Every person not being duly qualified according to the provisions of this Act, who shall practise medicine for remuneration or gain, either directly or indirectly, or who shall carry on the trade and business of a Chemist and Druggist, shall forfeit and pay for every such offence the sum of *Twenty Pounds.*

The penalty for employing an Assistant, not duly qualified according to the provisions of the Act, was stated at *Ten Pounds.*

Sec. 51.   In every case of the adjudication of a pecuniary penalty under this Act, and non-payment thereof, it shall be lawful for the magistrate to commit the offender to any gaol or house of correction within his jurisdiction.

Coupling the definition of the term *practising medicine* with the clauses inflicting a penalty or imprisonment, for practising without a certificate, it is clear that a Chemist would be liable to a penalty of twenty pounds for recommending ten grains of rhubarb, strapping a cut finger, or explaining to a customer the usual mode of taking any medicine, however simple or innocuous, and that summary imprisonment (or a ruinous law-suit) would be the result of non-payment.

The constitution of the governing body was also objectionable :—

A Council was to be elected in each kingdom every three years, twenty Councillors for each.   The several universities and medical bodies to send each one member to their respective Councils, the other members to be elected by ballot. Every medical practitioner to have a vote.

Hence the general practitioners, the number of whom preponderates over all other medical bodies, would have a proportionate majority of votes.

Each Council to elect three persons every five years to form a medical senate.   The senate to make bye-laws to regulate the education of students and the examinations for diploma of qualification to practise medicine, or to carry on the trade of a Chemist and Druggist.   The Council to appoint examiners annually.

Chemists and Druggists therefore would be under the jurisdiction of a body in which they were not represented, and in the election of which the Apothecaries had the largest number of votes.

Sec. 39.   All persons, being at present Chemists and Druggists, or Assistants or Apprentices, claiming the exemption within twelve months, to obtain licences, and not to be called upon to renew them annually, unless they desire ; if they renew them, their names are to be published in the respective medical lists, and not otherwise.

Thus a Chemist and Druggist who claimed the exemption, would lose his rank altogether, his name being omitted in the list ; and if he claimed to be registered, he would forfeit the only privilege to which he was entitled from having been in business before the passing of the Act.

A few other objections of minor importance might have been enumerated, but the above constituted the chief ground of resistance on the part of the Chemists.

The credit of drawing the attention of the trade to this bill is due to Mr. Farmar, Mr. G. W. Smith, and Mr. Baxter, who met several times to consider the subject, in company with a few of their friends.

The following is a report of one of the meetings held at the house of Mr. Farmar :—

> At a meeting of Chemists and Druggists, held Feb. 10th, 1841, to take into consideration the draft of a Bill recently proposed by Mr. Hawes,
>
> Mr. FARMAR in the chair.

Moved by Mr. G. W. Smith, seconded by Mr. Baxter, *and resolved,*

> "That this bill having been introduced into the House of Commons, and having for its object an entire change in the present method of conducting the business of a Chemist and Druggist, this meeting deems it expedient that a public meeting of the members of the trade be forthwith held, to take into consideration the tendency of the provisions of the said bill."

Moved by Mr. Thomas Kent, seconded by Mr. S. M. Mayhew, *and resolved,*

> "That a public meeting of the Chemists and Druggists of the metropolis be held at the Crown and Anchor Tavern, in the Strand, on Monday, the 15th instant, at eleven o'clock in the forenoon."

Moved by Mr. Warboys, seconded by Mr. S. Weatherby, *and resolved,*

> "That advertisements of the intended meeting be made in the *Times* and *Morning Chronicle* newspapers, and also that circulars be issued to as many of the trade as may be practicable."

Moved by Mr. W. Lowe, seconded by Mr. Thomas Kent, *and resolved,*

" That Mr. William Allen, of Plough Court, be requested to preside at the meeting."

" GEO. W. SMITH, *Secretary pro tem.*"

Mr. Farmar and his friends lost no time in waiting on as many of their brethren as possible, in order to obtain signatures to the requisition calling a public meeting. Although they met with but little encouragement they succeeded in obtaining a sufficient number of names, and issued the following circular :—

" We, the undersigned, having seen with considerable alarm some clauses in a bill recently introduced into the House of Commons, and appointed for a second reading on Friday, Feb. 19th ; such bill tending materially to injure the interests of Chemists and Druggists, do hereby invite a public meeting of the members of the trade, to be holden at the Crown and Anchor Tavern, in the Strand, on Monday the 15th instant, at eleven o'clock in the forenoon, to take into consideration the provisions of the said bill."

WM. ALLEN, HANBURYS and BARRY.
SAVORY, MOORE & CO.
JOHN BELL & CO.
GODFREY & COOKE.
W. B. HUDSON & SON.
CORBYN & CO.
PIGEON & SON.
HERRING BROTHERS.
HORNER & SONS.
ELLIS, LANGTON & CO.
BARRON, HARVEY & BARRON.
J. GIFFORD.
FISHER & TOLLER.
CHARLES DINNEFORD.

GEORGE GRINDLE.
JOSEPH SMITH.
JAMES STARKIE.
W. WILLMOTT.
R. YATE & SON.
HODGKINSON, STEAD & TONGE.
HOWARD & COLEMAN.
DREW, HEYWARD & CO.
THOS. MARSDEN & SONS.
EVANS & LESCHER.
JAS. METCALFE & SONS.
BAISS BROTHERS & CO.
ED. WINSTANLEY & SON.
RICHARD BATTLEY.

It is a singular fact, that those whose names were attached to the circular had taken no part in the proceedings, while the names of the original movers and acting men were omitted. The object of this selection was to enlist in the work those members, both of the wholesale and retail trade, whose interest it was thought desirable at once to secure, and whose names were extensively known throughout the country.

It was in this manner that several of the members of the Council of the PHARMACEUTICAL SOCIETY were induced to embark in an undertaking in which they had no desire to take a prominent part, but having been called together by the solicitations of others, and considering it their duty to unite with their brethren in any measures which, to the majority, might appear desirable, they found themselves obliged to continue their exertions in a manner which they had not at first anticipated.

At a large and influential public meeting of Chemists and Druggists, held at the Crown and Anchor Tavern, Strand, convened by advertisement, and held on Monday, February 15th, 1841, for the purpose of taking into consideration " A Bill to amend the Laws relating to the Medical Profession of Great Britain and Ireland," recently introduced into Parliament by Mr. Hawes,

Mr. GIFFORD in the chair,

A letter having been read from William Allen, of Plough Court, excusing his absence, but sanctioning his appointment as member of any Committee, it was

Moved by Mr. Bell, seconded by Mr. Keating, *and resolved*,

" That the provisions of this bill deeply injure the interests and lessen the usefulness of Chemists and Druggists, as well as affect the comforts and resources of the poorer classes of society, whilst the immediate and pressing wants of individuals would create a liability to informations, which would be a source of unceasing vexation."

Moved by Mr. Barry, seconded by Mr. Farmar, *and resolved*,

" That it is the opinion of this meeting, that Benjamin Hawes, as author of this bill, intituled ' *A Bill to amend the Laws relating to the Medical Profession in Great Britain and Ireland*,' should be requested to defer for one month the second reading, to enable the public and all parties interested to form their opinion upon its merits."

Moved by Mr. Walker, seconded by Mr. W. Ince, *and resolved,*

"That petitions be immediately presented to Parliament against Mr. Hawes' bill, especially against that clause depriving Chemists and Druggists of their right to prescribe and recommend medicines."

Moved by Mr. Wilkinson, seconded by Mr. Mayhew, *and resolved,*

"That the following be a Committee, with power to add to their number, for the purpose of watching and opposing the progress of this bill, viz. :—

WILLIAM ALLEN, F.R.S.	THOMAS WALKER.
JOSEPH GIFFORD.	THOMAS KEATING.
JACOB BELL.	EDWARD WINSTANLEY.
CHARLES DINNEFORD.	GEORGE WAUGH.
JOHN TOLLER.	THOMAS BUTLER.
JOSEPH SMITH.	SAMUEL M. MAYHEW.
RICHARD BATTLEY.	ROBERT FARMAR.
JOHN T. BARRY.	SAMUEL DE CASTRO.
JOHN ELLIS.	SAMUEL GREEN.
SAMUEL FOULGER.	EDWARD SIMKIN.
WILLIAM LOWE.	WILLIAM INCE.
CHARLES DAVY.	EDWIN BRIGGS.
EDWARD HORNER.	GEORGE BAXTER.
RICH. HOTHAM PIGEON.	J. S. LESCHER.
THROWER HERRING.	G. W. SMITH.
CHARLES BARRON.	RALPH STAMPER."
THOMAS HERRING.	

Moved by Mr. Dinneford, seconded by Mr. Austin, *and resolved,*

"That Mr. R. H. Pigeon be appointed treasurer, and subscriptions solicited from all the Chemists and Druggists of the United Kingdom."

Moved by Mr. Keating, seconded by Mr. Watts, *and resolved,*

"That a copy of these proceedings be printed, and sent to every member of the drug trade in town and country, and also be published in the newspapers."

Moved by Mr. Herring, seconded by Mr. Farmar, *and resolved*,

> "That the best thanks of this meeting be given to the chairman, for the official performance of his duties."

The above resolutions gave rise to a very animated discussion, and, although on minor particulars a little difference of opinion was occasionally expressed, there was but one individual present who stood up in support of the bill. This gentleman had been deputed by Mr. Hawes to attend the meeting, in order to explain any clauses in the bill which might require elucidation, and the able manner in which he performed the task deserves to be recorded. In a large assembly, in which considerable agitation and enthusiasm prevailed, in which the bill was denounced in no measured terms, and each sally of criticism was followed by applause, this champion stood up, unmoved, and in a calm and temperate manner, expatiated on the various clauses, for the purpose of proving that the bill, instead of being injurious, was, in fact, intended as a boon to Chemists and Druggists—that it was calculated to raise their standing in the profession, to increase their influence and extend their business. The meeting listened with as much complaisance as could be expected on such an occasion, under the impression that the speaker was the legal adviser of Mr. Hawes, but no change of sentiment was the result, as the data on which the chief arguments were founded were hypothetical, whilst the objections against the bill were felt to be unanswerable by all present, except the speaker.

Immediately after the meeting, the Committee assembled, and resolved that 3,000 copies of the resolutions should be printed and circulated, and the Report advertised. Mr. Alderman Thomas Wood was engaged as solicitor, and J. Sidney Taylor, Esq., was retained as counsel. A circular was drawn up to accompany the resolutions, calling upon the members of the trade to unite in raising subscriptions, and preparing a petition to Parliament. This appeal was answered by a voluminous correspondence from all quarters, accompanied by subscriptions from many places. The Committee met on the following day, February 16th, at the house of Mr. Pigeon, in Throgmorton Street, when a letter from

Mr. Ewart was read, stating that the second reading of the bill would not take place on the 19th. Mr. Pound was added to the Committee, and a Sub-Committee was appointed to draw up a petition, and also to wait upon Mr. Hawes.

An interview having been granted, the Sub-Committee detailed their objections to the bill, requested that the second reading might be delayed for at least a month, and that a clause should be inserted exempting Chemists and Druggists from the operation of the bill. Mr. Hawes introduced his friend Mr. Cooper, whom the Committee recognised as being the gentleman who had fought the battle so ably single-handed at the public meeting, and who it appeared was not a legal but a medical practitioner. Mr. Cooper acquiesced in the propriety of delay, and Mr. Hawes offered to expunge every clause in which Chemists were mentioned, but the insertion of a new clause, similar to that in the Act of 1815, was objected to.

At a meeting of the Committee on February 22, the solicitor reported that Mr. Hawes had withdrawn his bill, and also that the Colleges of Physicians and Surgeons, and the Society of Apothecaries contemplated the introduction of a bill for the regulation of the profession. A Sub-Committee was appointed, which met on the 5th of March, and instructed the Secretary to address the Colleges of Physicians and Surgeons, requesting an interview with each of those learned bodies.

The deputation waited on the College of Surgeons on the 9th of March, by appointment, and opened the discussion by inquiring whether the College was opposed to the principles of the bill of Mr. Hawes? and whether the three medical bodies were, as had been reported, preparing a bill in which the interests of Chemists and Druggists were concerned? The President replied that the College had petitioned against Mr. Hawes' bill; but did not intend to take any active measures on the subject of medical reform. It was their desire to confine their proceedings to their own department—pure surgery. They declined interfering in any way with Pharmacy, which they left in the hands of the Physicians, Apothecaries, and Druggists.

In their official capacity as Surgeons they did not pretend to be able to distinguish one drug from another, and trusted to those whose duty it was to prepare their prescriptions.

On the 8th of March the General Committee met, and the solicitor presented a copy of a modified bill just introduced by Mr. Hawes. This bill was considered no less objectionable than its predecessor; for, although the clauses relating to Chemists and Druggists had been expunged, no provision was made for the regulation of that body, and some parts of the bill were *indirectly* prejudicial. The solicitor was, therefore, instructed to prepare a petition against the bill for presentation to both Houses of Parliament. Mr. Morson was added to the Committee.

On the 10th of March the Sub-Committee adopted a form of petition, which was prepared for signature, and the Secretary was instructed to forward printed copies to every town in the kingdom, for the signature of the Chemists in their respective localities.

The Sub-Committee waited on the College of Physicians, by appointment, on the 10th of March, and was informed that the College had opposed the former bill of Mr. Hawes, and intended to oppose the one then before the House. The College had consulted with the Apothecaries' Company on the subject of a bill, but had not as yet come to any determination on the subject. The members of the College had no wish to interfere with Chemists and Druggists. They thought it evident that some adequate education and an examination should be instituted, and proposed to form a board in conjunction with the Apothecaries' Company for that purpose. To this the deputation objected, stating that a board composed of Physicians and Chemists would be mor satisfactory. The Physicians replied, that they had no desire to take an active part in the examination of Chemists, and their only reason for proposing to join in it was that they might satisfy themselves that it was efficiently conducted. They inquired whether the deputation had any definite plan to lay before them ; and being informed that the arrangements were not yet matured, they expressed their willingness to confer with the deputation at a future time when they were prepared with a definite proposition.

At a meeting of the General Committee, March 20, the Chairman (Mr. Gifford) reported that the metropolitan petition, with 604 signatures, had been presented to the House of Commons by Mr. Alderman Thompson, and that when the Speaker inquired whether any members had petitions to present against the bill, above half the House rose simultaneously, and a shower of petitions covered the table. The House was afterwards counted out. The Committee instructed the solicitor to watch the further progress of the bill. On the 2nd of April, Messrs. Savory, Squire, Hudson, and Alsop, were added to the Committee and also to the Sub-Committee.

During the numerous meetings of the Committee (of which the above is a considerably abridged report) the propriety of establishing a society was frequently suggested; but it was found impossible in an open committee to come to an unanimous decision on the details of so important a measure.

The subject, however, was not forgotten, and the members of the Committee saw plainly that nothing short of a permanent Association could secure the trade against a recurrence of the inconveniences and annoyances which it had from time to time experienced during the last half-century. An opportunity was within their reach which might not speedily occur again. A correspondence had been opened with the Chemists in all parts of the country on a subject in which all their interests were concerned; in the excitement occasioned by the threatened blow at their independence minor considerations were forgotten; and all appeared disposed cordially to unite in promoting the general welfare. So little intercourse had hitherto existed among the members of the body, that a degree of coolness and distrust had been unfortunately too prevalent; and the failure of all former attempts to form an efficient society had been, in a great measure, occasioned by the division of that influence which ought to have been united and directed with energy to this one object. But in the present crisis, jealousy seemed to be forgotten, and the necessity of union was so obvious that the first step appeared to be accomplished.

The ground upon which the late attempts had been made to interfere with Chemists and Druggists, had reference to their amount of professional qualification, although the arguments brought forward against them assumed a variety of forms, and were in many cases unjust and intemperate. However galling it might be to bear the taunts and impu-

tations, there was no escape while the fact was notorious that
no institution existed in this country for the systematic education and examination of Chemists and Druggists, and whilst
no proof could be advanced that each individual possessed the
needful qualification.

It was evident that Pharmacy must be placed on a more
scientific footing, and that some measures would speedily be
adopted for introducing an improved system of education. It
was, therefore, the policy of the Druggists to anticipate what
was about to take place, and instead of wasting their time in
fruitless controversy, to give a practical answer to all objections by establishing a system of government for themselves
which could admit of no reproach.

The prospect of attaining this object opened out a new field
of interest, and some members of the Committee who had
been in the first instance induced reluctantly to join it, by
the earnest solicitations of their brethren, entered into the
subject with increased spirit when the opportunity of raising
the professional character of their body presented itself. But
the task was one which required the most mature deliberation
and unwearied perseverance. The members of the Committee
were not unanimous either as to the details of the plan or the
mode of accomplishing it, and there was every reason to
anticipate still greater difficulty in amalgamating the various
opinions of the body at large on so intricate and momentous
a question.

On the 20th of March, 1841, several members of the Committee met at a Pharmaceutical tea-party, at the house of one
of their number (Mr. Bell, Oxford Street), and after having
discussed the subject in a friendly manner, agreed to a few
resolutions as the basis to the new society. Several other meetings of this unofficial character took place, at each of which
other members were added to the number, until twenty-four
of the Committee were unanimous on the general principles
of the Association. During these deliberations it was found
difficult to decide what relation the society should bear to the
medical profession, and whether it should be a body entirely
independent, or in some degree connected with the College
of Physicians or the London University. Some of the leading members of the profession were consulted on these points,
but so great a difference of opinion was found to exist, tha

the Committee abandoned the prospect of receiving any assistance from the profession, and determined to create an
independent body.

The abstract principles of the Association having been
maturely considered by the Sub-Committee, the subject was
referred to the General Committee on the 5th of April, and
the following resolutions were unanimously carried :—

"1st. That the permanent interests of Chemists and Druggists require that they shall immediately form themselves into
a society.

"2nd. That this Society be forthwith formed under the
title of the PHARMACEUTICAL SOCIETY OF GREAT BRITAIN.

"3rd. That the Society consist, in the first instance, of
such established Chemists and Druggists as shall voluntarily
come forward in aid of its objects and intentions.

"4th. That the object of the Society be,—To benefit the
public, and elevate the profession of Pharmacy, by furnishing
the means of proper instruction; to protect the collective
and individual interests and privileges of all its members, in
the event of any hostile attack in Parliament or otherwise;
to establish a club for the relief of decayed or distressed
members."

"5th. That at a general meeting of Chemists and Druggists, to be convened for the purpose of forming an outline
of the Society, a Committee be appointed to frame such laws
and regulations as may appear desirable for the attainment
of the objects intended, which laws, etc., shall be afterwards
discussed and completed at another general meeting of the
members.

In accordance with these resolutions a public meeting was
convened at the Crown and Anchor Tavern, on the 15th
of April, at which the Committee presented the following
report :—

Your Committee, immediately upon their appointment,
opened a communication with the Chemists and Druggists
of every town in England, and of some towns in Ireland and
Scotland, requesting the co-operation of the members of the
trade, and soliciting subscriptions to enable them to offer the
most powerful and effectual opposition to Mr. Hawes's bill ,
and your Committee had the satisfaction of receiving, not

only promises of support, but liberal subscriptions from many places.

Agreeably with the instructions of the general meeting, your Committee proceeded to the appointment of a deputation, for the purpose of conferring with Mr. Hawes, on the subject of postponing the second reading of his bill; to which request Mr. Hawes readily acceded, and also undertook to erase from the said bill every clause having special reference to the Chemists and Druggists.

Upon the introduction of Mr. Hawes's second bill, your Committee, acting under the advice of their counsel and solicitor, determined to offer it their most powerful opposition, as the provisions of the latter bill had an injurious power over the interests of the Chemists and Druggists equal with that of the former.

Your Committee, through their solicitor, thereupon required of Mr. Hawes that he should insert a protective and explanatory clause, which should render the bill totally inoperative upon the interests of Chemists and Druggists. To this Mr. Hawes has assented; and should the bill pass a second reading the said clause will be duly inserted.

Your Committee, however, are bound by parliamentary usage to offer an opposition to the second reading of the bill, and they have caused a petition to be presented in the House of Commons against the measure.

They have also sent a copy of the same to almost every town in England, requiring the members of the trade, in the various localities, to forward a petition, on their own parts, against the bill, and to instruct their representatives in the same opposition. Your Committee had the satisfaction of finding that, upon the second reading of the bill being attempted, a large number of petitions were presented against it, and the House was "counted out." Your Committee, though warranted in expressing an opinion that this bill will not pass, are yet aware of the undiminished necessity of watching any further attempts to accomplish that object.

In the progress of their proceedings your Committee ascertained that the College of Physicians, the College of Surgeons, and the Apothecaries' Company, had conjointly proposed obtaining some legislative enactment, by which the Chemists and Druggists were to be, for the future, placed under the government and control of these learned bodies, more especially of the Society of Apothecaries.

A deputation from your Committee, therefore, sought and obtained an interview with the College of Physicians and the College of Surgeons, respectively, and received from the former an official notification that it was their intention to introduce into their proposed measures of medical reform, a provision by which the Chemists and Druggists should henceforth be placed under some legislative control; and your Committee have, therefore, again assembled you for the purpose of receiving new instructions and enlarged powers to meet present and future circumstances.

Your Committee having considered the subject, are of opinion that the Chemists and Druggists are capable of self-government; they, therefore, recommend that the Chemists and Druggists of the empire should immediately form themselves into a permanent Association, to be denominated the "PHARMACEUTICAL SOCIETY OF GREAT BRITAIN," having for its object the union of the members of the trade into one body, the protection of the general interests, and the improvement and advancement of scientific knowledge. As the basis of such union, your Committee would recommend the adoption of education, examination, registration, and representation as involving beneficial results to the public in general, and to the Chemists and Druggists in particular; and offering to the existing medical corporations, and to the medical profession at large, a guarantee, that whilst the Chemists and Druggists are anxious to retain their present privileges, they are disposed to afford every public evidence of their fitness to exercise them.

JOSEPH GIFFORD, *Chairman.*

———

At a public meeting of the members of the trade, held at the Crown and Anchor Tavern, in the Strand, on Thursday, April 15th inst.,

R. H. PIGEON, Esq., in the chair,

the foregoing report having been read, it was

Moved by Mr. Payne, seconded by Mr. Wilkinson, *and re-solved,*

"That this report be received, and the best thanks of this meeting be given to the Committee for their past exertions."

Moved by Mr. Dinneford, seconded by Mr. Hudson, *and resolved,*

"That the report be printed, and circulated at the discretion of the Committee."

Moved by William Allen, F.R.S., seconded by John Bell, *and resolved,*

"That for the purpose of protecting the permanent interests, and increasing the respectability of Chemists and Druggists, an Association be now formed under the title of the ' PHARMACEUTICAL SOCIETY OF GREAT BRITAIN.' "

Moved by Mr. Morson, seconded by Mr. Davy, *and resolved,*

"That the present Committee be requested to frame laws and regulations for the government of the society, to be laid before the next meeting of the members for confirmation and adoption."

Moved by Mr. Savory, seconded by Mr. Gifford, *and resolved,*

"That the thanks of this meeting be given to Richard Hotham Pigeon, Esq., for the able and satisfactory performance of the duties of Chairman; and also for having afforded every accommodation to the Committee in their meetings at his house in Throgmorton Street."

Nearly 100 signatures were obtained at the close of the meeting to a declaration which stated, that the undersigned constituted themselves members of the PHARMACEUTICAL SOCIETY OF GREAT BRITAIN.

LIST OF COMMITTEE.

ALLEN, WILLIAM, F.R.S., Plough Court; ALSOP, ROBERT, 15, Sloane Square, Chelsea; BARRON, CHARLES, 6, Giltspur Street; BARRY, JOHN T., Plough Court; BATTLEY, RICHARD, 32, Lower Whitecross Street; BAXTER, GEORGE, 144, High Holborn; BELL, JACOB, 338, Oxford Street; BRIGGS, EDWIN, 48, Wigmore Street; BUTLER, THOMAS, 4, Cheapside; DAVY, CHARLES, 100, Upper Thames Street; DE CASTRO, SAMUEL, 25, Great St. George's Place, Knightsbridge; DINNEFORD, CHARLES, 172,

New Bond Street; ELLIS, JOHN, 225, Upper Thames Street; FARMAR, ROBERT A., 40, Westminster Road; FOULGER, SAMUEL, 133, Ratcliffe Highway; GIFFORD, JOSEPH, 104, Strand; GREEN, SAMUEL, 1, Harleyford Place, Kennington; HANBURY, DANIEL B., Plough Court; HERRING, THOMAS, 40, Aldersgate Street; HORNER, EDWARD, 20, Bucklersbury; HUDSON, WILLIAM B., 27, Haymarket; INCE, WILLIAM, 31, Southampton Street, Covent Garden; KEATING, THOMAS, 79, St. Paul's Churchyard; LESCHER, J. S., 4, Cripplegate Buildings; LOWE, WILLIAM, 47, Blackfriars' Road; MAYHEW, SAMUEL M., Camberwell Green; MORSON, THOMAS, 19, Southampton Row; PAYNE, CHARLES JAMES, 5, St. Martin's Court; PIGEON, RICHARD HOTHAM, 31, Throgmorton Street; POUND, MATTHEW, 198, Oxford Street; SAVORY, JOHN, 143, Bond Street; SIMKIN, EDWARD, 2, New Cavendish Street, Portland Place; SMITH, JOSEPH, 29, Haymarket; SMITH, GEORGE W., 125, Lower Thames Street; SQUIRE, PETER, 277, Oxford Street; STAMPER, RALPH, 140, Leadenhall Street; TOLLER, JOHN, 18, Conduit Street; WALKER, THOMAS, 48, Tooley Street; WAUGH, GEORGE 177, Regent Street; WINSTANLEY, EDWARD, 7, Poultry.

Immediately after the meeting, the Committee assembled, and ordered 5,000 copies of the report to be printed and circulated. Mr. G. W. Smith was appointed Secretary, conjointly with Mr. Farmar, and Mr. Payne was added to the Committee.

The consideration of the laws was referred to the Sub-Committee, and, on the 27th of April, a draft of the same, which had been prepared for discussion, was ordered to be printed: frequent meetings took place, during which every clause was discussed and canvassed in all its bearings; a variety of amendments were made, and, on the 25th of May, the LAWS were submitted to the General Committee in their complete state.

During the period in which the laws were in course of preparation, which occupied nearly two months, inquiries were not unfrequently made by those who were not on the Committee, respecting the progress of the Society, and surprise was expressed at the apparent cessation of the work which had been undertaken. The excitement which had been occasioned by Mr. Hawes's bill had in some measure subsided,

when that measure was withdrawn; the official correspondence had almost ceased, and it was feared that an impression
might prevail that the project was falling to the ground.

In order to keep up the interest in what was going on, and
to promote the good feeling which had recently been evinced
by the members of the trade, a pharmaceutical meeting was
held on the 11th of May, at 338, Oxford Street, to which
medical men as well as Chemists and Druggists were invited.
A paper, on the Constitution of the Pharmaceutical Society,
was read; and, at the suggestion of several persons present,
a few copies were printed and circulated. An opportunity
was afforded on the above occasion of explaining the measures
which were in progress for the establishment of the Society,
and the favourable reception which this explanation met with,
together with the good attendance at the meeting, more than
realized the objects for which it was held; and five other
meetings for the discussion of subjects relating to Pharmacy
were announced as an experiment, with a view to the permanent establishment of similar scientific assemblies by the
Society.

On the 25th of May, the General Committee having discussed and approved the laws which had been prepared by
the Sub-Committee, resolved to convene a public meeting of
the members, which was held at the Crown and Anchor, on
Tuesday, the 1st of June, and at which they presented the
following REPORT, together with the draft of the LAWS :—

Agreeably with your instructions, and in conformity with
the principles laid down in the last report, your Committee
have prepared the fundamental laws of the Pharmaceutical
Society in such a manner as shall leave to every one, whether
Principal, Assistant, or Apprentice, all rights and privileges
enjoyed by his predecessors; whilst regulations are proposed
which shall assure to the public and the profession the competence of such Chemists and Druggists as shall be members
of this Society.

The unanimity which prevails among Chemists and Druggists, upon the expediency and necessity of establishing an
Association for the purpose of protecting their interests,
induces the Committee to hope that the same unity of sentiment will prevail in carrying out the details of this important
measure.

The influence which Chemists and Druggists possess as a body when their efforts are combined, has been demonstrated in a manner which affords every encouragement to perseverance. It is equally manifest, that if they relax in their exertions, or allow any minor considerations to interfere with the zealous and harmonious performance of the duty which they owe to themselves, they will inevitably sacrifice their independence and be deprived of many of their existing privileges, by becoming subject to extraneous jurisdiction. It must be recollected that the Society is of a PUBLIC nature, and involves the prosperity of Chemists and Druggists as a body throughout the kingdom. It is only by the combined and continued efforts of individuals that a scheme so comprehensive and laborious can be effected ; and these efforts, to be successful, must be supported by all those who are interested in its accomplishment.

In drawing up the fundamental regulations of the Society, your Committee have carefully guarded against the possibility of those abuses which have often arisen in similar institutions; and while they have vested in the Council sufficient powers to render their services effective, they have made them entirely responsible to, and to be elected by, the members at large.

To Chemists and Druggists now established, this Society offers the means of extending pharmaceutical knowledge by the establishment of a recognised medium through which discoveries and improvements may be promulgated ; whilst the institution of a School of Pharmacy—the development of scientific acquirements, and the exhibition of existing talent will tend to confirm the confidence of the public, and remove our apparent deficiency as pharmacopolists, when compared with other nations.

To Assistants it will afford the means of practical improvement, and an opportunity of obtaining honorary distinction.

To Apprentices the Society offers an immediate recognition of their admission to the trade, and holds out a sufficient inducement for industrious and studious habits, by affording the prospect of participation in the elevated position and character which will hereafter appertain to those who practise Pharmacy.

The course of education proposed embraces only such subects as should be known by every person presuming to dispense prescriptions; and though at the outset it would not be stringently enforced, it will be the duty of the Council to extend the examination as circumstances may require.

By the regulations under the head of Education and Examination, all existing Chemists and Druggists have the opportunity of escaping any restriction or ordeal which may be imposed upon their successors; and in order to enjoy this exemption, nothing is demanded from them but that they shall unite in supporting an institution which the protection of their interests has rendered necessary.

The establishment of an examination in the classics for all future Apprentices, will ensure the possession of that preliminary education which is essentially necessary for the creditable performance of their duties, and their ultimate success as pharmaceutists; and the increased importance and respectability which will be conferred upon Pharmacy by means of this Society will induce many of the more wealthy classes to devote themselves to its pursuit.

In order to establish among the Chemists and Druggists of the empire a substantial and permanent bond of union, and also to supply a deficiency which has hitherto existed, your Committee recommend the foundation of a fund for the relief of the distressed, the widow, and the orphan; and, taking encouragement from the example and success of other bodies, they trust that this collateral object of the Society will obtain universal support.

The Committee have the satisfaction of stating, that a communication has been received from Paris, intimating a desire on the part of some of the leading members of the Society of Pharmacy in that city, to establish a scientific correspondence with " THE PHARMACEUTICAL SOCIETY OF GREAT BRITAIN ; " and overtures of a similar character have been made on behalf of the College of Pharmacy in Philadelphia. The Chemists and Druggists of Scotland and Ireland have also expressed considerable interest in the undertaking.

Your Committee, therefore, congratulate you on the circumstance, that, although the Chemists and Druggists of Great Britain united in the first instance merely for the purpose of self-defence, in support of their acknowledged rights, that union has resulted in the creation of a National Institution for the advancement of Pharmacy, which will be enabled to carry on a correspondence with similar institutions throughout the world.

The establishment of such correspondence, the formation of this Institution, and the successful result of the opposition to the bill of Mr. Hawes, will ever be regarded by your Committee as a gratifying recompense for their past exertions.

JOSEPH GIFFORD, Chairman.

R. H. PIGEON, Esq., took the chair,

And the report of the Committee having been read, it was

Moved by Mr. Savory, seconded by Mr. Morson, *and resolved unanimously,*

"That the report now read be adopted and printed for circulation."

The Laws of THE PHARMACEUTICAL SOCIETY having been submitted to the meeting, it was

Moved by William Allen, F.R.S., seconded by John Bell, *and resolved unanimously,*

"That the Laws now read be passed under their separate heads."

Moved by Mr. Keating, seconded by Mr. Dinneford, *and resolved unanimously,*

"That the Laws now read and passed be adopted as the Laws of 'THE PHARMACEUTICAL SOCIETY OF GREAT BRITAIN.'"

Moved by Mr. Hulse, seconded by Mr. Yarde, *and resolved unanimously,*

"That the several members of the Committee be the first Council of the Society, and do continue in office, exercising all the functions and duties provided by the Laws of the Institution, until the general meeting in May, 1842; from which period the Council shall consist of twenty-one members only, to be elected according to the Laws."

Moved by Mr. Smith, seconded by Mr. Butler, *and resolved unanimously,*

"That Messrs. Hallows, Redwood, Yarde, F. J. Bell, and Edwards be appointed Auditors."

Moved by Mr. Hallows, seconded by Mr. Edwards, *and re-solved unanimously,*

"That the thanks of this meeting be given to the Metro-politan Committee, for their earnest and successful exertions in support of the privileges of Chemists and Druggists, and especially for having laid the foundation of a *National In-stitution* for the elevation and advancement of Pharmacy."

Moved by Mr. Thomas Herring, seconded by Mr. Wilkinson, *and resolved unanimously,*

"That the thanks of this meeting be given to Richard Hotham Pigeon, Esq., for his efficient performance of the duties of Chairman."

R. A. FARMAR, ⎱ *Secretaries.*
G. W. SMITH, ⎰

On the 17th of June a pamphlet was published, entitled OBSERVATIONS *addressed to the Chemists and Druggists of Great Britain on the* PHARMACEUTICAL SOCIETY, *by Jacob Bell.* This was intended as a general answer to inquiries and animad-versions daily received by the author, in consequence of an extensive correspondence which he had opened on the subject; and above 2,000 copies were transmitted to various parts of the country during the interval between the appointment of the Council and the publication of their first official address.

Early in July the Council issued their first address to the Chemists and Druggists of Great Britain, of which upwards of 5,000 copies were circulated, and fresh members were daily added to the Society. In this, as on former occasions, the want of an authentic list was found to be a great disadvantage, as many Chemists and Druggists in the country, especially in small towns, received no intimation of what was going on, while several hundred letters were returned, the parties having left business, or the directions being incorrect. This is an additional proof of the advantage of a complete registration of the members of the body, which will, it is to be hoped, result from the formation of the Society.

The Address of the Council is inserted, as it completes the chain of documents connected with the subject, and may pro-bably be referred to with some degree of interest at a future time.

ADDRESS.

In entering on their official duties, the Council of the Pharmaceutical Society are most anxious to draw the attention of the Chemists and Druggists of Great Britain to the immediate necessity of uniting their strength and influence to meet the emergencies of the present crisis. They consider that in having successfully opposed the bills lately brought before Parliament, they have only commenced the duty which they are called upon to perform, and that the fear of injury on the one hand, and the prospect of substantial improvement on the other, ought to stimulate all their brethren to assist them in the important work which they have undertaken.

Chemists and Druggists have long had reason to regret the want of a union of their influence for mutual benefit and protection, and of a uniform education and internal government among themselves, as a means of substantiating their claim to public confidence; being conscious that as long as these defects exist, they may expect to be assailed by obnoxious imputations on the part of those medical reformers who are endeavouring to enforce a system of extraneous restrictions and supervision.

If "the trade" is to be protected merely *as a trade*, and Acts of Parliament professedly designed for its reformation are to be opposed solely on the ground of self-interest, the task of self-defence will be endless, and probably unsuccessful, while the exertions wasted on such struggles can reflect no credit on the spirit or integrity of those who are thus engaged; but if, aware that some regulations may be required, we endeavour to supply the deficiency which is urged as a pretext for hostile proceedings, we shall secure ourselves against the possibility of persecution.

The importance which Chemists and Druggists have obtained as a branch of the medical profession, the reputation which many among them have acquired individually in their own department, and the great accession of numbers which now swells their ranks, *demand* the establishment of some judicious regulations which shall place them in a safe and creditable position as *a body*.

Those among us who take a real interest in our scientific art, rejoice at the opportunity which is now afforded of

placing the "trade" of a Chemist and Druggist on a professional footing, and effecting a union of our scattered forces
for mutual benefit and advancement. By these means talents
which have hitherto lain dormant will be excited into action,
a harmonious intercourse will take the place of reciprocal
jealousy and distrust, and all the collective influence we
possess will become available in attaining the desired improvement among ourselves, and resisting encroachments or interference on the part of others.

The Council are particularly desirous of overcoming the
impression, that a voluntary society cannot effect these
objects. They consider that it will, in the first place, concen-
trate their power of self-defence, and be the means of distinguishing those who aspire to a high standard of qualification
from the careless and indifferent; and, secondly, that by
introducing a system of government conducive to the welfare
of the public, it will form a basis for any legislative measures
which may hereafter be adopted.

The Council wish also to call the attention of Assistants
and Apprentices to the advantages which they will ultimately
derive from the establishment of a society which will give
increased importance, character, and respectability to all its
members, which is especially calculated to advance and elevate
the rising generation, and which will give Associates increased
facilities in obtaining situations.

As a collateral but very important object of the Society,
the Council must particularly advert to the Benevolent Fund,
which, in their estimation, claims the support of every
Chemist and Druggist in the kingdom. In a body so
numerous as we have now become, and among whom we
must calculate upon the existence of a proportionate amount
of distress, or even destitution, the absence of any specific
means of mitigating the sufferings attendant on such cal-
amities is indeed to be deplored : and those who are duly
impressed with the uncertainty of worldly prosperity, and a
desire for the welfare of their fellow-creatures, will rejoice to
see Science and Benevolence going hand in hand in the great
work of improvement which is before us.

In conclusion, the Council recapitulate the general advantages contemplated in the Society ; namely, the union of
all the members of the body, for the purpose of self-govern-

ment and self-protection; the establishment of a uniform system of education, which will promote the advancement of science and the elevation of the profession of Pharmacy; the restraint which will be placed upon the incompetent for the benefit of the public; and, lastly, the alleviation of the sufferings of the unfortunate. In appealing to their brethren for assistance in the prosecution of this comprehensive undertaking, the Council are especially anxious to draw attention to the important, fact, that although the growth of the Society to maturity may be gradual, the rapidity of its progress is entirely dependent upon the number and assiduity of its supporters.

On Monday, November 1st, 1841, a meeting of the subscribers to the fund of 1814–15 was held at the Crown and Anchor in the Strand; Mr. Gifford in the chair. Among the subscribers present were Messrs. William Allen, Butterfield and Westwood. Several communications from the country were read, suggesting the propriety of presenting the balance in hand to the Pharmaceutical Society, and the following resolution was moved by Mr. Butterfield, seconded by Mr. Savory, and unanimously adopted:

" That the original object of this fund being the protection and advancement of the interest of Chemists and Druggists, this meeting of subscribers, convened by circulars and also by public advertisement, desires to recognise in the establishment of the PHARMACEUTICAL SOCIETY of Great Britain a permanent and legitimate means of accomplishing such object; namely, by a general union and organization for the protection of present privileges and the education and improvement of the future members of the trade. They, the said subscribers, do hereby authorize and instruct their sole surviving trustee, William Allen, Esq., Plough Court, to transfer to the Council of the said PHARMACEUTICAL SOCIETY of Great Britain, the whole of the funds he now holds in trust, to be used and appropriated by them, in such manner as shall be deemed best calculated to advance their noble and useful design."

The sum thus transferred, which had been accumulating during the last twenty-five years, amounted to £862 18s. 2d. This transfer connected the present association of Chemists and Druggists with that which had been for some time in a dormant state, but which had originated from circumstances similar to those which had led to the formation of the Pharmaceutical Society.

Although the objects of the two associations were the same, the manner in which it was proposed to attain these objects was, in some respects, different.   On the former occasion the proceedings of the trade were directed to a defensive resistance of threatened encroachments, and contemplated merely the preservation of accustomed rights and privileges by legal means and parliamentary influence.   In the establishment of the Pharmaceutical Society a more extended view of the subject was taken, and the more immediate source of alarm having been successfully combated, the extension of pharmaceutical knowledge and the further improvements in the qualifications of the trade individually and collectively, became the basis of the defence which was set up against future innovations or restraint.

Soon after the confirmation of the general laws of the Society, at the meeting of the members, the Council sent a copy of the same to the College of Physicians, with a letter requesting the favour of a conference.   It was some time before a reply to this communication was received, and it was evident from this circumstance, as well as from an answer received on a former occasion, that the College was not anxious to take an active part in the regulations relating to Chemists and Druggists.   It was desirable, however, that such measures should be adopted as would be likely to receive the sanction of that body, more particularly in reference to the mode of conducting the examination of members and associates, which was one of the most important duties undertaken by the Society, and one in which the experience of the members of the medical profession might have been a considerable advantage.

On the 18th of November, 1841, a deputation of the Pharmaceutical Society had an interview with a Committee of the College of Physicians, and explained, in general terms, the nature of the regulations for educating and examining Chemists and Druggists, which were under consideration, and in the completion of which it had been thought desirable and right to confer with the College.   The Committee appeared to concur in the opinion, that the course adopted by the

Chemists and Druggists was calculated to benefit the profession and the public, and undertook to take the sense of the
members of the College, at an early meeting of that body, and
to report the result to the Council of the Pharmaceutical
Society. On the 27th of November the following communication was received :

" College of Physicians, Nov. 27, 1841.

"The Royal College of Physicians of London has received
from the Council of the Pharmaceutical Society an address
and an outline of a plan for the education and examination
of Chemists and Druggists, etc.

"The College is sincerely desirous that Chemists and Druggists, on whom such large responsibilities rest, should not
dispense medicines without being previously examined; but
the College must have further time to consider how this may
be best effected, with due attention to the privileges conferred
by charter upon other bodies ; at the same time, having the
most earnest wish to assist the Chemists and Druggists for
the general good of the profession and the public.

In conclusion, the College begs to add, that the Committee charged with the duty of conferring with other professional bodies is proceeding with the inquiries and negotia-
tions in which it has been engaged, and hopes, at no distant
period, to be in a position to answer more fully.

(Signed)   "Francis Hawkins, M.D., Registrar."

It having been ascertained that the College was not likely,
at present, to co-operate or interfere in the matter, the
Council appointed a Committee to prepare a draft of the
regulations for the examinations, and, after mature deliberation, resolved, that the Board of Examiners should consist of
Dispensing Chemists, and that the College of Physicians and
the London University should be invited to depute respectively a representative to attend as a visitor.

To this invitation the College of Physicians sent a verbal
reply, through the medium of Dr. Frederick Farre, to this
effect: That while the College cordially approved of the
educational improvement contemplated in the formation of
the Pharmaceutical Society, and had watched with considerable interest the progress of that institution, the College

could not, without exceeding the powers conferred by its charter, officially depute any of its members to take a part in the proceedings of another society in the manner proposed. At the same time, the College would not object to the appointment of any of its members, in his or their individual capacity, to such office.

It having been intimated to the Council of the Pharmaceutical Society that the Senate of the London University was not likely officially to co-operate in the proposed examinations, the Council proceeded to the appointment of Examiners and made the needful arrangements for commencing operations.

During the first few months after the establishment of the Society, the proceedings were observed with some degree of distrust and suspicion by the members of the medical profession ; and this is not at all surprising, when we consider the nature of the controversies which have prevailed in times past, and which are briefly noticed in this epitome. But this prejudice appeared gradually to subside, as the object and tendency of the institution became more generally understood and appreciated. The scientific meetings, which were attended by many medical men, served to give a favourable impression, by demonstrating the advantage likely to result from the discussion of subjects relating to Pharmacy, in a mixed assembly of that description, and also affording an opportunity of defining the province of the Pharmaceutical Chemist in such discussions. The subjects introduced were generally of a practical nature, comprising the various operations of the laboratory and dispensary, and having no reference to medical and surgical practice, or to questions of a political character. The pharmaceutical meetings, therefore, enjoyed the sanction of the medical profession, and those who attended them expressed much satisfaction at the course of proceeding which had been adopted, and the spirit with which it was carried on. The introduction of these scientific assemblies, and the establishment of a school for the education of Pharmaceutical Chemists, may be considered as an important event in the history of Pharmacy, from which we may anticipate a great advantage.

The establishment of the Pharmaceutical Journal was an accidental circumstance. The first number was printed for gratuitous circulation, for the purpose of making known the object of the scientific meetings, and five other numbers were announced as an experiment. It very soon became evident that a periodical of this description was much required, and the only doubt which arose was, whether the Council should undertake the publication of a Journal, or sanction that which had been projected. It was thought by some members that the work should be conducted officially by the Society, or a committee appointed by the Council, but no definite plan having been matured for carrying this into effect, the work proceeded as before, with a few modifications in the arrangement, the Transactions of the Pharmaceutical Society being kept distinct from the other portions of the Journal.

In December, 1841, the Council of the Society, having been informed that the subject of Medical Reform was likely to come before Parliament during the ensuing session, thought it right to address the Secretary of State on the subject, requesting the favour of an interview. After some correspondence between Sir James Graham and the President, an appointment was made : a deputation attended at the Home Office, and was allowed the opportunity of explaining the grounds upon which the Society claimed the protection of the Government, and the circumstances which had led the Council to seek an interview. Sir James Graham stated, that the Government had not yet determined what course to pursue in reference to the medical profession, the subject being one on which it was not easy to legislate, and inquired whether the Society desired a royal charter of incorporation ? The deputation replied, that it was the intention of the Council to apply for this favour when their plans were more fully matured; but they thought it right to wait until they were in a position to prove, by an appeal to facts, that the measures which they proposed to carry out, in reference to their body, were calculated to promote the public welfare, and that, in granting a charter to the Society, her Majesty would benefit the community at large, no less than the parties to whom it was granted. The leading object of the Society being to regulate the education, and ensure the competence, of those who compound medicines, it was contended, that as soon as it could be shown that the means adopted were calculated to attain the end in view, the Council might, *on public grounds*, petition for the sanction and protection of her Majesty and the Government. The arrangements of the Society being as yet incomplete, the immediate object of the deputation was to solicit the privilege of being communicated with as the representatives of the Chemists and Druggists, in the event of any measures affecting that body coming before the Government. The subject having been fully and fairly discussed, Sir James Graham engaged that nothing should be done, in reference to the subject in question, without timely notice being given to the President of the PHARMACEUTICAL SOCIETY.

It has hitherto been considered a necessary consequence of the education of a Chemist that he becomes a medical practitioner. Our predecessors, the original Apothecaries, who were merely compounders of medicine, possessed very limited advantages in respect to education, and in proportion as they advanced in intelligence and knowledge they encroached on the Physicians, until they became to all intents and purposes medical men. When they established a Hall, and laid down a regular course of study for their apprentices, they were not content with instructing them in those sciences which relate to the compounding of drugs, but included in their curriculum surgery, physiology, anatomy, the practice of medicine and midwifery. By this means they supplied the public with a very useful class of medical practitioners, whose services are called into requisition by a large proportion of those patients whose situation in life does not admit of the regular employment of Physicians and Surgeons. But, by the same course, they left a gap to be filled up by another class of compounders of medicine.

From the foregoing account of the origin of Chemists and Druggists, it is evident that this result was brought about by the wants of the public, and, on reviewing the circumstances of the case, we are naturally led to the consideration of the position which Pharmacy occupies, or ought to occupy, as a branch of the medical profession.

Among the ancients the medical profession was divided into three classes. The first related chiefly to *Diet* and the treatment of disorders by regimen; the second was the *Pharmaceutical* department, relating to the use of medicines; the third comprehended the manual operations which come within the province of *Surgery*. These offices occasionally merged into each other, and were also subdivided, giving rise to various grades in rank as well as classification of labour. For instance, there were Αρχιτεκτονικοὶ, or *consulting Physicians;* Δημιουργοὶ, executive or Junior Physicians; Pharmacopolæ, vendors of drugs who did not prepare them, some of whom were also called περιοδευτοὶ, or ἀγύρται, *charlatans;* Pharmaceutribæ, *compounders and vendors* of drugs, who did not administer them; παντοπώλαι, καθολικοὶ and μιγματοπώλαι, *wholesale vendors of drugs, colours, perfumery, dyes, etc.;* ῥιζοτόμοι, *cutters of roots;* βοτανικοὶ, *collectors of herbs.* The cutting of roots was often performed with superstitious ceremonies, and those who followed this department were termed ἀποθῆκαι. There were also *barbers, corn-cutters, poisoners*, and other pretenders to medical art, whose separate functions it is unnecessary to particularize.

Although this classification differs from that which obtains at the present day in this country, it presents an analogy in some particulars. We have the first grand division into three classes, representing, in ordinary language, *Physic, Surgery,* and *Pharmacy.* Physicians and Surgeons are subdivided according to their rank, or the particular line of practice each individual embraces, but these details are foreign to our present subject. We have also a variety of grades and offices comprised in the third grand division, which is denominated Pharmacy.

This department merges into the other two in the case of the general practitioner, and it indeed appears impossible to maintain rigidly an *absolute* separation; but it is our present object to discuss the merits of PHARMACY in its isolated state, distinct from the practice of Medicine and Surgery, and comprehending every office or operation relating to the preparation and sale of medicines.

Although the preparation and compounding of drugs is considered a subordinate office, it is quite as important as any other office in the profession. This is so obvious as to require no demonstration, since remedies are the tools which the Physician employs, and on the efficacy of which he is dependent for success. Pharmacy in the present day embraces so many sciences, and has become so complicated from the discoveries which have recently been made, especially in Chemistry, that a complete knowledge of the subject can only be acquired by those who devote their exclusive attention to the pursuit. The science of Chemistry is alone sufficiently comprehensive to engage the whole time of those who are desirous of becoming acquainted with all its details. Whether we consider the simple elementary bodies (according to the present state of our knowledge), the mineral kingdom, and the endless combinations of the metals, or turn our attention to the more abstruse and mysterious peculiarities of organic structure, we are confused by the multitude of facts and the complication of theories which crowd upon us.

Explanations of phenomena are at one time universally received as plausible and satisfactory, and are afterwards proved to be entirely fallacious, while mysteries which have puzzled philosophers for ages, are sometimes unravelled by the discovery of a principle of nature which had been overlooked. These revolutions in chemical science give rise to changes in nomenclature, and improvements in the processes of the laboratory, which innovations involve the study of Pharmacy in increasing difficulty, and confer on the pursuit the character of a philosophical profession. It is the province of the Pharmaceutical Chemist to apply the various discoveries which are made in this science to his own peculiar department, and although it may not be necessary for every Chemist and Druggist to be practically acquainted with the details of ultimate analysis, the principles of Chemistry should be understood by every person who undertakes to prepare a prescription, and in many of the daily operations of Pharmacy a profound knowledge of the science is indispensable.

The range of the Materia Medica is too extensive to be embraced in the mind without a systematic study of all its minutiæ in the first instance, followed up by constant application. The variations in the quality of drugs, and the sophistications to which they are liable, increase the responsibility of the Druggist, and demand the utmost vigilance. In reviewing the history of Pharmacy in all ages, we find that fraud has always prevailed to a remarkable extent in this kind of traffic, which circumstance may chiefly be attributed to the facility of eluding detection, from the imperfect acquaintance possessed by the public of the nature and pro-

perties of drugs. The detection of adulterations is, therefore, one of the most onerous duties of the Pharmaceutical
Chemist, and it is one which requires, besides chemical knowledge, a practical acquaintance with the sensible properties of
all the substances used in medicine.

The science of Botany, although to a great extent comprised in the Materia Medica, alone affords occupation for the
whole life of those who are ambitious of attaining proficiency;
and even that amount of knowledge which every Chemist
ought to possess of the plants which are used in medicine
cannot be acquired without many years of study.

It is needless to enumerate the collateral branches of science
which might be comprised in a complete pharmaceutical education; enough has been stated to prove, that PHARMACY is
deserving of a separate and distinct place in the arrangement
of the medical profession, and that it is not likely to advance
as a science, and keep pace with other sciences, unless it be
followed by a class of persons who devote themselves exclusively to it. That Pharmacy is worthy of this exclusive
attention cannot be disputed, when we consider its object—
namely, the preparation of remedies for the relief of human
suffering—and also the mental acquirements which the performance of this office demands.

One of the disadvantages under which the art and science
of Pharmacy has hitherto laboured in this country, is the
false position which it occupies, and the prejudice which has
degraded it to the level of a mere trade. From this prejudice has arisen the notion, that the necessary result of
improving the character and education of the Chemist and
Druggist would be to convert him into a medical practitioner.
It has been shown that the system of education adopted
by the Apothecaries was *Medical* and *Surgical*, rather than
Pharmaceutical; and it is obvious, that the odium which
rested on Pharmacy as a TRADE, induced them to aspire to
medical practice as a PROFESSION.

But if proper encouragement were given to the followers of
pure Pharmacy; if this pursuit were held in the estimation
which it deserves, and which it enjoys in other countries; if
the same professional credit were attainable in this field of
labour which is within the reach of the members of other
professions, the inducement which now exists to encroach on

the medical practitioner would be greatly diminished, or cease altogether, and the science of Pharmacy might be expected to flourish.

It is scarcely necessary to observe, that this division of labour cannot be carried to the same extent in all localities. Many small towns and villages could neither support a Physician nor a Surgeon, and a Chemist and Druggist could not live without uniting some accessory business to the sale of drugs.   In this respect the position of small towns in the present day resembles that of the country in general in ancient times, when all persons connected with the medical profession were *General Practitioners*.   In the metropolis, and some other large cities, not only are the three grand divisions observed in the case of many individuals, but each "genus" is subdivided into a number of " species ; " for instance, in Pharmacy, we have *Operative Chemists, Dispensing Chemists, Manufacturing Chemists, Wholesale Druggists, Saline Chemists, Chemists and Druggists* who give their attention to *particular classes of preparations* ; others who cultivate the sale of *horse and cattle medicines* ; others who are *between wholesale and retail*, and supply Apothecaries with drugs.   The nature of the retail trade also varies according to neighbourhood and the rank of the customers.   Under these circumstances there is some scope for classification, and with reference to such a state of things, the medical profession in its broadest extent should be considered.   The division of labour having been regulated accordingly, the example may be followed in smaller towns to such an extent as is compatible with the amount of the population and the wants of the public.

The question which has always caused the greatest agitation in the profession is that which relates to the suppression of uneducated practitioners, and the prohibition of "counter-practice" among Chemists and Druggists.   Notwithstanding the loud protestations respecting the " welfare of the public," and the " credit of the profession," it is too evident that the controversies which have hitherto taken place have not been altogether disinterested, and that the desire to prevent *encroachments* on the one hand, and to escape *restrictions* on the other, has been the chief stimulus to action.   It cannot be denied that the public ought to be provided with *highly quali-fied practitioners in every department;* but whether the public should be *allowed to employ* unqualified persons or not, is a question on which opinions are divided.

Those who advocate the protection of the profession and the public by stringent laws, contend that no person should be allowed to practise in any department without having had a regular education, and passed an examination; and support this opinion by stating, that in justice to those who have been at the expense of passing this ordeal, they should possess the exclusive right of enjoying the emolument to be derived from it, and that by no other means can the public be secured against the danger and suffering which may result from ignorance in unqualified pretenders.

It is argued, on the other side, that it is *impossible* to suppress quackery by law; that the public have the option of selecting such practitioners as they prefer; and that provided no person be allowed to assume a title or rank which does not fairly belong to him, the responsibility of trusting to those who are not worthy of confidence rests with the patients themselves. It is argued, that from time immemorial, empirics have been encouraged and supported not only by the ignorant and unwary, but also by persons of rank and education *: and that the endeavour to restrain or put down an impostor or unqualified practitioner generally has the effect of giving him notoriety and increasing his practice. The reputation of St. John Long continued to increase until several of his patients died, under circumstances which exposed the fallacy of his theory and the recklessness of his practice; and this circumstance tended more to explode his theory than all the opposition which the medical profession could have offered, or the rigour which the law could have inflicted. It is also urged by those who oppose restrictions, that many of the remedies now in use and sanctioned by our Pharmacopœia have been derived from empirics.

The arguments which have been advanced in favour of restricting Chemists and Druggists from giving advice, apply more or less to the case of quacks and the proprietors of patent medicines, as it would obviously be absurd to prohibit the Chemists from recommending an aperient draught or a digestive pill to a patient who describes his symptoms, and at

---

* See pages 4, 5 and 6.

the same time to sanction the sale of secret medicines, with printed directions, announcing them as infallible specifics against a long list of disorders. It would be unjust to punish a man for recommending five grains of compound rhubarb pill of the London Pharmacopœia, while he might with impunity prescribe a box of Morison's pills or a bottle of Daffy's elixir. It is therefore necessary to view the subject in all its bearings, and to consider not only the responsibility attached to the practice of medicine, but the practicability and consistency of any measures which may be proposed for guarding against the evils complained of.

The Chemist is not supposed to possess the advantage of a medical education; but he is and ought to be acquainted with the properties and doses of medicines, and the ordinary mode of administering them. In this capacity his opinion is sometimes asked, in simple cases, and however unwilling he may be to interfere in any degree in medical practice, he cannot avoid occasionally giving his advice, without incurring the imputation of ignorance and losing the confidence of his customers altogether. It cannot be denied that this practice is sometimes carried beyond the limits which ought to be observed, but which it is impossible to define, and in some cases time may be lost while urgent symptoms are gaining ground for want of regular medical treatment.

It may happen that a patient suffering under an acute disorder consults a homœopathic doctor, who denouncing depletion under any circumstances, trusts to the imagined efficacy of an infinitesimal dose of charcoal or of pulsatilla, and neglects to resort to that treatment which the experience of the medical profession would dictate. The disorder increases: another globule is administered and repeated once or twice in the day. The patient dies, and the doctor attributes this event to some accidental circumstance which had interfered with the action of the medicine. Other medical men, not homœopathists, would probably take a very different view of the case.

Again: A patient of a delicate constitution consults a hydropathist, and dies of consumption, *in spite of* the damp sheets and drenchings of cold water, from which a cure was anticipated. In this case, also, opinions may differ as to the proximate cause of death.

Other patients, caught by a plausible advertisement in the newspaper, resort to some "infallible drops" or "vegetable pills," which they take according to the printed directions. Some of them may become worse, or even die, notwithstanding the "infallibility" of the medicine. It is sometimes said, in such cases, that the nostrum was the cause of death; but this cannot always be proved, and is of course denied by the promulgators of the specific.

The science of medicine (which has been termed the "*ars conjecturalis*") is involved in so much mystery, that even doctors occasionally disagree; and a patient, worn out by an obstinate disorder, is not unlikely to be attracted by the professions and promises of those who propose a new system, or advertise, as a wonderful discovery, a remedy which they describe as a specific. Sometimes a paragraph in the newspaper creates a great sensation, and induces hundreds of persons to undertake their own cure, according to the directions laid down.

At the time the cholera first appeared in England, this was the case to a remarkable degree. A paragraph was published, recommending, as a certain cure for this formidable disorder, a poultice of mustard and linseed meal to the feet, an embrocation of camphorated spirit to the pit of the stomach, and twenty or thirty drops of oil of Cajeput, Peppermint, or Cloves, in a glass of water, at stated intervals internally. Accordingly it was recommended that every person should keep in the house, in case of emergency,

> 1 lb. linseed meal,
> 1 lb. mustard,
> Half a pint of spirit of camphor,
> 1 oz. of one of the oils.

Orders flocked in from all quarters, and the Chemists were scarcely able to supply the demand. The price of Cajeput oil rose to about twenty shillings an ounce, the other oils advanced, though not in the same ratio. Some Chemists kept cases ready put up, containing "A complete set of all the articles required for Cholera," which were sold as fast as they could be filled. Various other remedies were recommended in the newspapers, each of which had its day; and while the doctors were discussing the mysterious nature of the disorder, the public eagerly bought whatever remedy was recommended. In fact, any person who happened to have a stock of an article on hand which could be made available, found it the best plan to advertise it as a remedy for cholera.

The circumstances attending the influenza on a previous occasion were somewhat similar, although the treatment was perhaps rather better understood. The remedies usually applied for were, a calomel pill and black draught, and a cough mixture. These articles were often demanded by patients, who, when advised by the Chemists to whom they applied to call in a medical man, persisted in doctoring themselves, and described the kind of medicines which they required.

A few years ago, the fame of Morison's pills extended throughout the kingdom. They were recommended for almost every disorder, and the circumstance of twenty or thirty pills being prescribed for a dose, was a novelty which gave additional notoriety to the Morisonian system, and threw the doctors into the shade. Some patients who had previously suffered from obstinate constipation, found benefit from this active treatment, and recommended it to their friends, and many others followed the fashion under the idea that the pills would purify their blood, and that because they cured one person they could not fail to be beneficial to another. At length, however, the traffic arrived at its zenith, several victims died of hypercatharsis, resulting from an excessive indulgence in the specific; Morison himself was among the number on whom it failed to produce the desired effect, and with him died his fame. Morison's "college of health" still exists, but it has lost its *Morison*.

In an article in the *Quarterly Review* of December, 1842, several other cases were noticed, in which certain fashions in medicine and pharmacy have sprung up, each in succession creating a considerable sensation, until the bubble burst.

The first delusion adverted to, is that respecting the king's evil, in which case royalty was implicated in the assumption of the magical power of curing scrofula by a touch, and this practice was sanctioned by some members of the medical profession. Care was taken, however, to try the efficacy of the charm only in cases in which a tendency to recover had manifested itself.

King George the First discontinued the practice altogether

Tar water, Mrs. Stephens's cure for the gravel and stone, Perkins's metallic tractors, and mustard-seed, successively enjoyed an ephemeral reputation, and in turn gave place to other fashions. Brandy and salt was extensively recommended as a specific in a great variety of disorders, by Mr. Lee and Mr. Vallance, who were so disinterested in their practice as to give away a considerable quantity of this invaluable mixture. The proportions used were six ounces of salt in a pint of French brandy, and it was used internally or externally, or both, according to circumstances.

The embrocation of St. John Long has already been alluded to; it was supposed to consist of a mineral acid, mixed with spirit of turpentine. Some said it contained arsenic; but this is only conjecture, as St. John Long did not trust it out of his own hands. Near the end of the year 1830 a Miss Cassian, who had symptoms of consumption, died while under the influence of this application, and her sister, who had not shown symptoms of the disorder, was brought to St. John Long, who recommended the same treatment by way of *prevention.* A severe wound was established in her back, her strength declined, violent sickness and other alarming symptoms ensued. Sir Benjamin Brodie was called in, but unfortunately too late to avert the fatal result. These cases, and a few others which terminated unsuccessfully, shook the reputation of St. John Long, but he continued to practise as an infallible consumption doctor until he fell a victim to consumption himself.

The system which has acquired the greatest notoriety is Homœopathy, which, in its relation to Pharmacy, deserves a few remarks. The founder of this system, Dr. Hahnemann, was a Physician in Dresden, and being unsuccessful in his practice, and also in literary pursuits, to which he resorted in order to make ends meet, turned his attention to the study of human nature, and promulgated a theory which was destined to make him a great man. We are told that a secret was suddenly revealed to him, by "the star of truth," on which he founded his method of curing diseases. The law of nature, to the discovery of which he lays claim, is this—"*Similia similibus curantur,*" which being interpreted reads thus:—A medicine which has the power of producing any disease, will cure that disease, if it already exist in the system. As two similar diseases cannot exist together, the artificial disease drives out the other, and then spontaneously subsides. Thus ipecacuanha is given to allay sickness, jalap to arrest diarrhœa, etc., etc. But the most remarkable feature in this mode of practice consists in the administration of doses so inconceivably small as to be invisible by the naked eye, and incomprehensible to the human understanding. Great importance is also attributed to the manipulation of the remedies. The *Pharmacopœia Homœopathica*, by Dr. Quin (1834), contains explicit directions on this subject, and each article is described separately; with the dose, the antidote, and the duration of the effect. No compounds are introduced, each medicine being administered in its isolated state, sugar of milk or spirit being selected as the menstruum, on account of their possessing no medicinal properties which could interfere with the desired effect. Porcelain or glass mortars are recommended, and some descriptions of stone or marble are prohibited, because they are said to contain a portion of magnesia, or other substance, which might be injurious.

Each substance is directed to be prepared in various degrees of attenuation. To produce the *first attenuation*, one grain is to be triturated for six minutes in a mortar, with thirty-three grains of sugar of milk, it is then to be detached from the mortar, and again triturated for four minutes. Each of these operations is to be repeated a second time. To this powder thirty-three grains of sugar of milk are to be added, and the friction repeated in the same manner; after which a third portion of thirty-three grains is to be added, and the ceremony having been repeated, the first attenuation is attained. To produce the *second attenuation*, one grain of the above is to be triturated in the same manner with ninety-nine grains of sugar of milk. This process is continued with strict attention to all its details until the *thirtieth* attenuation is produced, each attenuation occupying half an hour, and reducing the product to one hundredth of the strength of the former attenuation. The exact period and method of trituration is considered to exercise an important influence on the efficacy of the remedy: according to Dr. Hahnemann "the brute matter of medicines becomes spiritualized by friction and concussion." Liquids are prepared in the same proportions, one drop of the juice of a plant, or solution of a substance, being agitated with ninety-nine drops of the menstruum, which dilution is carried on to the requisite number of attenuations.

One of the most interesting preparations in the Homœopathic Pharmacopœia is the Tincture of Sulphur, which is prepared as follows:—five grains of sulphur having been washed with spirit of wine and dried, are shaken in a bottle with a hundred drops of spirit of wine. The bottle is allowed to stand twenty-four hours, that the sulphur may subside. One drop of the supernatant fluid is added to ninety-nine drops of alcohol. This constitutes the first attenuation, and the process of dilution is repeated thirty times. *Dose*, one, two, or three drops of the thirtieth attenuation. *Duration of the effect*, thirty, forty, or fifty days. *Antidotes*, camphor, pulsatilla, sepia, nux vomica.

Another interesting preparation is *Graphites* or Plumbago. This substance is purified by washing, first with water, then with nitric and muriatic acids, and is diluted *secundum artem*. The *dose* is two or three globules of the twenty-second, twenty-fourth, or thirtieth attenuation; the *duration of the effect*, forty-eight days; the *antidotes*, arsenic, nux vomica and wine.

In some instances globules of sugar of milk, prepared by the confectioner, are wetted with very attenuated solutions of active substances, and afterwards dried. By this means it may be supposed that a considerable degree of subdivision is attained. When one of these globules is dissolved in a tumbler of water, and a teaspoonful taken for a dose, it can scarcely be expected that an antidote would be required. It is indeed surprising that any efficacy should be attributed to these inconceivably minute doses, but when we see instructions gravely and explicitly laid down in a Pharmacopœia, with the doses, effects, and antidotes, how can we doubt the fact?

According to the homœopathic system, bleeding, and indeed depletion of any kind, is prohibited; perfumes, coffee, aromatics, fermented liquors, spirits, and many other articles are denounced; and in any case in which a substance is administered homœopathically, the patient is enjoined to take particular care that none of that substance is taken in the diet. For instance, if salt (chloride of sodium, or *natrum muri-*

aticum, as it is called homœopathically) be the remedy employed, it is said that salt taken in the usual way would interfere with its action; if charcoal be prescribed, charcoal tooth-powder must be avoided, lest a few particles should accidentally be swallowed. Particular instructions are also given respecting regimen, exercise, etc., which are said to be essential to the proper action of the homœopathic remedies. *

Dr. Hahnemann tried the efficacy of his system on himself, his family, and friends, and performed a variety of experiments, which occupied above twenty years, before he fully developed his valuable secret to the public. As the result of these investigations, he details the various symptoms produced by the remedies employed, and this statement is truly astonishing. We are told that charcoal produces upwards of 600 symptoms, sulphur 1000, pulsatilla 1100, nux vomica 1300, etc. These symptoms are minutely described in the works which have, been published by Dr. Curie and others on the subject.

The following is a specimen:—

Graphites, according to "The Star of Truth," relieves—†

"A buzzing in the head, eruption of crusts behind the ears, confused noise and tingling in the ears, ulceration in the corners of the mouth, dry crusts in the nose, dislike for baked food, weight in the stomach, blowing up of the lower part of the belly, escape of wind in too large quantity, false voice in singing, night cough, gout knotty in the fingers, cold feet in the night in bed, burning heat in the feet, suppuration of the toes, cramps in the ham, tendency to sprain the loins, plucking pain in the limbs, drowsiness at night, foolish dreams in sleep, ill-humour, aversion to work, and many other symptoms."

The Lycopodium is said to cure—‡

---

* It may not be out of place to notice the Sympathetic Powder of Sir Kenelm Digby, which had great reputation for curing wounds, and which was eulogized in a discourse before a learned assembly at Montpelier (1658). The weapon which had inflicted the wound was anointed with ointment, and sprinkled with the powder several times a day. The wound itself was directed to be brought together, carefully bound up, and not disturbed for seven days, at the end of which time, *provided the powder had been regularly applied to the weapon*, the cure was generally effected in the wound.

† Dr. Curie's Practice of Homœopathy, p. 287.   ‡ P. 293.

"Attacks of tearing pain in the top of the head, in the forehead, temples, eyes, and nose; head-ache in the exterior of the head during the night; piercing and scraping pain; suppuration from the eyes; disagreeable impression produced by organ-music; warts in the nose; ulcerated nostrils; repugnance for brown bread; risings of fat; canine appetite; dry snoring cough; nocturnal pain in the elbows; cramps; a turning back of the toes in walking; itching; old ulcers of the legs; painful plucking of the limbs; thoughts preventing sleep; a capricious and irritable temper; morose, unsteady mind; a tendency to seek quarrels," etc., etc.

Among the symptoms to be relieved by Carbonate of Ammonia are—*

"Hardness of hearing, with suppurations and itchings in the ears; pain in the nape of the neck; chronic unsteadiness of the teeth; swelling of the interior of the mouth; asthma; cough, with shooting pains in the sacrum; pain in a wrist which had been injured a long time previous; cramps in the feet; great weakness in the limbs; sweating; anxiety," etc.

Muriate of Soda is given to relieve— †

"Head-ache, in which it seems there are strokes of a hammer; crusts on the scalp; button-like eruption on the forehead; pain as of internal ulceration of the jaws in chewing; sour risings; contraction of the throat, with flow of water into the mouth; immoderate appetite for dinner and supper; perspiration in the face while eating; empty risings after having eaten; jolting in the head; incapability of thinking; splitting, tearing, and lancinating head-ache; plucking pains in the forehead; shutting of the eyes in the morning; whirling in the stomach; noises in the left side of the belly; pain, like that caused by a dislocation of the hip; inconvenience from eating bread; irritability, disposing to anger; sadness; great propensity to take alarm; leanness; a tendency to twist the loins," etc., etc.

The above is a very scanty selection from the prodigious list of symptoms produced (and therefore cured) by some very simple remedies.

On pursuing this extraordinary catalogue of sensations and sufferings, the reader is naturally led to inquire, How was so

---

* Dr. Curie's Practice of Homœopathy, p. 267.   † P. 303.

wonderful a discovery made?—by what process of reasoning, induction, or experiment, was the connection between cause and effect established? It was in the attainment of this end that Hahnemann, his family, and his friends, Franz, Hornberg, Stapf, etc., sacrificed about twenty years of their lives in a series of tedious experiments, the mode of conducting which is thus described by Dr. Curie :

" The essential conditions of these experiments are : that the experimenters be in perfect health; that they scrupulously adhere to diet which is merely nutritious, and in no way pathogenic; that they carefully avoid the use of fermented liquors, wine, spirits, spices of every kind, coffee, strong tea, acid fruits, all vegetables, except those of a farinaceous and mild description : that they shun all fatigue, bodily and mental, all excess, and even excitement; and that they previously note every habitual symptom by which they are affected." *

These conditions being implicitly observed, every symptom or sensation which follows each dose is recorded, and, according to the law " *similia similibus curantur,*" the statement is taken to represent the therapeutic action of the remedy. When we see how numerous and distressing these symptoms are, it is clear that the ordeal through which the enthusiastic experimenters passed, must have been such as few constitutions could have outlived.

The action of these minute doses on the nervous system when administered therapeutically is thus described, in contradistinction to the " violent and dangerous operation " of medicines administered in the ordinary way :

" By the homœopathic method, those medicaments for which the system has the greatest aptitude are brought into contact with the papillæ of the tongue, which is found to be sufficient in all cases to produce the desired effect; and in some, smelling alone is enough. They thus touch directly the sentient roots of that nervous tree, through which their power is conveyed to the whole system."†

It is a rule in Homœopathy never to administer more than two kinds of medicine in a day, as it is considered that all substances act better in a simple state, and that the effects of any remedy would be materially impaired or modified by ad-

---

* Curie's Principles of Homœopathy, page 104.　　† Page 154.

mixture. It is usual to give a dose every four or five hours, but in acute cases as often as every two hours.

Dr. Curie informs us that *

"Homœopathy, which may appear easy of attainment at first, because it is founded on a few clear and simple principles, presents increasing difficulties as the student advances in his career, because, in proportion as he advances, the difficulties are more clearly defined, and because the choice of the exact remedy for each individual case requires a serious study, to which the routine practitioner of the old school is unaccustomed."

He observes that "Allopathy," namely, the common or established practice, "has long been known to the world by its acknowledged want of all principle in the administration of medicine, its utter uncertainty, its excessive costliness, its hazards, and its failure;" † and that "Homœopathy forms a new era in medical science, destined to dispel the darkness, errors, and uncertainty in which therapeutics have been hitherto enveloped; its principle is a law of nature, unerring and immutable—a principle on which alone can be established the future progress and improvement of the healing art." ‡

The promulgation of this extraordinary doctrine by Dr. Hahnemann was followed by grievous persecution on the part of the medical profession in Germany, which had the effect of giving him notoriety, and his cause was espoused by the Duke of Anhalt Cöthen. By degrees the system gained ground, not only in Germany, but in other nations in Europe, and in course of time it was imported into England, where it is extolled as infallible by many votaries. The system has also been introduced into Veterinary practice, and we are told that it is infallible in curing the *Distemper* in *Puppies*.

The circumstance that every theory, however puzzling to reason and common sense, has its supporters, is thus accounted for by Dean Swift :—

"Let us therefore now conjecture how it comes to pass, that none of these great prescribers do ever fail providing themselves and their notions with a number of implicit dis-

---

* Curie's Principles of Homœopathy, page 159. † Page 12.
‡ Curie's Practice of Homœopathy, page vi.

ciples. And I think the reason is easy to be assigned, for there is a peculiar *String* in the harmony of human understanding, which, in several individuals, is exactly of the same tuning. This, if you can dexterously screw up to its right key, and then strike gently upon it, whenever you have the good fortune to light among those of the same pitch, they will by a secret necessary sympathy strike exactly at the same time. And in this one circumstance lies all the skill or luck of the matter, for if you chance to jar the string among those who are either above or below your own height, instead of subscribing to your doctrine, they will tie you fast, call you mad, and feed you with bread and water." *

But Homœopathy, Pharmacy, and indeed the science of medicine in all its branches, has lately been threatened with entire extinction by the discovery, on the part of Priessnitz, of Graeffenberg, of the virtues of cold water, which is recommended as a panacea. In addition to the internal administration of vast quantities of this beverage, it is applied externally in a great variety of ways. Damp sheets were formerly avoided with the most scrupulous care. It is now discovered that patients may sit in a cold-bath for a considerable time, envelope themselves in wet sheets, and retire to a dripping bed, not only with perfect safety, but with a very beneficial effect! These ablutions are directed to be repeated more or less frequently, and are either topical or general, according to the circumstances of the case. The symptoms of a *crisis* are severe boils and eruptions in all parts of the body, which, although troublesome at the time, are said to be indicative of approaching convalescence. This system is practised by persons who are not medical men, and who, in fact, have little or no pretensions to medical knowledge, but who nevertheless undertake the treatment of any patients who may happen to present themselves. Large establishments are fitted up in different parts of the country, and the speculation is found to be particularly profitable.

The conductor of one of these mansions was formerly a Chemist and Druggist, who having thrown cold water on his creditors a few years ago, evaporated for a time, and reappeared in the capacity of a water-doctor in another part of

---

* Tale of a Tub. 7th edit., page 115. A.D. 1727.

the country.   Several other persons have visited Graeffenberg for the purpose of acquiring a knowledge of this new system, and following in the wake of the inventor, who has risen from the station of a peasant to that of an oracle.

In giving an historical account of the theories and systems relating directly or indirectly to Pharmacy, it would be foreign to the purpose to enter minutely into the merits of each ; but it may perhaps be allowable to quote one other passage from *The Quarterly Review*, as it explains in a few words the comparative value of remedies in general :

" The union of a broken bone, and the healing of a simple wound, are the results of a natural process.   The recovery from many internal complaints is the result of a natural process also.   Under such circumstances, the best evidence of the skill of the physician or surgeon is, that he merely watches what is going on, taking care that nothing may obstruct restoration, and avoiding all further interference. But it is his duty also to learn what unassisted nature can do and what she cannot do, and, where her powers are insufficient, to step in to her assistance and act with promptness and decision.   It is just at this point that danger arises from faith in pretended remedies.   If they have the virtue of being in themselves innocent, no harm can result from their use where nothing is wanted or nothing can be done ; but it is quite otherwise on those occasions which call for active and scientific treatment ; and we have good reason to say that many individuals have lost their lives from trusting to their use under these circumstances." *

There is another subject, which, although not exactly connected with Pharmacy, is as much in place in a pharmaceutical treatise as in any other, inasmuch as it relates to one of the most powerful " *sedatives* " with which we are acquainted.   The subject alluded to is Mesmerism. This science, art, or mystery, having been roughly handled on the continent, has taken refuge in this country, and is cultivated by a considerable number of philosophical investigators.   We may pass over the conjuring tricks with mesmerized water, nickel, and sovereigns ; the development of phrenological indications by mesmeric "passes," the power of

* Brandy and salt, Homœopathy, Hydropathy, page 103.

reading with the forehead and elbows, and other marvellous exhibitions which have astonished a section of the public. The only part of the subject which comes within our province, is the *sedative* effect of mesmeric manipulations, thrusts, or "passes," which are said to have the power of tranquilising more effectually than any preparation of opium, producing an entire insensibility to pain,'and thus disarming surgical operations of their usual torture.

On a recent occasion, the Medical and Chirurgical Society admitted for discussion at one of their meetings the case of a man whose leg had been amputated while he was "in a mesmeric trance," * and who afterwards declared that he had been unconscious of the operation. The subsequent dressing of the part affected was performed under similar circumstances, and with the same success. This was *primâ facie* a strong case; but some of the mesmerists present, as if afraid of gaining a victory, launched out into the phenomena of mesmerized water, and the faculty of reading with various parts of the head, which feats were said to have been performed in the presence of THREE ARCHBISHOPS. This of course produced laughter, and weakened the main argument.

The anti-mesmerists on the other hand (with two or three exceptions) seemed scarcely disposed to give the case fair play, expressed regret that it had been admitted for discussion, rejected the evidence of the patient in reference to his insensibility to pain, and treated it as an attempt at imposition. At the same time they cited, in illustration of their remarks, the cases of other patients in which sensation was lost or impaired in morbid states of the system, forgetting that the evidence of this insensibility was derived from the *declarations and conduct* of these patients, which, in the case of the mesmeric patient, they would not admit as evidence at all. This mode of treating the question tended to impress the audience more favourably towards mesmerism than the defence of the mesmerists themselves.

Within a day or two of this discussion a pamphlet appeared in print, containing a full, true, and particular "*Account of a*

---

* A lawyer officiated as mesmerist on the occasion, whilst a surgeon amputated the limb, and the paper was the joint production of the two operators.

case of SUCCESSFUL AMPUTATION OF THE THIGH, *during the* MES-
MERIC STATE, *without the knowledge of the patient, read to the*
ROYAL MEDICAL AND CHIRURGICAL SOCIETY OF LONDON *on Tues-
day, the 22nd of November, 1842.*"

One great obstacle to the advancement of science is the prejudice which prevails in favour of *preconceived opinions* on one
side, and *new theories* on the other, which conflicting influence
frequently divides the scientific world into opposing parties,
and checks that dispassionate investigation and discussion,
which would be more in accordance with a candid desire to
arrive at the truth.

When a new remedy is introduced to the notice of the profession, it generally has " a run " in the first instance. Those
who are prone to be sanguine in such matters, probably attri-
bute to it more merit than it deserves, and are too indiscriminate in its employment. Disappointment in the effect ensues
in some cases, and the fame of the medicine subsides. Those
who are averse to innovation, instead of giving it a trial, note
down the instances in which it has been unsuccessful, and
condemn it. In this manner many articles in the Materia
Medica have at various times been almost discarded by the
profession, simply because they failed to realize the expectations which had been raised, and having fallen into disrepute,
their actual merit or value has not been correctly estimated.

The theory of the action of remedies on the system is not
sufficiently understood to enable us to predicate what will be
the effect of a substance hitherto unemployed, and therefore
recourse must be had to experiment in most cases, in order to
determine the value of new remedies. In this respect quacks
possess an advantage over regular practitioners, since, having
no character to lose, they are not subject to the same pruden-
tial restraint, and, therefore, although they may often do
mischief, they occasionally make discoveries which are ultimately beneficial to the profession.

Even regular medical men sometimes incur the persecution
and reproaches of the profession, when they adopt a more bold
and speculative practice than their neighbours, of which the
case of Dr. Greenfield will serve as an illustration. The
following are the leading particulars, taken from a work by
the doctor himself, which was written in Latin, and translated
by John Marten, surgeon (1706). The dispute arose from

the employment of Cantharides, by Dr. Greenfield, as an internal remedy in "iscuries, stranguries, ulcers of the bladder," etc., which was considered by his brother practitioners to be *Mala Praxis*. The doctor informs us, that among other researches on the subject, he tried the effect of the medicine on dogs, in the presence of the President and Censors of the College; and he states—

" To one of which dogs I had administered Cantharides alone, and to the other corrected with Camphir; besides I undertook to produce as evidence of the wonderful vertue and effects of Cantharides, women (of whom I have very many) cured with the use of it, as also Physitians of our own College, who were eye-witnesses of the same, but it was preaching to a dead wall, all was to no purpose, they refuse, reject, and disdain, all that could be offered in my defence,

> And since no reason could be brought,
> With private fraud they make it out ;

for they gave a particular and pleasing attention and credit to the railings and calumnies of three women, sworn clandestinely and privately in my absence, and denied me the liberty to hear their examination, or to make any reply thereto, though often requested ; but sent me away wholly ignorant of what was done. But about fourteen days after, committed me to NEWGATE, the common gaol for THIEVES and ROGUES, by vertue of a certain warrant under their hands and seals, charging me guilty of MALE PRACTICE."

After his liberation Dr. Greenfield wrote the work from which the above extract is taken, which is entitled a TREATISE *of the safe, internal use of* CANTHARIDES *in the Practice of Physick*. The author describes the virtues of the remedy, quotes various ancient authorities in its favour, and points out the effect of Camphor in moderating the irritant property of Cantharides. The translator, in a poem which precedes the Preface, commends the doctor in these words :—

> " Justly the conqueror's proud bays he claim'd ;
> The small but dread CANTHARIDES he tam'd ;
> Taught the cool CAMPHIRE's well-mixed sovereign balm
> The fierce CANTHARIDES' hot rage to calm."

Although the internal employment of Cantharides, by Dr

Greenfield, at that period, exposed him to much obloquy and persecution, the remedy is now in frequent use, and the tincture is ordered in the Pharmacopœia and other works on medicine, with directions respecting the dose and mode of administration.

From the facts above stated, relative to the various modes of practice which are allowed and sanctioned by law, the great discrepancy in the notions and practice of medical men, and the disposition of the public to resist any restraint upon individual judgment in the matter, it is obvious that the line of demarcation between the regular and irregular practitioner is by no means clearly defined, and consequently that "the protection of the public and the profession against the effects of ignorance," by legislative measures, is extremely difficult.

Reverting to the subject of the PHARMACOPŒIAS, we ought to notice that of the Dublin College, which is of less ancient origin than those of London and Edinburgh. A *Specimen Pharmacopœiæ* was published in 1794, and another in 1805, which were circulated among the members of the College only, and the first Dublin Pharmacopœia was printed for general circulation in 1807. This work, which had been several years in course of preparation, was chiefly compiled by the late Dr. Percival, who was then Professor of Chemistry in the University, and who acted under the *surveillance* of a Committee of the College. About six years afterwards Dr. Percival commenced a series of experiments preparatory to the production of a new edition: in this task he was assisted by Mr. Donovan, who is now well known as a Professor in Dublin, but after the lapse of two years, Dr. Percival finding the undertaking onerous at his advanced period of life, abandoned it, and was succeeded by Dr. Barker, who had come into office as Professor of Chemistry. A committee was appointed to assist Dr. Barker, but the new edition did not appear until the year 1826. Shortly afterwards, Dr. Barker published an English translation, with notes and commentaries on the several processes. This, however, only embraced the Chemical department, and a second part containing the Galenical portion was produced by Dr. Montgomery. The Dublin Pharmacopœia is but little if at all circulated in England, but the processes are quoted in Thomson's Dispensatory, which is familiar to most Chemists in this country.

Dr. Christison's Dispensatory was published in the year 1842. In this work the plan of other dispensatories is essentially deviated from. Instead of its subjects being divided into several parts, and each topic treated of under several distinct heads, every special topic is exhausted under a single head, so that the observations on any one article of the Materia Medica constitute, as it were, a complete treatise. Thus, for instance, that portion of the work which, in the Pharmacopœia, is classified as " *The Preparations*," is distributed in different parts of the volume, each formula being given under the article in the Materia Medica which forms its basis. The several substances are arranged alphabetically.

Gray's Supplement to the Pharmacopœia has enjoyed considerable reputation as a book of reference. The first edition was published in 1818, the sixth in 1836. It contains a notice of almost every substance used in medicine, the preparations of the Pharmacopœias, patent medicines, etc., and although each subject is treated of in general terms, and with very little detail, the Chemist seldom has occasion to refer to the work without finding some allusion to the article on which he desires information.

Among other works on Pharmacy may be noticed Dr. Paris's Pharmacologia, of which the first edition was published in 1812, and the ninth is just published. This is a very useful book, both to the Medical Practitioner and the Pharmaceutical Chemist; and we need no further proof of its value than the number of editions which have been required by the profession.

Thomson's Elements of Materia Medica and Therapeutics; Rennie's Supplement to the Pharmacopœia; Brande's Manual of Pharmacy, and the Dictionary of Materia Medica, by the same author; Dr. Christison's Treatise on Poisons; Dr. Kane's Elements of Practical Pharmacy; Dr. Stephenson's Medical Botany; Dr. Lindley's Flora Medica; Dr. Alexander Ure's Compendium of Materia Medica, Dr. Lane's Compendium, and Dr. Bellingham's Materia Medica, are among the most important works which have been produced in Great Britain.

But the most remarkable work which has appeared in this country in the department of Pharmacy is Dr. Pereira's Materia Medica. It comprises 1900 closely printed pages, and contains a scientific and explicit description of every article in the Materia Medica, with 365 woodcuts, and innumerable references to other works, both British and foreign. The chemical constitution of substances, the botanical characters of plants, the therapeutic action of remedies, the history of every variety of drug, and the various opinions and theories on each subject, are detailed in a manner which indicates complete practical knowledge, as well as the most laborious scientific research.

It is worthy of remark, that until lately we have had no periodical devoted to the subject of Pharmacy. The first work of this description was *The Chemist*, which was commenced in 1839. The *Pharmaceutical Journal* originated at the time of the establishment of the Pharmaceutical Society in 1841; since which period the *Annals of Chymistry and Practical Pharmacy* and the *Chemical Gazette* have appeared.

From the circumstance of four journals of a Pharmaceutical character having sprung up and met with encouragement within so short a space of time, we may infer that the desire for information is extending itself in the profession, and we may hope that this periodical diffusion of knowledge will be attended with a beneficial result.

It is quite clear that the advantage of improved education and scientific intercourse among Pharmaceutical Chemists cannot be too highly appreciated, and in order to understand the manner in which an attention to measures of this description affects the general interests of our body, it is only necessary to observe the change in our position and prospects which appears to have been effected since the establishment of the Pharmaceutical Society.

At the time that Mr. Hawes undertook to set the profession in order, he was supported and urged forward by the advocates of a system, liberal on the one hand and restrictive on the other. According to the plan laid down, a new order of medical men was to be raised up on the basis of the general practitioner, and although Mr. Hawes did not contemplate the annihilation of the existing medical institutions, his measures were calculated indirectly to undermine their influence, and reduce their power, by creating another channel open to all, by which professional rank and honour might be attained. While the profession was to be thus thrown open, and purged from what are termed its "corruptions," it was also to be protected, by means of stringent prohibitions against unqualified practitioners, enforced by heavy penalties.

These latter measures were chiefly levelled against the Druggists; and were designed, among other objects, to settle the knotty question respecting " counter practice," which has been a subject of dispute from the time of the Apothecaries of the sixteenth century to the present day. It was not supposed that the Druggists could make any effectual resistance on the occasion, as it was considered proverbial that they were a disunited body—that they had no representative government, or means of concentrating their influence. On the other hand, Mr. Hawes and his party were backed by a large and influential association, the ramifications of which extended throughout the empire, and which had the means of creating a sensation by directing the power of the members into one channel, when a simultaneous effort was found desirable. A notion prevailed to a considerable extent in the profession, that the interests of the two parties were at variance, that in order to elevate and protect the Medical Practitioner, it was necessary to subdue and restrain the Druggist. This *prejudice* had been handed down during nearly two centuries, and the jealousy which existed on both sides had been a bar to any mutual accommodation or dispassionate argument between the two parties. The medical journals, and even the daily papers, were constantly advocating some effectual legislative measures, and quoting cases illustrative of the ignorance and misdeeds of the Druggists. Although these arguments were frequently one-sided, and the cases highly coloured, they were seldom answered, except, perchance, in an occasional anonymous letter, the pungency of which was taken out during its passage through the press.

Pharmacy stood in a precarious condition. Its real representatives—those on whom had devolved the chief responsibility of preparing and compounding medicines, were calumniated on every hand, and threatened with extraneous control, and a variety of restrictions. Even their right to dispense prescriptions was called in question,* and they held their other privileges on an uncertain tenure. Yet they possessed no means of defence or representation, and although

* *Lancet.*

they were all sensible of the disadvantages of their anomalous position, none felt called upon to act for the general welfare.

In this state of affairs, the bill of Mr. Hawes came before Parliament, and the Druggists suddenly roused themselves from their state of apathy, and arranged a plan of defence. The effect of this vigorous movement has already been described; but when they had warded off the immediate cause of alarm, the Druggists did not fan the flame of opposition, by keeping up an acrimonious controversy and raising a political faction. They endeavoured to trace the evil to its source, and having discovered that their weakness proceeded chiefly from the want of regular education, as well as the absence of unity among themselves, they turned their attention to the intellectual improvement and organization of the members of their body.

In proportion as these measures advanced, the opposition subsided; a more harmonious feeling sprung up, not only among the Druggists themselves, but between the Druggists and the medical profession. We have now (1843) almost completed our arrangements for the education of our members, the examinations have commenced, a form of representative government is in operation, and our right to regulate the concerns of our own body is undisputed.

This change of circumstances naturally leads us to conclude, that the professional and scientific improvement of the Pharmaceutical Chemist is not incompatible with the interest or friendly relation of the Medical Practitioner; in fact, we have reason to hope that a continuance of the line of conduct which has hitherto been attended with success, will promote an increase of harmony among all parties, and thus prevent a recurrence of those mercenary and political controversies which disgraced the profession during the last century.

When the Council of the PHARMACEUTICAL SOCIETY had brought their arrangements to a state approaching to completion, and felt prepared to prove, by what had been already done, that much public benefit might be expected from the plan which the Society had laid down, they drew up a petition to Her Majesty, which was presented on the 5th of November, 1842, praying for a Royal Charter of Incorporation. Sir James Graham undertook to give the subject his mature attention, and intimated that he should consult some of the leading members of the profession, and take other means for forming his opinion as to the *public* utility of the PHARMACEU-TICAL SOCIETY, before he could give a definite answer.

On the 1st of December, the Secretary of the Society received an official communication from the HOME OFFICE, requiring his attendance, and was informed that the petition having been favourably received, the draught of the proposed charter might be prepared in due form for the consideration of the Secretary of State. No time was lost in taking this step, and the charter having been prepared by Mr. Alderman T. Wood, and Mr. Serjeant Talfourd, was approved by Sir James Graham, and also by the Attorney and Solicitor Generals, with a trifling and unimportant alteration. It appeared, however, that a " CAVEAT " had been lodged by some party who suspected that the Society would apply for a charter, and who was desirous of opposing it.* But the twelve months during which period such caveat remains valid had just expired, and, as it had not been renewed, it fell to the ground; and, on the 18th of February, 1843, the PHARMACEUTICAL SOCIETY OF GREAT BRITAIN became a COR-PORATE BODY.

This event is important—being the first public recognition of the Chemists and Druggists as the representatives of Phar-macy. It cannot henceforth be said that the Chemists and Druggists have no political existence; and, consequently, in the event of any legislative enactments being proposed in which their interests are concerned, they may now claim not only to be heard, but to be consulted. By virtue of their charter, they possess the power of regulating the education and admission of members, and thus providing the public with qualified practitioners in Pharmacy, while they establish an ostensible distinction between the members of their body and

---

* It is not improbable that this was the result of the following sugges-tion contained in the leading article of the *Lancet*, of December 4th, 1841, p. 333:

" The Privy Council should be admonished of the application which may be made for a charter by the Chemists and Druggists ; and, finally, they (the Apothecaries) should pray to be heard, by counsel, before such a charter receives the sign-manual of the QUEEN."

It happened, however, that the Council of the PHARMACEUTICAL SOCIETY were aware that the proper time for applying for a charter had not then arrived.

unqualified persons. In case of any grievance affecting the individual members in any district, or in any part of the country, and rendering an appeal to the legislature desirable, there is an effective and efficient channel through which such appeal can be made; and it may be supposed that the Council of an incorporated Society, representing so large a body as the Chemists and Druggists of the United Kingdom, would possess the advantage of an amount of influence which might, on a great variety of occasions, be beneficially exerted. We have seen, by the specimens already quoted, what would, in all probability, be the nature of a medical bill brought into Parliament by parties who have no community of interests or circumstances with Chemists and Druggists, and who have, on former occasions, endeavoured to introduce measures of a stringent and oppressive character. We have seen that about twelve months ago measures were taken to restrain the progress of that body, and to impede the acquirement of that political influence which a charter would afford. And we need no stronger proof of the propriety and policy of the course which the Chemists and Druggists have lately adopted, than the fact, that although it must have been clear to every one that, in the natural course of events, application would be made for a Royal Charter, and although any individual might, at a trifling expense, have lodged a fresh caveat, and thus, to a certain extent, thrown an obstacle in the way of its being granted, yet the proceedings of the PHARMACEUTICAL SOCIETY having been confined to the improvement and regulation of the Chemists and Druggists, and divested of any political or party spirit, there was not in the whole medical profession one man, within the last twelve months, whose conscience would allow him to oppose a measure the tendency of which was so obviously beneficial to the public and creditable to the profession.

In conclusion, it may be as well to recapitulate the moral which may be drawn from our past history, namely, that *political controversies and mercenary disputes are injurious to the interest and character of all parties—that the most effectual method which any class of men can adopt for securing their political rights, and advancing their professional standing, consists not in disputation and warm argument, but in a steady and persevering attention to intellectual improvement, and the establish-*

ment of such regulations as are calculated to ensure collective privileges by increasing the amount of individual merit.

The members of the PHARMACEUTICAL SOCIETY are following in the footsteps of the original Apothecaries. We have the opportunity of profiting by the experience of our predecessors, taking advantage of their example where the result has shown its wisdom, and avoiding any errors into which they may have fallen. Those who are sincere in the desire for the advancement of our own legitimate profession, which is pure PHARMACY, will perceive the importance of confining our attention as much as possible to that pursuit, by which course we shall not only be more likely to attain the object in view, but shall also conciliate the other branches of the profession, and establish an amicable and harmonious relation among all parties.

[END OF THE FIRST PART.]

THE PROGRESS OF PHARMACY, FROM 1841.

IN tracing the progress of pharmacy in this country from the time at which it became a separate occupation, first in the hands of the apothecaries, and afterwards of chemists and druggists, the author of the foregoing Historical Sketch has depicted some of the various phases of the practice and administration of medicine, including pharmacy, during a period of about three centuries, prior to, and including the early steps which were taken towards, the establishment of the Pharmaceutical Society.

Another period, of shorter duration, but not less productive of important changes affecting the cultivation and progress of pharmaceutical knowledge, and the interests of those engaged in its application, has since elapsed, and it has fallen to the lot of another author to record the events of this period of about a third of a century, during which the Pharmaceutical Society has passed through its early development and has finally been established on a permanent basis by legal enactment.

The circumstances which led to the association in 1841 of the leading chemists and druggists of London and most of the provincial towns of Great Britain, have already been described. Called together for the purpose of self-defence, they became sensible, while successfully warding off the danger with which they were then threatened, of causes which exposed them unnecessarily to aggression from without, and of sources of internal weakness by which they were deprived of much of the usefulness and influence which rightly belonged to those engaged in the exercise of their profession.

The committee who, by their active exertions, had prevented the passing of Mr. Hawes's bill, taking advantage of a concurrence of favourable influences, succeeded in laying the foundation of a Society of Chemists and Druggists the record of whose proceedings will comprise the most important part of the history of British Pharmacy during the period to which we are referring. Some of the events attending the founding of the Pharmaceutical Society have been narrated, but to give distinctness and continuity to this part of our Historical Sketch, we purpose briefly to recapitulate the leading facts, and to accompany them with reflections the expression of which has been justified by subsequent events and the lapse of time.

The first formal step towards the establishment of the Pharmaceutical Society was taken at a meeting of the members of the trade on the 15th of April, 1841. On that occasion the committee, consisting of forty of the leading chemists and druggists of the metropolis, who had been appointed two months previously, to watch and oppose the progress of Hawes's Medical Bill, or at least such parts of it as injuriously affected the interests of chemists and druggists, presented their report, in which they described the successful result of their efforts as far as related to the bill in question; but at the same time they explained that other legislative measures were in contemplation, and had received the sanction of the Colleges of Physicians and Surgeons and of the Society of Apothecaries, which would place the chemists and druggists under the government and control of those bodies and especially of the Society of Apothecaries. Under these circumstances the committee recommended the immediate formation of a Society of Chemists and Druggists, to be called the Pharmaceutical

Society of Great Britain, having for its object the union of the members of the trade into one body, the protection of their general interests, and the improvement and advancement of scientific knowledge. The committee recommended that education, examination, registration, and representation, should be made the basis of such union, as involving beneficial results to the public in general, and to the chemists and druggists in particular; and offering to the existing medical corporations and to the medical profession at large, a guarantee that whilst the chemists and druggists were anxious to retain existing privileges, they were disposed to afford every public evidence of their fitness to exercise them.

The report of the committee was cordially received by the meeting, and a resolution, moved by William Allen, F.R.S., of Plough Court, and seconded by John Bell, of 338, Oxford Street, was unanimously adopted, to the effect, " that for the purpose of protecting the permanent interests, and increasing the respectability, of chemists and druggists, an Association be now formed under the title of the Pharmaceutical Society of Great Britain."

The same committee was requested to frame laws and regulations for the government of the society, to be submitted to a subsequent meeting for confirmation and adoption. Within a fortnight after the date of this meeting a draft of the proposed laws, which had been drawn up by a sub-committee and frequently discussed, was submitted to a public meeting of the members of the society on the 1st of June, and the laws, then finally settled, were adopted as the laws of the Pharmaceutical Society of Great Britain. In accordance with these laws the society was to be governed by a council, consisting of twenty-one members, to be elected every year in May, but a special resolution was passed appointing the forty members of the committee who had already performed so much good service members of the first council, with authority to act as such until the following May. William Allen was elected president; Charles James Payne, vice-president; Richard Hotham Pigeon, treasurer; and George Walter Smith and Robert A. Farmar, joint honorary secretaries of the society.

From this date, namely the 1st of June, 1841, the society was fully organized, and we may here briefly review the

L

means and influences which had contributed to this result.
The movement from which the suggestion to form a society
of chemists and druggists originated, was that connected with
the opposition to Mr. Hawes's bill.   The prime movers in
that opposition were Mr. Robert A. Farmar, of 40, Westminster Road; Mr. George Baxter, of 244, High Holborn ; and
Mr. George Walter Smith, at that time an assistant to a
wholesale druggist.   The meeting at Mr. Farmar's house, on
the 10th of February, 1841, has been noticed in an earlier
part of this history.   Those who took part at that meeting,
and especially the three gentlemen just named, undertook the
duty of calling on the more prominent and influential members of the trade, both wholesale and retail in London, and
trying to interest them in the subject.   The three active
pioneers in the agitation thus commenced, although originators of the movement, made no attempt to put themselves
into a more prominent position than that of zealous agents
and assistants, ready to perform the time-consuming work so
requisite and yet so unproductive of distinction, in movements
of this description.   By their means men of higher mark and
greater influence were induced to take the foremost ranks in
the powerful array of well-known members of the trade who
formed the London committee.   The character of this committee, and the disinterestedness of those who brought the
members of it together and stimulated them to action, contributed much to the successful result of their operations.   It
was important that the measures adopted should have the
sanction and support of all the leading drug-houses, both
wholesale and retail, and accordingly we find among the
requisitionists of the first public meeting, held at the Crown
and Anchor, on the 15th of April, the names of Allen, Hanbury & Barry ;· Savory, Moore & Co. ; John Bell & Co. ;
Godfrey & Cooke; Corbyn & Co. ; Hudson & Son ; Fisher &
Toller; Winstanley & Co. ; Richard Battley ; Charles Dinneford; George Grindle ; Joseph Gifford, and other old ,estab-
lished retail firms ; and those of Pigeon & Son ; Herring
Brothers ; Horner & Sons ; Ellis, Langton & Co.; Barron,
Harvey & Co. ; Baiss, Brothers & Co. ; Evans & Lescher ;
Hodgkinson, Tonge & Stead ; Drew, Heyward & Co., and
other wholesale houses.   These were names that could not
fail to carry weight, but the names of those who called the

requisitionists into action do not appear in the list. They were satisfied to give the benefit of their labour in carrying out the dry details of organization, while those who inherited or had created great reputations, lent the influence of their names as an efficient motive power to put the machinery into action.

Credit was especially due to Farmar and Smith for having discerned and called attention to the true import of events that were occurring at this time in connection with the practice of pharmacy, and for having judiciously turned some of those events to account in furthering the attainment of objects which many of their brethren, whose easy circumstances made them less disposed for agitation, were no less anxious than they were to see accomplished. But mere assent to the propositions made, unquestionable as these might be, and great as might be the influence of those who gave the sanction of their approval to them, would have failed to accomplish what was required, notwithstanding all that a few active workers were doing, had it not been for the enthusiastic devotion of the best energies of a man endowed with the qualifications of wealth, position, a cultivated mind, and sound judgment, who made the establishment of the Pharmaceutical Society, and the elevation of chemists and druggists to the highest rank of pharmaceutical chemists, the object of his life's work.

Jacob Bell, the eldest son of the founder and proprietor of one of the largest dispensing establishments in London, had recently become a partner in his father's business, the sole management of which was passing into his hands. He occupied a position, with regard to the character of the business he had come into, which left nothing that he could desire in that respect. He had taken advantage of all available means to fit himself by study and practical work for the exercise of the responsible duties he had undertaken. He commanded the confidence of the medical profession and the public, and as far as he was individually concerned there was no prospect of any advantage resulting from the measures contemplated for raising the qualification of the body of chemists and druggists. In this respect he and others with whom he was associated could not have been actuated by selfish or personal motives, yet all joined in promoting what was considered to be for the general good. At the first meeting of the first council of the society a vote of thanks was passed "to Mr. Jacob Bell, of Oxford Street, for his zealous exertions in establishing the Pharmaceutical Society," and this was ordered to be engrossed on vellum. But with a modesty characteristic of the man, he at once declined to accept so formal a recognition of his services, and in place of the engrossed vote of thanks to himself he suggested and carried into effect the issuing of an engraved certificate of membership, to be supplied to those who joined the new society. He was authorized to obtain a design for this certificate, his known taste for the fine arts and acquaintance with several of the most eminent artists of the day, fitting him especially for such a duty, and the design which was subsequently approved and adopted was executed by his friend, Mr. H. P. Briggs, R.A.

With a president who was not merely a chemist by name, but a successful cultivator and teacher of the science and practice of chemistry, and who was known throughout the civilized world, and admitted to personal communication with men of the highest rank and position, as an esteemed promoter and patron of benevolent and educational institutions; with a vice-president of sterling worth and more than average ability, who was respected by all who knew him, and placed in the foremost rank among his compeers as a zealous and talented advocate of their cause; with councilmen comprising the most influential members of the drug trade, representing every department of the business; and lastly, with two secretaries who had well merited the position they occupied, it might be thought that the society was provided with an efficient staff of officers equal to the carrying out of all its objects. But no just estimate could be formed of the requirements in those days for effecting such a social revolution as was contemplated, by a reference only to the better mutual understanding that has since arisen among the same class. Prior to the establishment of the Pharmaceutical Society there was no social or professional intercourse among chemists and druggists,—no medium of communication,—no common principle of action, or bond of union. Trade jealousies, suspicion and distrust, prevailed to such an extent as to render it difficult to bring the members of the trade together or to induce them to join in any common object. It required a man of independent means, disinterestedly devoted to the work, with tact, temper, and powers of persuasion, to overcome the difficulties of the undertaking, and such a man was Jacob Bell.

Although possessed of the means to some extent of mixing in fashionable society, for which at an earlier date he had manifested a disposition, he was not inclined to throw off his business connections or to despise the shop which had made him, in a pecuniary sense, what he was. He had formed the acquaintance of many artistic, literary, and scientific men, including some of the celebrities of the day in those departments, and especially among medical men and artists. But he also cultivated the acquaintance of his pharmaceutical brethren. On the 25th of March, 1841, he gave what he called a pharmaceutical tea party at his house of business, 338, Oxford Street, to which he invited chemists and druggists, and medical men ; and the desirability of establishing a Pharmaceutical Society was talked of on that occasion as it also had been previously. In the discussion of this subject, whenever it occurred in his presence, Jacob Bell took a prominent part, and manifested the deep interest he took in the project. Until the foundation-stone of the new society had been laid on the 15th of April, the name of Jacob Bell appeared less frequently than that of his father in connection with the proceedings of the associated chemists and druggists; but the son having now identified himself as leader of this movement, the father, who was retiring from active participation in business, left to his more energetic partner all future action in connection with the establishment and operations of the Pharmaceutical Society.

Henceforth, when the name of Bell occurs in this historical account, unless otherwise distinguished, it will relate to Jacob Bell, who had become a moving spirit, originating, actuating, or organizing measures tending to the furtherance of the general interests of the body to which he belonged, and of the association which had been formed of the members of that body.

The pharmaceutical tea party of the 25th of March was followed by a series of monthly meetings at Mr. Bell's house, the first of which was held on the 11th of May; and as the new society had now been founded, these were ostensibly meetings of the society, to which the members, together with medical and other scientific men who took an interest in the subject, were invited for the purpose of reading and discussing papers relating to the'practice of pharmacy. Although instituted and conducted by Mr. Bell on his sole responsibility and at his expense, these meetings were designed and intended as an experiment, for the purpose of illustrating the advantage of scientific discussion, and as a starting point for meetings of a similar description which it was hoped the Pharmaceutical Society would carry out, with the twofold object of bringing the members of the society together, and of inducing them to communicate and discuss matters of practical or scientific interest relating to their daily occupations. At the first meeting Mr. Bell read a paper " On the Constitution of the Pharmaceutical Society of Great Britain." This sketch was followed at the next meeting, on the 9th of June, by papers " On the Rise and Progress of Pharmacy," by Mr. Morson ; " On Hippuric Acid and its Tests," by Dr. Alexander Ure ; and " On the Preparation of Medicinal Extracts," by Mr. Redwood.

These first meetings sufficiently indicated the probable success of the experiment. Mr. Bell's rooms were crowded, and men pursuing the same occupation in the same street or neighbourhood, who had never before exchanged a friendly greeting, were here hustled together, brought face to face and warmed into recognition, at the meetings or in the refreshment room of their generous host.

But the question arose, what was to be done with the papers read at these meetings ? There was no journal devoted to pharmacy in which they could be published, and by means of which the beneficial influence of the social gatherings in Oxford Street might be extended to districts beyond the reach of Mr. Bell's invitations, and to numbers greater than his house, though not his liberality, could entertain. It was seen from the first, that some channel for the publication of the proceedings at the pharmaceutical meetings was much wanted; and with the view of providing for this requirement, and also of furnishing a medium of communication between the members and others interested in the society, Mr. Bell started a monthly publication, the first number of which appeared in July, 1841. It contained the papers read at the first two meetings, and was entitled " The Transactions of the Pharmaceutical Meetings." Subsequent meetings furnished matter, but not sufficient matter, for succeeding numbers of this publication. In the second number, which appeared on the 1st of August, the title was changed to " Pharmaceutical Transactions : " other papers besides those produced at the July meeting were introduced, and the work now began to assume more of the character of a scientific journal.

Mr. Bell was not only the proprietor of this publication, but took the position of editor, for which he possessed considerable aptitude. In his early youth, while at school, he had manifested much fertility of imagination and readiness and power of expressing his ideas,—qualifications which developed themselves in successful literary competitions with his schoolfellows, and also in the establishment and maintenance for some time, principally by the use of his pen, of a manuscript school journal, devoted to the humorous treatment of schoolboy incidents, which were often cleverly illustrated with pen-and-ink sketches. This tendency to indulge, and power of excelling, in graphical representations of events, was evidenced during his apprenticeship in the production of an illustrated journal or diary, in which daily events were recorded ; but unfortunately this artistic representation of trivialities was destroyed by him at a later period when his attention was devoted to subjects of greater importance.

The establishment of a journal devoted to the interests of pharmacy and the Pharmaceutical Society was an object that could not have failed, under any circumstances, to enlist the zealous advocacy and assistance of Mr. Bell. The proposition for such an undertaking, however, had originated with himself, and he was prepared to find the means of submitting it to a fair and ample trial. With no small qualification for the purpose, he undertook the duty of editor, and the leaders were all, or nearly all, written by him, while other parts of the journal were under the immediate management of the sub-editor, Mr. Redwood, who acted in that capacity from the commencement of the work until at Mr. Bell's death a change was made, when Mr. Redwood took a more prominent part as editor.

It had been proposed by Mr. Bell that the monthly pharmaceutical meetings should be held at his house until the society had a habitation of its own, and this arrangement was adhered to. The first of these meetings having been held on the 11th of May, 1841, they continued to be similarly held at 338, Oxford Street, until the 12th of January following.

The meetings of council and of committees were meanwhile held at the houses of members of council, and especially at the house of business of the treasurer in Throgmorton Street, where the Defence Committee had been originally accustomed to meet.

But a fixed residence for the society had now become necessary, and numerous inquiries for such resulted in the selection of 17, Bloomsbury Square, where there were vacant rooms affording the requisite accommodation. In December, 1841, the council, on the recommendation of a committee, agreed to take this house at a rent of £240 a year, subject, however, to the occupation of some of the rooms by two tenants, who were jointly to pay the society £60 a year for them.

The first meeting, a meeting of council, at which the president was present, was held in the newly acquired premises on the 6th of January, 1842, and arrangements were made for holding an evening meeting of the society there on the 12th of January, at which the president was to deliver an address.

The premises in Bloomsbury Square, although in the first instance only taken from year to year, with the option of having a lease, seemed likely to afford the required accommodation for carrying out the contemplated operations of the society. But the step thus taken engendered other arrangements. In the place of two honorary officers who had hitherto performed the secretarial duties, Mr. George Walter Smith was appointed resident secretary at a salary. Alderman Thomas Wood had already been appointed solicitor for the society.

Thus provided with a house and executive officers, the business of the society was promptly entered upon. An address from the president, who was unable to attend personally, was read at the evening meeting held on the 12th of January, in which he remarked that the arrangements relating to the establishment of the School of Pharmacy, the regulation of examinations, and the appointment of examiners, had for some time claimed the attention of the council. These appear to have been looked upon at that early stage of the society's operations as among the most important of the

means by which the objects of the association were to be
attained. While, as the president remarked, the council were
thus "concerting measures for the early adoption of a complete and well digested plan " of education and examination,
evidence was afforded of their earnestness in promoting this
object by the commencement at once of a series of evening
lectures introductory to the subjects on which it was proposed
to establish and maintain courses of systematic instruction.
On the 16th of February Dr. Anthony Todd Thomson delivered an introductory lecture on Materia Medica, which
was followed by lectures—on the 2nd of March, by Dr.
Andrew Ure, on Chemistry ; on the 16th of March, by
Mr. Redwood, on Pharmacy; on the 30th of March, by
Dr. Pereira, on modern discoveries in Materia Medica; on
the 20th of April, by Mr. Fownes, on Organic Chemistry ;
and on the 11th of May, by Dr. A. T. Thomson, on Botany.

During the time that these preliminary lectures were
being delivered, arrangements were made for commencing
courses of systematic instruction in Botany, Materia Medica,
Chemistry, and Pharmacy, and professors were appointed in
each of those subjects, Dr. A. T. Thomson in Botany, Dr.
Pereira in Materia Medica, Mr. Fownes in Chemistry, and
Mr. Redwood in Pharmacy. Dr. Thomson commenced his
course on Botany on the 17th of May. The other courses
were commenced in the following October.

A board of examiners was appointed, and the College of
Physicians and the University of London were consulted as
to the best arrangements for conducting the examinations ;
but these bodies, although invited to do so, declined to send
representatives to be present as visitors at the examinations.
The society was as yet too young and undeveloped to justify
the expectation of recognition and assistance in such form
from those bodies. Encouragement to proceed was, however,
offered by many distinguished members of the medical profession and other scientific men.

A deputation from the council waited on Sir James
Graham, the Home Secretary, to explain the objects and proceedings of the society, and point out the claims it would
have, when its plans were brought into full operation, for the
countenance and support which the Government might afford
by granting a charter of incorporation.

While the council was thus laying the foundations of the society on a broad basis, and actively promoting its development, it was obviously necessary to provide a constituency that should give it moral and substantial support adequate to the carrying out of all the contemplated objects in an efficient manner. It was only by such means that the society could be established in popular favour, and that it could obtain the looked-for assistance from Government and the legislature. The object sought, however, was not easily to be accomplished among a class of men hitherto unorganized and unaccustomed to combined action. One of the objects which had been contemplated in starting the *Pharmaceutical Journal* was that of providing a medium of communication among chemists and druggists, and a means by which they could be appealed to and corresponded with on subjects affecting their common interests. But even journalism was then in its infancy; the penny postage-stamp and newspaper had not yet created such an appetite for a knowledge of passing events as would ensure attention to appeals in this form. A personal appeal was necessary, and Mr. Bell, at his own cost, undertook the duty of making such appeal. He visited different parts of the country, for the purpose of bringing the members of the trade together, in towns where such meetings had rarely or never before occurred, and where, as in London, druggists were accustomed to look upon each other with jealousy and distrust. The mere act of bringing them together and inducing them to discuss questions affecting their interest was an important step towards the social improvement of the body. They could hardly refuse to assemble when invited to meet one of their brethren, a man well known by name, who had come from a distance on such a mission.

Soon after the society was started, in 1841, Mr. Bell made a flying visit to towns in the south-west of England, the result of which he summed up as follows:—" In every place there are a few who take a lively interest in the advancement of our profession; there are a few who are satisfied with our present state of mediocrity, and are indifferent about any improvement; but the majority appear to hesitate on the threshold, unwilling to come to a hasty decision, but convinced of the necessity of some regulations, and only waiting to see a commencement before they enter the field."

Similar visits were subsequently made to other parts of the country; in fact, wherever it was thought that good could be done by such means, Mr. Bell was ready to devote himself to the work; and the unostentatious and disinterested zeal he manifested on these occasions gained for him a cordial welcome and attentive consideration of the subject of his mission.

The progress made in obtaining members was by no means unsatisfactory, although it scarcely realized the anticipations of some of the most sanguine promoters of the movement. Thus the number of members and associates, which in September, 1841, was 450, and at the end of that year was about 800, had increased to 1958 when the first annual meeting of the society took place in May, 1842. When it is considered that a member's subscription was then two guineas and an associate's one guinea a year, it will be admitted that strong inducements must have been brought to bear upon the body of chemists and druggists throughout the country to cause within a few months so great an accession of subscribers to a new and as yet imperfectly developed association. The rapid growth of the society was no doubt mainly due to the prevalence of a consciousness, among those to whom the appeal was made, of the existence of professional weakness for which a remedy was required, and to a feeling of confidence in the capabilities of those who had undertaken to provide and apply the remedy.

On the 17th of May, 1842, the first anniversary meeting of the society was held at the Crown and Anchor Tavern, with the president, William Allen, F.R.S., in the chair. The council presented what was considered to be a very satisfactory report, showing a balance in hand of £1026, and £3000 stock invested. Some progress had been made towards fitting and furnishing the house in Bloomsbury Square, but much yet remained to be done in that direction. The library and museum were not formed, and the requisite provisions for the School of Pharmacy were incomplete. The regulations which the council had adopted for the examinations, which were to come into operation on the 1st of July of that year, were submitted to the meeting. The Board of Examiners was to consist of the president and vice-president of the society with eight dispensing chemists; a physician and a

professor in some department of medical science were to be
invited to attend as visitors. There was to be a minor examination for associates, and a major examination for members.
Every person presenting himself for examination was required
to produce testimonials of having been apprenticed to or regularly educated by a vendor of drugs or dispenser of medicines.
The text book of examination was to be the Pharmacopœia
of the London College of Physicians, and questions were to
be submitted with reference to Chemistry, Materia Medica,
Botany and Pharmacy, as embodied in that work. The candidate was required to translate medical prescriptions, and to
demonstrate his acquaintance with practical pharmacy.
He was also required to know the antidotes for common
poisons. There was a preliminary examination for apprentices
to be passed previous to the execution of their indentures.

In all these proceedings the prominence given to provisions
for promoting and extending pharmaceutical education might
be considered to indicate what was felt to be the prevalent
feature of weakness in the then existing body of chemists and
druggists. There were very few members of the body who
were not sensible that their professional acquirements were
in some respects imperfect; yet it could not be said that the
duties performed by chemists and druggists in the preparation
and sale of medicines were in general badly performed. In
every district where a demand for such existed there were
men who had grown with the occasion, and who were filling
as best they could the positions for which their natural and
acquired abilities adapted them; but in most cases these were
self-educated men, their knowledge was practical rather than
scientific, it related to the special requirements of their
particular positions, and having been picked up as wanted
was liable to fail them when new requirements arose. They
necessarily took much on trust, and were not unfrequently
imposed upon; they knew as much as appeared to be required
for their daily occupations, but if taken beyond that on any
subject in materia medica, chemistry, or pharmacy, they
would speedily break down. They were conscious of their
own shortcomings, and as fitting occasions presented themselves they were generally ready to fill up the most prominent
gaps in their educational curriculum. When they had entered
the business there were no schools at which they could

obtain systematic instruction in subjects directly bearing upon the practice of pharmacy, and feeling now the loss they had sustained through that deficiency, they were anxious not only to provide better means of instruction for those who were to follow them, but to do so in such a way as to offer at the same time facilities for extending their own qualifications.

Among the stimulants to these proceedings might be mentioned one which, emanating as it did from no unfriendly quarter, added to the general feeling that there was room for improvement. A series of articles appeared in the *Pharmaceutical Journal*, entitled "Illustrations of the state of Pharmacy in England," written by a man who had for some time held a prominent position in the almost unoccupied field of pharmaceutical literature. The author, Mr. Richard Phillips, had sprung from the rank of chemists and druggists, but, having devoted himself to the study of chemistry, had attained to the position of lecturer on that subject at St. Thomas's Hospital. He had given a good deal of attention to the subject of the adulteration of drugs, and had offered some evidence on this subject before a committee of the House of Commons in 1834. Previously to that date he had distinguished himself by the publication of severe criticisms upon the London Pharmacopœia, but he was afterwards engaged by the College of Physicians, to prepare subsequent editions of the work, a translation of which he published with explanatory notes. The purport of his communications to the *Pharmaceutical Journal* was to show that medicines sold by London druggists frequently did not correspond in strength and composition with those under the same names ordered in the Pharmacopœia. To enable him to do this he collected samples from different shops and published the results of his examination, without however giving the names of those who had supplied them. The mineral acids, the alkalies, sweet spirit of nitre, salvolatile, and other medicines, were thus tested, and the results certainly did not appear to reflect much credit on the state of pharmacy even in the metropolis. There was obviously room for improvement, and it was the object of the originators of the Pharmaceutical Society, and the tendency of the educational arrangements adopted by them, to effect such improvement.

Movements in the direction of education were not confined to London. In several provincial towns attempts were made, by means of lectures or in some other way, to afford to members as well as apprentices or junior students means for acquiring or extending a knowledge of some of the branches of science included in a sound pharmaceutical education. Bath appears to have taken a prominent part, soon after the starting of the society, in promoting the cultivation of pharmaceutical knowledge, by the formation of a branch association, for discussing subjects relating to pharmacy, and providing lectures for students. Similar arrangements were also made at Manchester, Liverpool, Birmingham, Bristol, Exeter, Norwich, Newcastle and elsewhere.

The examinations for the admission of members and associates were to have come into operation, according to the regulations of the council, in July, 1842, but no candidates presented themselves until nearly the end of the year. On the 15th of November, the first associate by examination was admitted, and another was similarly admitted on the 20th of December. There were as yet no candidates for the major examination, nor did any pass until February, 1844.

The society was now in full operation, and its promoters having obtained for it an adequate amount of support to justify the conclusion that it fairly represented the views and objects of the members of the trade throughout the country, the time was thought to have arrived when a further important step might be taken.

On the 5th of November, 1842, the council presented a petition to the Queen praying that she would be graciously pleased to grant to the Pharmaceutical Society a charter of incorporation; and in less than a month, on the 1st of December, the secretary of the society was requested to attend at the office of the Secretary of State, where he was informed that the draft of a charter might be submitted for consideration.

Something more than a mere flutter of agitation was created among the officials in Bloomsbury Square by this announcement. No time was lost in preparing the required document, which after a few conferences and due legal revision received the sanction of the Government and the authorization of the Crown.

The date of the charter is February 18th, 1843. This forms an important epoch in the history of the Pharmaceutical Society; for although the charter gave no legal power to the society that was not previously possessed, it greatly increased its influence by showing that its objects, and the means by which they were proposed to be attained, were approved of and sanctioned by the Government. And even beyond this the objects of the society and the means of attaining them were defined and limited, which gave a character of stability to a body otherwise subject to change. The charter sets forth in the preamble that the society was established "for the purpose of advancing chemistry and pharmacy, and promoting an uniform system of education of those who should practise the same; and also for the protection of those who carry on the business of chemists and druggists; and that it is intended also to provide a fund for the relief of the distressed members and associates of the society, and of their widows and orphans." The defined objects of the society are therefore threefold; namely, education and protection for all, and relief to the unfortunate and distressed.

As soon as the charter was obtained, further progress was made towards completing and issuing the engraved certificate of membership, the design for which had some time previously been made by Mr. Briggs, R.A. As this document was intended to partake of the character of a diploma, it was important that it should proceed from a publicly recognised and incorporated body, and the filling in of the terms in which the society should be described in it was therefore deferred until the granting of the charter.

The society had something now to present to its members in return for the support they had so liberally afforded. In this respect the granting of the charter and issue of the diploma came opportunely at a time when there was a tendency to a little reaction from the feeling of enthusiasm which had brought members together under the apprehension of danger. Threatened attacks upon the interests and independence of the trade were no longer heard of. A body had been organized capable of resisting such if they should again appear. There was a sense of relief from danger which, following the excitement of action, caused some to relapse into their wonted indifference, and others to view with critical if not unfriendly

disposition the proceedings of the council.   Some thought
the subscription to the society unnecessarily high, and objected
to be called upon to provide the means of investing capital as
well as defraying the expense of creating an educational
establishment, the benefits of which would be experienced by
their successors more than by themselves.   There were a few
even who took exception to the position occupied by Mr. Bell
as proprietor and editor of the *Pharmaceutical Journal*, the
organ of the society, while he was at the same time a member
of council.   But although there were murmurs of discontent,
they neither spread nor did they assume a definite form.   In
fact, the council consisted of men who were held in such high
respect throughout the trade and among those outside the
trade who took an interest in pharmacy, that their influence
and the confidence placed in their judgment were sufficient to
prevent any public expression of dissatisfaction with the policy
adopted.

It would probably be within the truth to say that the druggists of London, wholesale and retail, who at this time formed
the council of the Pharmaceutical Society, have never, either
before or since, been surpassed among the same class in the
power and influence they possessed. This might, perhaps, be to
some extent ascribed to the prevalence of defective professional
education among the body to which they belonged.   As there
had been no regular system of education among chemists and
druggists, there was much professional ignorance or incom-
petency, and the few who through superior natural abilities
or exceptional means had overcome the difficulties caused by
the want of proper systematic training, acquired high reputations and obtained especially the confidence of the medical
profession.   The council of the society at this time consisted
entirely of London druggists, and mostly of those who occupied
prominent positions.   It was important at the starting of the
society that its representatives should have influence outside
the body to which they belonged, and a council consisting of
known London men was therefore appointed ; but with a view
to the carrying out of the important object of raising up a
class of educated and qualified pharmacists, capable of efficiently
performing the duties required of them in every town throughout the country, it was necessary to ensure the support and
enlist the co-operation of a large country constituency, and this

could only be done by extending representation to country districts.

At the second anniversary meeting, held in May, 1843, a financial report was presented, which showed an income of more than five thousand a year, and an invested capital of nearly six thousand pounds. Some allusion was made to the annual subscriptions paid by members and associates to the society. The council in their report say they " do not think it necessary to recapitulate the arguments which have been so often stated, but they still adhere to their original opinion, after another year's experience, and are satisfied that all the comprehensive objects of the society cannot possibly be carried out if any modification beyond that which the bye-law committee have suggested be at the present time insisted on, particularly in the prospect of very considerable expense being incurred in watching the progress and provisions of the forthcoming Medical Bill." No explanation appears to have been given or asked for with reference to the allusion thus made to a modification of the annual subscription, but it may be assumed that the bye-law committee were chiefly influenced by the feeling frequently expressed that the subscription was unnecessarily high, and that they had therefore suggested a modification such as was adopted two years afterwards.

At this meeting two country members were elected into the council.

It was understood that Sir James Graham, the Secretary of State, intended to introduce a bill into Parliament for effecting certain reforms in the medical profession. Attempts had been repeatedly made by those connected with different branches of the profession to initiate legislation for the removal of admitted evils; but unfortunately the profession was divided against itself, and no sooner was a measure introduced by one party than it was opposed and defeated by another. The Government, it was thought, might be more successful in satisfying the wants without exciting the jealousies and fears of the various parties interested. This position of the question had tended to allay much of the alarm previously existing among chemists and druggists, and there was therefore a great absence of excitement on the subject and a corresponding diminution in the ardour of some of those who had been

M

induced to support the society as a means of defence against aggression.

Almost the only grievance at this time, originating from without, was that caused by a few prosecutions for the sale of spirit of wine. It had become so much the practice for the public to apply to druggists for small quantities of spirit when required for burning in lamps or for other domestic purposes, and these sales had been so long passed unnoticed by the excise, that those engaged in them were taken by surprise when they found that by every such transaction they subjected themselves to a heavy penalty. The council readily undertook to intercede with the authorities at Somerset House on behalf of those who had been informed against, and subsequently they applied to the Government on the same subject. All, however, that could be done was to get a reduction of the penalties incurred, for the law was clear and its infraction undoubted.

While there were indications of some falling off in the enthusiasm which had previously brought members together, this was by no means general, and it chiefly affected those who viewed the society as a political agent. There were still evidences of much zeal manifested in the measures that were adopted for promoting the study of pharmacy and branches of science bearing upon its advancement. Thus, in addition to the ordinary educational lectures, a course of evening lectures was commenced in the early part of this year, on Polarised Light, by Dr. Pereira. These lectures were published in the *Pharmaceutical Journal*, and afterwards in a separate form. The subject was one which at that time was rarely studied by and had received but little attention from chemists. It was looked upon as an abstruse subject which admitted of few if any important practical applications, and was considered therefore more suited for those engaged in abstract philosophical research than for practical chemists and pharmacists. But Dr. Pereira, in his usual lucid style, while he made the subject intelligible and popular, showed and illustrated its various useful applications, and demonstrated the importance of its study to the scientific pharmacist.

The lectures in Bloomsbury Square were attended by classes ranging in number from seventy to ninety, and often including members as well as associates of the society. Those

who thus availed themselves of the instruction provided were
small in number as compared with those to whom it was
offered, nor could it be said that they consisted of such as
most required instruction. In fact they came from the better
class members of the trade. With many, perhaps the majority, of those who had entered the business, it was not merely
scientific or professional knowledge that was wanted, but also
the very rudiments of school knowledge, and persons in this
position were disinclined to enter the lists with better trained
competitors. A feeling also appeared to prevail, and considering all the circumstances it could not be wondered at, that
the instruction the Pharmaceutical Society was providing for
its students was in excess of what was required. The majority
of those who called themselves chemists and druggists had no
just claim to the former of these appellations, nor could they
in the full sense of the term be called pharmacists ; they were
dealers in drugs and chemicals just as grocers are dealers in
tea, sugar, and vinegar, without knowing anything of the
real nature of the articles in which they dealt. It might be
said of most of them that they rarely saw a physician's prescription, and therefore had little occasion for a knowledge
of dispensing. There were the great dispensing establishments to which physicians were in the habit of recommending
their patients, where dispensing was understood, and it was
among these and the higher class of chemists and druggists
that pharmaceutical education was most appreciated. All
honour to the worthy band of distinguished pharmacists who
laid the foundation for an educational system which, bringing
the required knowledge equally within the reach of all, was
calculated to undermine the pre-eminence of the great
historic houses.

Even books and periodical publications, conveying educational knowledge in the department of pharmacy, were at
this time wanting. The Pharmacopœia, published as it was
in Latin, would have been a sealed book to many who were
supposed to use it, if it had not been for an English translation. This, together with Gray's Supplement, which gave
brief information on many subjects, including the means of
adulterating drugs, and two or three works on Materia Medica
and the Practice of Medicine, often constituted the professional
library of a first class establishment where apprentices were

trained for the business.   Truly the study of pharmacy under
such circumstances was the pursuit of knowledge under difficulties.   Yet a few men with minds cast in a peculiar mould,
after groping in this abyss, succeeded in working out an
education of their own, and these, rising above the common
level, assumed prominent positions in various parts of the
country.

There were two journals, the *Lancet* and the *Medical Times*,
devoted to the interests of the medical profession, which occasionally admitted articles relating to pharmacy, and a journal
which had been started about a year or two before the commencement of the Pharmaceutical Society, under the title of
The Chemist, regularly devoted some of its pages to the subject of pharmacy; but there was but little sympathy manifested
in any of these publications with the promoters of the great
work undertaken by the pharmaceutical body.   Fortunately
this body possessed within itself and among its members an
amount of power and influence equal to the accomplishment
of its objects.   Of its best men, however, it was destined to
lose one at the close of this year, 1843.

On the 3rd of January, 1844, at a meeting of the council,
the following minute was passed :—

" That the council desires to record its deep and unfeigned
regret at the loss which the society has sustained on the decease of the late revered president, William Allen, F.R.S.

" Formed as the society was for the public benefit generally,
and for the welfare of that branch of the profession of medicine of which he was so distinguished a member, it was by
universal consent that he was solicited to allow himself to be
placed at the head of it, that under his wise and kindly superintendence its scientific and benevolent designs might be
carried out.

" The council is anxious to bear testimony to the zeal he
ever manifested in all the concerns of the institution, to the
encouragement it has derived from his advice, whenever his
health and numerous avocations enabled him to afford his presence or opinion ; and it sincerely trusts that the same harmony
which his beneficent spirit could not fail to infuse, will ever
continue to pervade its own meetings, and the general intercourse amongst the members."

William Allen was the son of Job Allen, a member of the

Society of Friends, and a silk manufacturer in Spitalfields. Having shown a taste for chemical and other pursuits connected with medicine, he was placed in the pharmaceutical establishment of Joseph Gurney Bevan, in Plough Court, Lombard Street, where he served an apprenticeship, and subsequently succeeded to the business. He attended several courses of lectures delivered at the medical schools on subjects relating to chemistry and pharmacy, and devoted much time to the study of these subjects by rising very early in the morning. After succeeding to the business he was joined by Luke Howard, the title of the firm being Allen & Howard. In addition to the retail business in Plough Court, they established a laboratory at Plaistow for the manufacture of chemicals, but at the expiration of the partnership the business in Plough Court reverted again to William Allen, and Luke Howard took the manufacturing business, which has since become the well known concern of Howards of Stratford. At a later period, and for more than a quarter of a century, William Allen occupied the position of lecturer on Chemistry and Experimental Philosophy at Guy's Hospital, having been associated in the chemical part of the course first with Dr. Babington, and at subsequent periods with Drs. Marcet and Bostock. During the period of his connection with Guy's Hospital, he accepted the chair of Experimental Philosophy at the Royal Institution, which he held for several years. He thus became intimate with Sir Humphry Davy; but his most intimate associate and friend was William Haseldine Pepys, with whom he was for several years engaged in chemical investigations, some of which were communicated to the Royal Society, of which learned body he became a fellow in 1807. The first of the papers communicated by Allen and Pepys to the Royal Society related to the quantity of carbon in carbonic acid (CO_2), and to the nature of the diamond. Their experiments tended to establish the accuracy of Lavoisier's previous statements with reference to the former subject, and to confirm Smithson Tennant's results in regard to the latter. As opposed to the representation of Guyton de Morveau, who assumed that carbonic acid gas contained 17·88 per cent. of carbon, they showed that the proportion of carbon was 28·6 per cent. They also arrived at the conclusion that the diamond was pure carbon. Subsequent papers gave the results of investigations relating to respiration, in which some points previously unknown were determined. These investigations afforded evidence that the authors were careful experimenters, who carried out their researches in a truly philosophic spirit.

But much of William Allen's time was occupied in the pursuit of objects other than those of experimental philosophy. He was a great philanthropist engaged in promoting and extending religion, charity, education, and civil liberty throughout the world. It was in connection with his labours in this direction that he acquired the world-wide reputation which rendered his services to the Pharmaceutical Society when struggling into existence of so much value.

As it now became necessary to elect a new president, the council at once proceeded to raise Mr. Charles James Payne, the late vice-president, to that position, and at the same time made Mr. John Savory, of Bond Street, vice-president.

The subjects which particularly claimed the attention of the council after this change, were the preparation of new bye-laws, rendered necessary by the granting of the charter, and the much debated question of what the annual subscription to the society should be. There was much and increasing dissatisfaction with the regulation that required the same payment from London as from provincial members, and imposed a subscription of a guinea a year on associates and apprentices. The committee who were engaged in revising the bye-laws had recommended an alteration of these terms, but it was not proposed to bring this into operation immediately. It was obvious that there would be considerable expense incurred in Bloomsbury Square in fitting up and extending the library, museum, and various provisions for teaching, so as to make them creditable to the institution and adequate to the carrying out of the objects contemplated. There was therefore a strong feeling entertained by leading members of the council that something ought to be laid by while the higher subscription continued, which might be drawn upon afterwards if the income should fall off. Already there were two new sources of expenditure talked of; namely, a laboratory for practical instruction for pharmaceutical students, and an Act of Parliament to strengthen the hands of the society. The council therefore, and especially the president, who was indefatigable in his attention to the business of committee and other meetings, had several perplexing questions before them. After some deliberation it was decided, in addition to the educational lectures, to fit up a small laboratory in which to give practical instruction to a few of the students who were anxious to have the means, while studying at the school, of filling up the whole of their time. There were schools on the continent, such as that under Professor Liebig at Giessen, where this kind of instruction in chemistry and pharmacy was given, to which English students sometimes resorted, but hitherto there had been no similar school in this country, and the attempt now made to establish one was quite an experiment. Accommodation was provided for ten students, and the full number speedily presented themselves as applicants for admission. The laboratory was opened in October, 1844, under the direction of the Professor of Pharmacy.

This year had commenced with the announcement of the loss of the first president of the society, a loss which could not have been otherwise than severely felt by a young institution, but the members thought they were fortunate in having a man so well able to fill the vacant place as Mr. Payne was admitted to be. This opinion was fully justified as long as the new president had health and strength enough to fulfil the duties of the office, but before many months had elapsed his health so completely gave way that he felt it his duty to resign the presidency, an event that was soon followed by his death. The society thus lost the services of its first two presidents within the short space of a year.

Charles James Payne was born on the 28th of January, 1794, at the house of his maternal grandfather, an apothecary, in Titchfield Street, Oxford Street. He was an only child, and lost his father at an early age; but was placed by his mother under the care of the Rev. Dr. Hamilton, of Hemel Hempstead, with whom he remained from the age of seven until he had completed his fifteenth year. At fourteen he was apprenticed to Mr. Burkitt, of Fleet Street, but did not commence his London life until a year afterwards. In this situation he remained six years. He attended the usual routine lectures, among which were those of Abernethy, and he obtained the Botanical prize in 1811.

At the age of twenty-one he took up his freedom, and became a member of the Apothecaries' Company: after which he went to Mr. Winstanley in the Poultry, where he remained for two years and a half.

In May, 1817, Mr. Payne opened a chemist's shop in St. Martin's Court, Leicester Square. He could not be said to have ever practised as an apothecary, although he had the necessary qualification. He considered and represented himself to be a chemist and druggist, and acted as such.

The first occasion on which Mr. Payne united with his brethren in any public proceedings was in the year 1839, when meetings of the chemists and druggists were held for the purpose of promoting the closing of shops on Sundays. Having adopted this custom himself ever since the year 1826, and having had satisfaction in doing so, he was anxious to prevail upon others to act in the same way.

At the meeting of the trade, which was held at the Crown and Anchor Tavern on the 15th of February, 1841, a gentleman made some observations which were received with approbation by all present, and which showed that the speaker was an eloquent and zealous advocate of the independence and established privileges of chemists and druggists. The clear sound reasoning and judgment evinced in those remarks made a deep impression, and although few present were aware at the time who the speaker was, he was soon discovered to be Mr. Payne, of St. Martin's Court. A short time afterwards he was induced to allow his name to be placed on the committee then acting on behalf of the chemists and druggists, and from that time until the state of his health obliged him to retire from office, he was one of the most indefatigable members of the committee and afterwards of the council. The estimation in which he was held by his brethren is forcibly expressed in a testimonial, engrossed on vellum, which is suspended in the council-room of the society, and a copy of which was presented to his daughter, an only surviving child. The testimonial is as follows:—

" PHARMACEUTICAL SOCIETY
OF
GREAT BRITAIN,
17, BLOOMSBURY SQUARE, LONDON.

" At a meeting of the Council held on the 6th November, 1844, it was unanimously resolved that the Council wishes

strongly to express its deep sense of the loss the Society has
sustained by the decease of

MR. CHARLES JAMES PAYNE,

whose unremitting zeal, indefatigable and disinterested exertions, urbanity of manners, judgment, and moral worth, so
eminently manifested in the discharge of the several offices of
president, vice-president, and member of the Council, conferred
on the Institution a lasting and substantial benefit.   Mr.
Payne was ever the advocate of the cause of the Chemists and
Druggists, and in an especial manner interested in the welfare
of the less fortunate members of the body.

"In the arduous labours attending the establishment of the

PHARMACEUTICAL SOCIETY,

in laying the foundation of the Benevolent Fund, and in promoting the

EDUCATIONAL OBJECTS OF THE INSTITUTION,

the extent of his zeal would only be fully estimated by those
who were associated with him.   To perpetuate the recollection
of the debt of gratitude the Society owes to so valuable a
member, the Council has directed that this MEMORIAL, engrossed on vellum, be presented to his daughter, and a copy
of the same be suspended in the Council room."

After the resignation of Mr. Payne, Mr. John Savory had
been elected to the presidency, and Mr. Thomas N. R. Morson
was made vice-president of the society.

The most important subject of discussion at this time in
medical circles was the bill recently introduced in Parliament by Sir James Graham, for regulating the practice of
medicine and the qualifications of those engaged in it.   This
was a measure of a very sweeping nature, which was based
upon the recognition of a new principle in medical legislation.
It was assumed by Sir James Graham that quackery cannot
be prevented by Act of Parliament, and that the prosecution of
unqualified practitioners is impolitic and unavailing.   The
new bill proposed to repeal the Apothecaries' Act, and every
other enactment which empowered any authorities to inflict
penalties for irregular practice.   There was to be free trade in
medicine to the fullest extent, and the public were simply to
judge for themselves whether they should employ qualified or
unqualified practitioners.   But at the same time inducements

were to be offered for the acquirement of qualifications by granting to qualified men the exclusive privileges of holding certain appointments and filling official positions of honour and profit, as well as of recovering professional charges by legal process. Only qualified men also were to be exempted from liability to serve on juries. A system of registration of qualified practitioners was to be established, and penalties imposed on those who assumed titles implying qualifications they did not possess. These regulations, as well as those for insuring efficient medical education and examination, were to be placed under the control and management of a Council of Health and Medical Education.

There was nothing in this bill calculated to interfere with the privileges of chemists and druggists, or in any way to affect the practice of pharmacy. It was not therefore likely to excite alarm or induce opposition among the pharmaceutical body ; but it was far otherwise with the medical profession, among whom a strong opposition was manifested. It soon became evident that the bill could not pass without considerable alteration. Even chemists and druggists hardly viewed with satisfaction the extreme free trade principles upon which the measure was based,—principles which, if applied to pharmacy, would destroy the hopes of those, a daily increasing number, who were looking to the prospect of future legislation for protection from the encroachments of unqualified dealers in drugs and dispensers of medicines. For the present, at any rate, druggists were allowed to pursue their course undis-turbed, and they wisely continued with increased energy to carry out the system which had been introduced for educating and improving the qualifications of the members and students of their body. It was in this way only that they could either expect to retain an independent position free from the exercise of control by one of the other medical corporations, or to obtain increased power and privileges.

In addition to the lectures and the ordinary scientific meet-ings, which had been successfully established, a laboratory for practical instruction in chemistry and pharmacy was about to be opened in Bloomsbury Square, and now the council, on the recommendation of Dr. Pereira, also appointed a scientific committee for the promotion of pharmacological knowledge. The immediate object contemplated in the formation of this committee was the elucidation of the natural history and origin of substances used in medicine. "Many points," said Dr. Pereira, "remain to be settled, questions to be answered, and uncertainties to be resolved, with reference not only to exotic, but even to indigenous products; not merely to rare, but also to some of the commonest drugs; not simply to modern, but also to some of the oldest articles of the Materia Medica."

"No country in the world," he said, "possesses so many facilities for carrying on inquiries such as those to which I here allude, as Great Britain. Her numerous and important colonies in all parts of the world, and her extensive commercial relations, particularly fit her for taking the lead in investigations of this kind, Moreover she is peculiarly interested in such inquiries. From her extensive possessions in different parts of the world, we draw a very large portion of the substances now used in medicine. By the establishment of a committee on pharmacology in the mother country, an opportunity would be obtained of bringing into notice the various medicinal substances produced in the different portions of this great empire. In this way substances now unknown to, or little employed by us, might be brought into use, and in some instances, perhaps, the produce of our own colonies might be advantageously substituted for that of other countries. Furthermore, in those cases in which British products are inferior to those of other countries, this committee might be able to ascertain the causes of the inferiority and suggest the means of removing them. In these and other ways then, I apprehend that such a committee would prove useful in a commercial, as well as a scientific point of view. It might be made the means of declaring to the remotest part of our colonial possessions the wants of the mother country, and conversely, of making known to England the capabilities of the different portions of the British Empire."

This appeal from so eminent a professor induced the council at once to appoint a committee, consisting of the following members of the society:—

JOHN SAVORY, *President.* | T. N. R. MORSON, *Vice-Pres.*

ROBERT ALSOP.	THOMAS HERRING.	J. S. LESCHER.
JACOB BELL.	EDWARD HORNER.	R. H. PIGEON.
HENRY DEANE.	ROBERT HOWARD.	PETER SQUIRE.
DANIEL HANBURY.	WILLIAM INCE.	GEORGE WAUGH.

And of the following honorary members and other scientific men :—

JAMES S. BOWERBANK, F.R.S.	T. HORSEFIELD, M.D., F.R.S.
W. T. BRANDE, F.R.S.	RICHARD OWEN, F.R.S.
J. F. DANIELL, F.R.S.	JONATHAN PEREIRA, M.D.,
F. J. FARRE, M.D.	F.R.S.
GEORGE FOWNES, Ph.D., F.R.S.	RICHARD PHILLIPS, F.R.S.
THOMAS GRAHAM, F.R.S.	J. F. ROYLE, M.D., F.R.S.
J. E. GRAY, F.R.S.	A. T. THOMPSON, M.D., F.R.S.

T. REDWOOD, *Hon. Secretary.*

The first meeting of this committee took place on the 25th January, 1845, when sub-committees were appointed for carrying out the several objects contemplated.

It was evident that the scientific and educational proceedings of the society were being actively promoted. The laboratory for practical instruction had proved so successful that a proposition for building a new laboratory on a larger scale in the basement of the premises was entertained by the council and ultimately adopted. But while a considerable outlay was thus being incurred, the income derivable from subscriptions was at the same time curtailed by the operation of a new bye-law which came into operation this year, 1845, in accordance with which the subscription of London members was reduced to one guinea and a half, and that of country members to one guinea, while the subscriptions of associates were lowered to half a guinea in town and country. By this change a source of much discontent among the supporters of the society was removed; and it was at the same time hoped that the number of members and associates would be increased so that the income of the society should not fall off to any serious extent. It was not thought prudent, however, by the council to continue the usual annual grant to the Benevolent Fund until the effect of lowering the subscriptions was known. Some of the members took exception to this, and thought the council were economising in the wrong direction.

Attempts were made to induce chemists to shorten the hours of business by closing their establishments at an earlier hour in the evening, and especially by closing on the Sunday. Some reference was made to this subject at the

annual meeting in 1845, but here and elsewhere the movement met with but little sympathy. The argument adduced,
that it was desirable to afford assistants and apprentices
time for study, was not generally appreciated; indeed, there
was much indifference manifested, both by employers and
employed, in acknowledging the necessity for, or even the
benefits of, the education that was being provided at so much
expense. Those who witnessed at that time, and who after
a lapse of many years, and from higher ground, can look
back at the listless state of contented ignorance that prevailed,
are alone able to estimate the difficulties that had to be
contended with in introducing and maintaining an efficient
system of sound practical and scientific training for students
in pharmacy.

The most efficient stimulant to movement among the dry
bones was the prospect of interference from without. Whenever this presented itself there were evidences of some vitality,
and indications of a desire to become what most intelligent
men considered that a chemist and druggist ought to be.
But since the introduction of Sir James Graham's bill the
fear of legislative interference with druggists had died away,
and a feeling of undue confidence in the intentions of the
Government, and in the tendencies of the legislature, had
induced a partial return to that sense of security and state
of inaction which had originally prevailed before 1841.

Meanwhile the three medical corporations were disputing
the claims to support of Sir James Graham's Medical Bill.
The general practitioners were mostly opposed to it, but
even among this class there were great differences of opinion,
and there seemed to be little chance of even the Government
being able to carry a measure that should be satisfactory to
themselves and to the bulk of the medical profession. This
was the state of the question when a sudden change took
place in the Government bill. To appease the outcry of the
apothecaries a clause was introduced into the bill which
was more completely restrictive than anything contained
in the old Apothecaries' Act of 1815. It was to the following
effect :—

"And be it enacted, that every person who, after the
passing of this Act, shall act or practise as an apothecary
in any part of England or Wales, without having been re-

gistered by the said Council of Health as a General Practitioner in Medicine, Surgery, and Midwifery, shall for every
such offence forfeit and pay the sum of twenty pounds, to be
applied to the use of the said College, to be recovered by
action of debt in any of her Majesty's Courts of Record in
Westminster."

This soon brought the Chemists together again at a public
meeting held at the Crown and Anchor, at which Mr. T. N.
R. Morson presided. Resolutions were passed strongly
objecting to the bill in its modified form, and calling upon
chemists and druggists throughout the country to petition
against it. A deputation from the council appealed to the
Home Secretary, and received assurances of a somewhat
satisfactory nature. The obnoxious clause, it was found,
had originated with the Apothecaries' Company, but a promise was given that it should be reconsidered. Petitions
were now pouring into Parliament against this attempt again
to interfere with the rights and privileges of chemists and
druggists, but the result of the reconsideration of the subject
by the Home Secretary in communication with the solicitor
of the Apothecaries' Company, was that a further clause was
introduced exempting chemists and druggists from the effects
of the Act, in the same way as this had been done in 1815.

This was considered satisfactory, and further opposition
to the bill was withdrawn as far as chemists and druggists
were concerned. But greater difficulties than those arising
from the opposition offered by the Pharmaceutical Society
stood in the way of medical legislation. The members of the
different sections of the medical profession were still at
variance on this subject; and after many attempts had been
made at reconciliation or compromise, all of which proved
abortive, the Government bill was withdrawn without any
prospect being held out that further efforts would be made in
the same direction.

Medical legislation having thus collapsed, the question came
to be frequently asked among chemists and druggists, why
is there no attempt made to get an Act for regulating the
practice of pharmacy? While the Medical Bill was before
Parliament, it was understood that if the Government succeeded in carrying their measure, they would probably follow
it up with another bill relating to pharmacy; but there was

now but small chance of such a result. The question of the desirability of promoting a Pharmacy Bill was considered in the council, but it was decided that the time for making any public movement had not yet arrived. While the society was steadily pursuing its legitimate objects of training and organizing a body of qualified pharmacists who should fill with credit the positions assigned to them in connection with the administration of medicine, it was preparing the way in the most efficient manner for any steps it might be thought desirable to take towards increasing by means of legislation the power and usefulness of the body it represented.

Among the means adopted by the society for promoting pharmaceutical education was the extension of laboratory instruction, and with this view the new laboratory had been constructed which was opened at the commencement of the session in 1845. It afforded accommodation for twenty-one students, and every place was almost immediately filled. The arrangements of this laboratory, and the accommodation provided in it for students, were far superior to those of the laboratory used throughout the previous session. It was still limited in extent, but was otherwise all that could be desired for the purpose for which it was intended. Indeed it was adopted as the pattern from which the Birkbeck laboratory in University College was shortly afterwards fitted up.

The Pharmaceutical Society is entitled to the credit of having been the first institution in which provision was made in this country for carrying out a system of instruction in chemistry and pharmacy by practical operations in which the students were engaged throughout the day under the instruction of a professor. The example thus set was shortly afterwards followed by the commencement of a class in connection with the College of Chemistry in temporary premises in George Street, Hanover Square, under Professor Hofmann, and this was followed by the opening of the Birkbeck laboratory under Professor Fownes.

The Scientific Committee of the Pharmaceutical Society was doing some good work, chiefly through the personal contributions or exertions of Dr. Pereira. At the pharmaceutical meeting held in July, 1845, four papers emanating from the committee were read: on the Manufacture of Palm Sugar in India, by Mr. Stevens; on the Origin of Samovey Isinglass, and on the Circular Polarisation of several Terebinthinate Substances, by Dr. Pereira; and on Some Vegetable and Mineral Productions of New Zealand, by Mr. W. Brown. At a subsequent meeting an interesting paper was read, on the Cultivation of Rhubarb for Medicinal Purposes at Banbury, by Mr. W. Bigg.

A paper on the Formation of a National Pharmacopœia, read at one of the meetings of the society by Mr. Peter Squire, serves to show what the direction of opinion was at that time on an important subject relating to pharmacy. The attention of the medical profession had, as Mr. Squire pointed out, been for many years directed to the desirability of having a national Pharmacopœia for Great Britain and Ireland, in place of the three separate pharmacopœias issued by the London, Edinburgh, and Dublin Colleges. Some efforts had been made to attain this object by the London College previously to the publication of their Pharmacopœia in 1836, but in that attempt they had not succeeded. The discrepancies existing between the three British pharmacopœias had been pointed out, and these individually had often come under discussion, but still they were allowed to exist, each college acting in accordance with the judgment formed by itself and its advisers, without reference to what was done by the other colleges. The consequence was that medicines bearing the same name as ordered in the three pharmacopœias sometimes differed in composition and strength to a sufficient extent, in the case of powerful medicines, to be a source even of danger. Mr. Squire, with the view of forcibly impressing upon those interested in the subject the importance of providing a remedy for this evil, set out the formulæ of the three pharmacopœias in columns, side by side, so as to show how far they agreed or differed. The time had not yet come for the fusion of the three pharmacopœias into one, but Mr. Squire's labours aided those who ultimately effected the much wished-for result.

Excise informations and prosecutions were sources of frequent trouble to members of the trade in different parts of the country. At one time it was for evading the payment of stamp duty on medicines that required to be stamped; at other times, for selling small quantities of spirit of wine for other than medical purposes, without having a licence for doing so. In these cases fortunately there were officials in

Bloomsbury Square ready to help unfortunate delinquents where help was right and available, and there were also, fortunately, sometimes cases in which the society by affording aid was enabled to justify its claim to support. The officers of excise appeared to be more active than they had usually been in endeavouring to ascertain the extent to which spirit was sold and used by chemists and druggists, and on this account complaint was made to the authorities at Somerset House of what was considered to be unnecessary interference with transactions which had hitherto passed unnoticed and were looked upon by most druggists as tacitly sanctioned, if not strictly legal. Inquiry into the state of the law relating to the sale of spirit showed, indeed, that strictly speaking a druggist subjected himself to a penalty by selling spirit of wine, whatever the purpose might be for which it was required, and although proceedings were not generally instituted when only small quantities of a few ounces were sold, or when it was sold for strictly medical purposes, yet even in these cases the Inland Revenue Board retained the power of inflicting the penalty if there were reasons for suspecting that the indulgence afforded was being abused. There were probably suspicions at this time that some unfair dealings were taking place, and this may have caused increased activity among the detective officers, some of whom made an important discovery in July, 1845. It was then discovered that a complete and extensive illicit distillery existed in one of the suburbs of London, where large quantities of spirit had for years been produced, most if not all of which was sold by chemists and druggists in the form of sweet spirit of nitre. Seizures of large quantities of spirit in all its stages of production and conversion into spirit of nitre were made in different localities both in town and country, from which it was evident that the public revenue had been defrauded to a great extent. There was no evidence to prove that the druggists through whose hands this illicit spirit was supplied to the public, excepting perhaps a few wholesale dealers, knew anything of the history of the spirit of nitre they were selling, but the circumstances were sufficient to excite suspicion, and to justify the adoption of precautionary measures for protecting the revenue.

About the middle of the following year, 1846, a bill was

N

introduced into Parliament which, if passed, would have had
the effect of placing the chemists and druggists under the
inspection of the excise in a way that was considered highly
objectionable. By this measure it was proposed that every
person keeping or using a still or retort, and every wholesale
dealer in spirit mixtures, should be required to take out a
licence and pay two guineas annually, or in default of doing
so they would be subject to a penalty of fifty pounds.   The
sale of spirit mixtures in quantities of more than a quart
would constitute wholesale dealing.   The rooms or buildings
in which spirit mixtures were kept were to be specially
licensed for the purpose, and were to be subject at all times
to the inspection of excise officers.   Druggists in fact, by this
measure, would have been brought as completely under the
inspection of the excise as public-house keepers are.   It was
felt that such an infliction would have been degrading and
intolerable, and a strong opposition was therefore offered to
the measure, in which both wholesale and retail dealers took
part.   The result was that the Government at last gave way,
and the bill was cut down to one for licensing the use of
stills and retorts for distilling spirit mixtures.   The duty
payable for such licence was reduced to ten shillings, and the
authority for excise officers to enter and inspect premises was
omitted.   Provision was also made for the use of stills and
retorts for experiments in chemistry, without payment of
duty, on permission being obtained ; and stills used exclusively
for other purposes than that of distilling spirit mixtures were
exempted from the operation of the proposed regulations.

In this modified form the measure was considered to be
as little objectionable as it could be made without entirely
destroying its efficacy, and further opposition to it ceased.
After the passing of the bill, however, it was found, in the
practical working of the Act, that the concessions made in
passing it had been carried rather too far, and in 1861 an Act
was passed by which the excise were empowered at any time
to visit the premises of persons licensed to keep or use stills
or retorts, with the view of ascertaining the purposes for
which they were used.

Although there was a considerable number of chemists and
druggists throughout the country who sincerely and zealously
advocated and supported the objects of the Pharmaceutical

Society in promoting the cultivation and general advancement of pharmaceutical knowledge, yet it cannot be denied that a much larger number were indifferent to these objects, and that even among the members of the society, who never constituted more than about a third part of the entire body of chemists and druggists, there were many, perhaps the majority, who, except on political grounds, were but lukewarm advocates of the cause. By these the question was frequently asked, What do I gain by subscribing to the Pharmaceutical Society? When any danger threatened the craft, or difficulties assailed individuals, under circumstances in which the efforts and influence of an organized association could render efficient aid, the advantage of belonging to the Pharmaceutical Society was acknowledged; but when the danger had passed, and there was no immediate prospect of a recurrence of troublesome questions affecting trade interests, the force of attachment to a society which entailed annual payments gradually diminished, and there was an increased tendency to find fault with the way in which the institution was managed.

Then among the better informed members of the trade, including those who had now become thoroughly educated, it was felt that without some legislative protection in the exercise of their professional duties, against the interference of such as had no claims to qualification, they were unable to realize the substantial advantage to which they were entitled

Under these circumstances the difficulty of maintaining the society was becoming a matter of serious consideration, and the importance of strengthening its position by an Act of Parliament was acknowledged by its best friends. The council began to think that a movement in the direction of pharmaceutical legislation might be made with advantage. Mr. Bell especially advocated this view, and made attempts at a definition of what the kind of legislation was that being attainable would be efficacious.

The sort of measure that was most desired was thought to be unattainable. It was considered to be inconsistent with the principles of modern legislation that the same corporate body should be an educating and an examining body, with the power of granting degrees or diplomas giving legal authority for the performance of professional duties. This opinion was in great measure founded on the knowledge of what had occurred with reference to the London University in Gower Street. That institution was originally intended not only as a college for educational purposes, but also as an examining body for granting degrees. But when application was made for a charter it was decided that one of these offices must be relinquished, and the founders accepted a charter for it as an educational body, resigning the office of granting degrees to the University of London, which was created for that purpose, while the name of the institution in Gower Street was changed to University College. It was assumed that the objection urged in that case would equally apply to the case of the Pharmaceutical Society if an attempt were made to obtain legal authority to combine the two functions of education and examination.

It was represented that the difficulty might be overcome by either of two methods: first, the society might confine its functions to those of examining candidates and granting diplomas, while a new body, under the title of the College of Pharmacy, might be established as an educating body; or, secondly, the society might continue to be an educating body, and resign the functions of examination, etc., to the College of Pharmacy. The latter alternative appeared to be the preferable one, and accordingly a bill was drafted embodying that object.

By this bill it was proposed to found a College of Pharmacy, which was to be limited in its operation to England and Wales. The Secretary of State was in the first instance to appoint a provisional council consisting of five or more chemists and druggists for carrying the Act into operation, and this council was to appoint a provisional registrar. Then every person who within one year after the passing of the Act should produce a certificate signed by two magistrates stating that such person was at the time of granting the certificate engaged in business as a chemist and druggist in some part of England or Wales, and every person who should produce a certificate from the council of the Pharmaceutical Society stating that he was a member of that society, would be entitled to be registered by the provisional registrar as a pharmaceutical chemist and druggist, and all persons so registered would become members of the said College of Pharmacy. At the end of the twelve months allowed for effecting this registration the list of persons registered would be published, and the constituency thus formed would be called upon to elect from among themselves a council consisting of twenty-one members, who would be the council of the College of Pharmacy. This council, one-third of whom would go out of office, but might be re-elected, every year, would have the appointment of a board of examiners for conducting examinations in classical knowledge, botany, materia medica, pharmaceutical and general chemistry, and toxicology, and no person thereafter would be entitled to be registered as a pharmaceutical chemist and druggist, or to be admitted a member of the College of Pharmacy, unless he produced a certificate of competent skill and knowledge from such board. Then there was to be a provision that any person in future who should prepare, compound, or dispense any medicine for sale or gain, unless he could prove that he was engaged in business as a chemist and druggist before the passing of the Act, or was registered under the Act, would be subject to the payment of a fine of not exceeding ten pounds.

This arrangement would not interfere with any of the rights and privileges of those who were already in business, nor was it intended to interfere with the Pharmaceutical Society, excepting with regard to its power of examining candidates, and granting certificates of examination.

The draft bill was submitted to the fifth annual meeting of the society, in 1846, and although some doubts were expressed as to whether the proposed new institution, the College of Pharmacy, would not injuriously affect the interests of the Pharmaceutical Society, no serious objection was raised to the measure.

A deputation from the society subsequently waited on a committee of the College of Physicians with the view of ascertaining the opinion entertained by the College respecting the bill, a copy of it having been previously sent them. At this interview it was stated that the College would perhaps be disposed to favour the appointment of a joint board of examiners, partly nominated by the College of Physicians and partly by the College of Pharmacy. This raised a new and important question in relation to the subject which could not be determined without mature deliberation. A second interview took place about a month afterwards,

when the subject was again discussed, especially with reference to the name and functions of the proposed College of
Pharmacy, the constitution of the board of examiners, and
the manner of enforcing the provisions of the Act so as to
ensure the efficient performance of the duties of pharmacists.
The suggestion which had been made for the appointment
of a joint board of examiners seemed likely to be a source of
some difficulty in coming to a final arrangement that should
be satisfactory to the parties immediately interested.

In the year 1846 great interest was excited among medical
men and pharmacists, as well as generally among the public,
by the introduction of a method of producing insensibility to
pain while important surgical operations were being performed.
This was effected in the first instance by the inhalation of
the vapour of ether. Drs. Warren and Morton, of Boston,
United States, introduced this method of operating in the
year above named, and it was adopted in this country towards
the latter end of that year, among others by Mr. Liston, the
eminent surgeon of University College Hospital. An opportunity was thus afforded for chemists to exercise their ingenuity in devising the best method of vaporising the ether
so as to bring it into a suitable state for inhalation. Mr.
Squire was one of the first to devote attention to this part of
the subject, and to construct an efficient apparatus for the
production and administration of the vapour. The ether, of
course, was vaporised by diffusion into atmospheric air, and
for the production of the best anæsthetic effects it was found
necessary to have the air fully charged at a temperature not
too low. This was introduced into the lungs by the mouth,
while the simultaneous introduction of air through the nose
was prevented by compression of the nostrils. Mr. Squire's
apparatus was used with perfect success by Mr. Liston in the
first capital operation performed under the influence of ether
vapour in this country, but in some subsequent cases the
effects were not so satisfactory, in consequence of due care not
having been taken to prevent the admixture of air with the
vapour. It was found that if too much diluted with air, the
ether vapour produced excitement unattended by complete
insensibility to pain.

Pure washed ether was used in these experiments; but the
use of ether was soon afterwards superseded by that of

chloroform, a substance previously almost unknown, so much so indeed that some difficulty was experienced, when it was first proposed to be used for this purpose, in ascertaining how it was to be produced, and what its physical and chemical properties were. A solution of it in spirit had been previously used in medicine under the name of chloric ether, and this had been tried as a substitute for ether in the production of an anæsthetic vapour, having been first suggested and supplied for that purpose by Mr. Jacob Bell; but in this diluted form it had but little effect. When subsequently the composition of chloric ether was made known, and pure chloroform was produced by a process just then published in a new edition by Mr. Redwood of Gray's "Supplement to the Pharmacopœia," it was used with great success by Dr. Simpson, of Edinburgh, and was preferred in many respects to ether. Several other agents, resembling chloroform in composition, have been tried for producing anæsthesia, but none of these has superseded chloroform.

In the introduction of the practice of applying anæsthetics in the form of vapour, by inhalation, we have the commencement of a new era in practical surgery, which has been characterized by the cessation and avoidance of a great amount of human suffering previously contingent upon most surgical operations of importance.

It was the duty of the qualified pharmacist to seek out and prepare the best chemical compounds for the production of these anæsthetic effects, and it was not inconsistent with his position that he should assist in producing and applying the vapour, as these involved the exercise of some amount of chemical knowledge and manipulative skill; but his taking part in such operations was liable to excite suspicion among members of the medical profession, who might suppose that it indicated an intention or desire to interfere with the legitimate duties of the apothecary. Thus we find the *Lancet* at this time insisting on the necessity of limiting the education of those engaged in pharmacy to strictly pharmaceutical knowledge, and defining the province of the pharmaceutical chemist to be "materia medica, the knowledge of all the articles it contains, or the raw material of physic, in all that relates to purity, preservation, and preparation; the knowledge of the pharmacopœias, or of the modes in which the

raw materials are combined according to the judgment of the
official bodies who preside over its construction; and the
perfect comprehension of prescriptions; these, with improvements or even discoveries in pharmacy."

In the article in which this representation was given of the
legitimate province and scope of the professional education of
the chemist and druggist, objection was taken to the fact of
toxicology being openly grafted on the pharmaceutical courses
of chemistry, botany, and materia medica as provided by the
Pharmaceutical Society. It was further objected that the
parties who supplied "this kind of partial information—this
little knowledge, which in medicine, so pre-eminently, is but
a dangerous thing," were physicians, public lecturers, who were
teaching the same thing at the same time to medical students.
The answer to these objections was that a certain amount of
the knowledge of therapeutics and toxicology was required
by the qualified pharmacist, and that only this amount was
taught at the lectures in Bloomsbury Square. It was hardly
to be wondered at, however, nor can it now be regretted, that
the proceedings of this society and of its promoters were
closely and jealously watched and frequently criticised.

At a much later period, in 1859, Dr. George Wilson, of
Edinburgh, a good authority on such subjects, took a very
different view from that expressed in the *Lancet*. In treating
of the education of pharmaceutical chemists, he represented
the following three things as essential in the knowledge
required by the qualified pharmacist:—

" 1st. A thorough familiarity with the appearance and
sensible properties, such as odour, colour, taste, and the like,
of every important drug or medicine, natural or artificial,
whether derived directly or indirectly from the mineral,
vegetable, or animal kingdom.

" 2nd. A knowledge, the greater the better, of the chemical
nature or composition of all the important drugs or medicines.

" 3rd. A general acquaintance with the physiological action
or influence on the living body of the chief medicines in use.

"This last requirement," Dr. Wilson said, " may seem to
some less justifiable than the others. None however, I
imagine, will deny that he cannot be considered an educated
pharmaceutical chemist, or even a safe dispenser of drugs,
who does not clearly understand why certain of them are

grouped together as narcotics, others as diaphoretics, others as anæsthetics, and so on."

It may further be stated that the founders of the Pharmaceutical Society had at an early date in its history insisted on the importance of a knowledge of the action of the antidotes for, and the means of detection of, poisons as qualifications for the educated pharmacist; and they were only deterred from prominently representing this department of knowledge as forming a distinct feature in the instruction given in their school from a fear of appearing to grasp at too much and trenching in any way upon the province of the medical practitioner. That the course pursued by them from the beginning has been right, is evidenced by the fact that no alteration has at any time been required to be made in it, and all opposition or objection has gradually died out. What the supporters of the society had chiefly to contend with, was not so much opposition from those outside their domain, as indifference and dissatisfaction among the body of chemists and druggists for whom so much was being done, and even among the members and associates of the society itself. The attendance at the lectures fell far short of what had been expected, and it was partly made up of men who had long been established in business, but who, during their pupilage, had no means afforded them for obtaining scientific instruction in the branches of knowledge appertaining to their professional occupation. Men of this description formed bright examples; they were the backbone of the society, by which alone it was supported and enabled to withstand the dispiriting effect of cold indifference through a long period of struggling existence. While this was going on, complaints were frequently made of the cost of the educational department of the institution, but the council persisted in keeping up the character of the school by the employment of eminent professors. The most successful part of the teaching arrangements was that conducted in the laboratory for practical instruction, this department being generally full, and testimony being repeatedly afforded by the board of examiners and others to the value of the instruction thus supplied to pupils. The time, however, had now arrived when there were other laboratories conducted on principles similar to those adopted in Bloomsbury Square, as regards the method of conveying laboratory instruction.

The new laboratories of the College of Chemistry, in Oxford Street, were completed in 1847, when the school was transferred there from the temporary apartments it had previously occupied in George Street, Hanover Square. The College of Chemistry was founded in July, 1845, under extensive aristocratic patronage, with Prince Albert as president. It was designed to occupy a position distinct from that of the school of the Pharmaceutical Society, its objects being much wider, comprising the applications of chemistry to the arts and manufactures generally, and therefore including its application to pharmacy. But although it met some of the requirements of a pharmaceutical education, they were not provided for in other respects. At first starting, and during several years of its early existence, the College had to contend against many difficulties, arising in great measure from injudicious officialism and the adoption of too florid a representation of the benefits that were said speedily to flow from its operations. When it was found that these were not likely to be realized, notwithstanding the matchless genius and talent of its professor, and the good work done by students, its original supporters fell off, while heavy debts accumulated, and at length the institution had to be kept up by a subsidy from Government.

Great and frequent as were the complaints of want of adequate support afforded to the Pharmaceutical Society, there was at least the satisfaction of finding that its school was as well attended as other similar schools, and that instead of accumulating debts, the society was yearly increasing its invested capital.

At University College, the Birkbeck laboratory, which was started about the same time as the College of Chemistry, was placed under the direction of Mr. Fownes, who was appointed Professor of Practical Chemistry. Mr. Fownes had for some time been suffering from incipient disease of the lungs, which had latterly rendered lecturing painful and difficult to him; and after receiving his new appointment he was advised to relinquish lecturing; accordingly, in 1846, he resigned the professorship of chemistry to the Pharmaceutical Society. This necessitated a new appointment in Bloomsbury Square, and Mr. Redwood undertook the duties previously performed by Mr. Fownes, the lectures on chemistry and pharmacy being united into one course.

The years 1847–48 were prolific in speculation and discussion on the subjects of both pharmaceutical and medical legislation, but no real progress was made in the substantial furtherance of either.   The council of the Pharmaceutical Society met with little encouragement to persevere in promoting the formation of a College of Pharmacy, the prevailing opinion being, that it was unnecessary and undesirable—that the idea under which it had been suggested was a mistaken one, and that all the objects contemplated might be effected through the medium of the Pharmaceutical Society.   Endeavours had been made to modify the Pharmacy Bill as first drawn, so as to meet the views of those who had objected to some of its provisions, and especially for the purpose of introducing the suggested arrangement of a joint board of examiners in which the College of Physicians should take part; but while on the one hand serious difficulties stood in the way of adopting this latter suggestion, so there appeared to be equally serious objections to the provisions of the bill which contemplated the formation of a new institution, the College of Pharmacy.   These features of the bill had been proposed under the impression that such an arrangement would be less likely to meet with opposition than one by which the Pharmaceutical Society should be made the sole medium of carrying out a system of education and examination connected with the granting of certificates giving exclusive privileges.   But in addition to the prevailing opinion among members of the Pharmaceutical Society that the establishment of a second institution, for no other purpose than that of doing part of the work which the society was authorized by its charter to perform, would be detrimental to the interests of the society, there was found to be a very general feeling among those unconnected with the society, including the College of Physicians, in favour of leaving the arrangements both of education and examination in the hands of the Pharmaceutical Society.

Under this view of the subject another bill was drafted, which was submitted to the members of the trade, and to others interested in it.   This bill resembled the former one in most particulars.   It provided for the registration of all persons who were then engaged in business as chemists and druggists, and for the examination and registration of those who should be entitled to commence business after a certain date. The clauses restricting the practice of pharmacy to those who had either passed an examination, or had been in business before the passing of the Act, and imposing penalties for infringing these regulations, were the same as those contained in the previous bill. In fact, the only essential difference was, that by this bill the Pharmaceutical Society, unaided by any other institution, was to be made responsible for the carrying out of the required objects, subject, however, in some respects, to the approval of the Secretary of State.

In drafting this and also the previous bill, the chief object had been to reduce crude ideas to a definite form, so that those who discussed the subject might have a specific proposition with all essential details before them. There was no immediate prospect of its being brought before Parliament, for although attempts had been made to interest members of Parliament in its favour, no one had been found who seemed disposed to take it up. The general public had not had their attention directed to the subject; the medical profession as a whole were not fully cognisant of all its bearings, or were fearful of its tendencies; and members of Parliament, as well as the Government, required to be stimulated from without before they would move in a subject they did not thoroughly understand. It was necessary, therefore, as far as possible to create an interest among all these parties in the promotion of the contemplated object.

The machinery of a well organized society was put into action for accomplishing what was required. The local secretaries throughout the country were set to work to get petitions signed by various classes of the public, in which the necessity for a systematic training of those engaged in preparing and dispensing medicines was expressed, together with a desire that some means might be adopted for insuring the qualification of all persons engaged in dealing with dangerous drugs. Petitions to this purport were soon poured into Parliament, some of which were signed by the highest medical authorities, including the president, censors and consiliarii of the College of Physicians, and the president and council of the College of Surgeons.

In pursuing this course advantage was taken of the excitement caused by the occurrence of some fatal accidents which had been caused by the administration of medicines by incompetent men. Attention had also been repeatedly directed to the incautious manner in which poisons were often supplied to the public.

In November, 1847, a deputation from the council of the Pharmaceutical Society had an interview with Sir George Gray, the then Secretary of State, in which they pointed out the evils resulting from the want of any legislative provision for insuring a safe and efficient exercise of the important duties required to be performed in the sale and preparation of medicines, and endeavoured to obtain a recognition from the Government of the desirability of legislating in that direction. No reference was made to any particular measure, but a hope was expressed that the Government would be willing to assist in furthering the object which the Pharmaceutical Society was endeavouring to carry out; and to this extent they received an encouraging assurance, although unfortunately it was coupled with a statement that pharmaceutical legislation should follow, not precede, medical legislation.

The difficulties which had for many years been experienced in the attempts to carry any satisfactory measure of medical reform acted as a discouragement to members of Parliament to take up the subject of pharmaceutical legislation; and there seemed but little prospect, therefore, of any effective movement being soon made towards the passing, or even the introduction, of a bill for that purpose.

Mr. T. N. R. Morson was president and Mr. Peter Squire vice-president at this time.

Thus, with relation to pharmacy, ended the year 1848. The following year commenced with a register of deaths among some of the early promoters and scientific officers of the Pharmaceutical Society. John Bell, the founder of the celebrated house of John Bell & Co., of 338, Oxford Street, and George Fownes, F.R.S., the first Professor of Chemistry to the Pharmaceutical Society and author of the well-known and popular manual of chemistry which still bears his name, both died in January, 1849; and a few months afterwards the same unsparing messenger summoned away another of the professors of the school of pharmacy, Dr. Anthony Todd Thomson.

The life of John Bell was one from which some useful lessons may be gleaned, although there was nothing of a very striking character presented in its incidents. The worthy founder of a great house and parent of a distinguished son owed his success in business to the strict integrity which characterized all his transactions, and the firmness with which he persisted in carrying out the dictates of his conscientious convictions. He was not a man of great talent, and he was mistrustful even of the powers he possessed. But he had a fixed determination to do what he believed was right. During his apprenticeship he had gained an insight into practices which were then of frequent occurrence among druggists, and which he determined to discountenance at any sacrifice. He opened his shop in Oxford Street with a small capital, and many doubts as to his means of making a business and keeping out of debt. He was naturally cautious and very timid, so that difficulties and slight reverses easily discouraged and alarmed him ; but nothing could induce him to swerve from a firm adherence to the principles which guided his conduct, and which, as they became known, gained for him the confidence of the public and insured his success. The shop was opened in 1798. On the first day his receipts amounted to ten shillings, but in giving change he was cheated out of half a guinea, a result which so discouraged him that at night he would not light his lamps until a friendly neighbour came in and consoled him. The balance of accounts at the end of the first year showed a loss, but then came a steady succession of years of increasing prosperity. There was no longer any occasion for the shopboy, John Simmons, to find occupation at the back of the shop in pounding a dusting-cloth in the bell-metal mortar in order to maintain a semblance of business activity, and at the same time to inform passers-by, through the ringing sound of the mortar, that physic was compounded there. The shopboy grew to be the laboratory man, who has since been immortalized by Hunt's water-colour drawing of " The Laboratory," engraved by J. G. Murray and published by McLean, and the master became one of the most successful dispensing chemists in London. John Bell was married in 1804, and his eldest surviving son, Jacob, was born in 1810.

Allusion has already been made to the interest taken by

John Bell in the proceedings connected with the establishment of the Pharmaceutical Society. He died at his residence at Wandsworth, at the age of seventy-five.

George Fownes was the son of a glover in Coventry Street,
Leicester Square. He was born on the 14th of May, 1815.
Having received his education, first with Dr. May, of Enfield,
and afterwards at Bourbourg, near Gravelines, he was apprenticed to his father and remained in that capacity until he
attained the age of twenty-two. But for many years previously
he had shown a liking for the study of chemistry, and together
with Mr. Everett, the lecturer on chemistry at Middlesex
Hospital, Mr. Henry Watts, who has since distinguished
himself in scientific literature, and Mr. Robert Murray, for
many years associated with Newman, the philosophical instrument maker of Regent Street, he contributed to form
a philosophical class at the Western Literary Institution in
Leicester Square, where he cultivated the talent he had manifested for pursuing scientific researches, and was encouraged
by his associates to look to scientific pursuits as affording
him more congenial occupation than that in which he was
engaged in the glover's shop. On the recommendation of
Mr. Murray, his father was induced to place him under the
tuition of Mr. Everett at Middlesex Hospital, where he remained for two years, with the exception of three months
spent at Giessen under Professor Liebig. He afterwards
became assistant to Professor Graham at University College,
and remained there for twelve months, or until he undertook
the appointment of lecturer at the Charing Cross Hospital.
His health had never been strong, and close confinement to
investigations and studies in a badly ventilated laboratory at
Charing Cross contributed no doubt to hasten the development of disease in his lungs, which ultimately terminated his
life. With an active and intelligent mind, however, and a
sound judgment, although often ailing, he was enabled to do
much good work. He frequently lectured at the Royal
Institution, and on the retirement of Mr. Everett from the
chair of chemistry at Middlesex Hospital, Mr. Fownes succeeded to it, perhaps imprudently, for at the same time he
was lecturing at Bloomsbury Square, and so much exertion
of the voice often severely taxed his strength.

As a lecturer he was clear, methodical, and painstaking;

but his reputation was chiefly founded on the successful results of his researches in connection with the artificial production of the alkaloids, for which the Royal Society awarded him their gold medal. He was elected a fellow of the Royal Society in 1845.

In 1844 he published the first edition of his "Manual of Chemistry," which, as a text-book for chemical students, was at that time the most explicit, concise, and yet complete work in the English language; and to this its great popularity may be ascribed. He had previously gained the Acton prize for his essay entitled "Chemistry as exemplifying the wisdom and beneficence of God."

He relinquished his duties as lecturer partly in 1845 and wholly in 1846, still retaining his position of Professor of Practical Chemistry in the Birkbeck laboratory at University College. But the state of his health becoming worse he was advised to try the effect of a sea voyage, and he accordingly went to Barbadoes in 1847. This proved of no avail, and after his return he gave up work entirely, and patiently submitted to the inevitable result of his malady. He was thus cut off in the thirty-fourth year of his age.

An incident or two may be mentioned here. Mr. Fownes was introduced and recommended as professor to the Pharmaceutical Society by Mr. Morson, who had formed the acquaintance, and entertained a high opinion of the talents, of this young but as yet unknown chemist. Mr. Morson's house was the resort of many men of rising and also of mature talent, who were accustomed to hold a sort of scientific service there on Sunday evenings. It was on the occasion of a visit paid by Mr. Fownes to the house of his friend in Southampton Row that he observed among some chemical curiosities in a cupboard a bottle labelled "oil of bran"; and being told that it had been prepared by distilling bran with sulphuric acid and water for a speculative gentleman whose expectations in reference to it had not been realized, he expressed a desire to have some of it for examination. His wish was complied with, and from this he produced his furfurine, one of the best defined of the artificial alkaloids.

Many scientific foreigners when in London, being either known to or introduced to Mr. Morson, were often at his house, and this was especially the case about the period to which we are referring. Liebig, Mitscherlich, Rose, Guibourt, Robiquet, Cap, and other celebrities were guests at Mr. Morson's house, and were taken by him to the Pharmaceutical Society, in which they were induced to take a lively interest.

The influence which these visits, and the resulting favourable opinions expressed both here and abroad, were calculated to exert on the prosperity of a young institution may be more correctly estimated now than they were at that time. Some of the former students of the school may look back with interest to the visits of Professors Liebig and Rose, who went through the laboratories and conversed with the students on the various operations in which they were engaged. Liebig especially left his mark behind, for two or three of the processes usually conducted by students in the laboratory were modified at his suggestion, and in that form were kept up for many years afterwards.

Dr. Anthony Todd Thomson, F.L.S., died in July, 1849. He was born in Edinburgh in 1778, and received his education there, principally in the Edinburgh College. Having acquired the qualifications for a general practitioner he came to London, passed an examination at the College of Surgeons, and commenced practice in Sloane Street. This was in the early part of the present century, and prior to the passing of the Apothecaries Act of 1815. While he was thus engaged as a general practitioner he took an active interest in promoting the adoption of an improved system of education among apothecaries, and in seeking legislation to aid that object, in which he was associated with Burrows, Kerrison, and Mason Good, who, in common with himself, were then general practitioners, but afterwards became physicians. Dr. Thomson's name appears frequently in connection with those proceedings in the earlier part of this Historical Sketch. In 1826 he removed from Sloane Street to Hinde Street, Manchester Square, and he then became a member of the College of Physicians. Shortly afterwards, in 1828, University College, then called the London University, commenced its operations, and Dr. Thomson was appointed Professor of Materia Medica and Therapeutics. He was a man of infinite labour, and endowed with a great capacity for work. In his early morning hours as well as at night he found time for literature, while throughout the day he kept up a large medical practice.

He was the author of the "London Dispensatory," which in its day had a great circulation, and of the "Conspectus of the Pharmacopœia," the circulation of which was still greater. But these were not his only literary productions; he published a mass of scattered papers, chiefly, but not entirely, of a medical character. Botany had been a favourite study with him, and as far back as 1810 he was lecturing on Medical Botany, his being the only course on that subject in London at that time.

Reference has already been made to Dr. Thomson's appointment as Lecturer to the Pharmaceutical Society, but we should fail to do justice to the memory of this distinguished professor if we did not more fully represent the benefits he conferred on the society, and we do so in the words used by the present writer when the circumstances were fresh in his recollection.

Approving of the objects for which the society was founded, and being enthusiastic in the cultivation of those sciences which form the basis of a pharmaceutical education, Dr. Thomson came forward in the most kind and liberal manner at a time when the infant institution stood most in need of such encouragement. He attended the meetings, contributed original papers, took an active part in the scientific discussions, delivered lectures gratuitously, and lost no opportunity that presented itself of promoting an undertaking in the probable success of which even the originators were not sanguine, and which was considered by some members of the profession to be a project almost chimerical.

Dr. Thomson, with that energy and penetration which characterized him through life, disregarded obstacles and difficulties, and keeping his eye steadily fixed on the ultimate object, threw his tact and experience into the scale, inspired the founders of the society with increased confidence, and stimulated them to persevering exertion. The society was indebted to many professional friends for cordial support and encouragement at that period, but the name of Dr. Thomson stands high on the list of those who may truly be designated as "friends in need," and who may be compared to sheet-anchors in rough weather.

When the School of Pharmacy was founded, Dr. Thomson accepted the office of Professor of Botany, which he retained until the time of his decease. By means of his influence he obtained for the students the privilege of admission to the gardens of the Royal Botanic Society, in the Regent's Park, where most of the lectures were delivered. In addition to the lectures officially comprised in the course, he voluntarily devoted the intermediate mornings to demonstrations or peripatetic lectures in the gardens, thus more than doubling the number of lectures, and contributing greatly to their practical utility. This early walk in the gardens he considered a recreation rather than a toil; and nothing appeared to give him greater satisfaction than the appeals of his pupils for information, evidencing their interest in his favourite subject.

In the summer of 1848 Dr. Thomson, both in mind and body, seemed to be as strong as ever.

He was accustomed to rise at six in the morning, walk up to the Botanical Gardens in the Regent's Park, deliver his lecture to the students of the Pharmaceutical Society at seven o'clock, then return and see patients till half-past twelve. At one o'clock he went to the hospital, and at three lectured on medical jurisprudence (this was during the summer months). After this lecture he visited patients till a late hour, when he returned home to dinner. Nor was his work yet over; for after dinner he devoted several hours to literature. In January, 1849, he caught a severe cold, the effects of which he never threw off entirely. Two attacks of bronchitis were followed by pneumonia and finally pleurisy, from the effects of which he died, in his seventy-second year.

The society at this time could ill afford to sustain such losses as had recently occurred among those who had largely contributed by active work and the influence of their reputation to promote its advancement. An uneasy feeling appeared to exist among many of the members, and there were frequent murmurings of complaint, although it rarely assumed any definite form or open expression. Sometimes it was, that nothing was being done towards getting an Act of Parliament, without which the society could be of no real benefit to those who were contributing to its support; sometimes, that there was useless expenditure of the society's funds in rearing up a class of young men who were inspired with high-fangled notions that placed them above their occupations; sometimes, that the council, being principally drawn from the great drug houses of London, had little knowledge of, or sympathy with, the requirements of country trade; sometimes, that the *Journal*, the official organ of the society, was exclusively under the control of one member of the council. In common with most other similar institutions, the society, in fact, began to encounter the difficulties arising from internal dissension, which seemed to increase with the growth of substantial prosperity.

Even the educational department was suffering from depression, and statements were sometimes made to the effect that young men, after incurring the expense of studying in Bloomsbury Square and passing the examinations there, found it difficult to obtain situations, and were often objected to by employers because they were thought to be conceited and disposed to set themselves above their masters.

But there was no possibility of retreating from the system of education and examination which had been established as the recognised fundamental principle of the Pharmaceutical Society.

Some of the past and present students of the school, thinking that it might be desirable to endeavour to infuse increased interest into the cause, suggested the holding of a Pharmaceutical School Dinner, which was approved of by the President and members of the council, and supported by friends of the society, both members and non-members.

Mr. Squire was at this time the President of the society, having been elected after the anniversary meeting in May, and Mr. William Ince was Vice-president.

Dr. Thomson's last illness having commenced while the Botanical lectures were being delivered, in the summer of 1849, and his death having occurred before their termination, Mr. Bentley, who was at that time Lecturer on Botany at the London Hospital, undertook to finish the course; and he was afterwards appointed to fill the vacant office of Professor of Botany.   He had been a student in Bloomsbury Square when the society commenced, and from his early youth he was an enthusiastic botanist.

The professors, of course, were among those who strongly favoured the projected dinner, which was held on the 17th of July, at the London Tavern, and proved a great success: Dr. Copland, F.R.S., occupied the chair.

An incident occurred at this time which served to show that while dissatisfaction existed among some of those connected with the society, it did not pervade the student class, or those who, having been in that capacity, were now reaping the satisfaction of feeling that they were entitled to command the confidence of the public as qualified and examined pharmacists. A testimonial engrossed on vellum, and accompanied by a handsome tea-service of plate, was presented by seventy-two students of the laboratory to the Professor of Chemistry and Pharmacy, " as an expression of the high estimation in which he is held by those pupils who have pursued their studies under his superintendence."

These were among the evidences of the existence within the society of feelings of approval of what was being done and of a desire to aid in promoting the good work; but at the same time there were evidences of a less satisfactory nature. An anonymous circular, purporting to emanate from a committee, the composition and location of which were kept secret, alluded to and dealt with the proceedings of the council and the management of *The Pharmaceutical Journal* in a spirit of decided hostility, tainted with indications of an acrimonious feeling.

In this as in previous cases in which a disposition had been manifested to get up an opposition party, there was a want of sufficient manliness on the part of those who propagated disparaging statements affecting the management of the society, to avow themselves openly and substantiate or defend their allegations. Still it was evident that there were troubled spirits abroad who were capable of fomenting discord.

The question was often asked, How are we to allay this chronic irritation? The best means of overcoming any slight amount of dissatisfaction within the society, when there was no obvious cause for it other than impatience of delay in the realization of expected benefits, had usually been found to consist in proving the value of association, by the successful defence of the body or its members from some real or threatened attack from without; or by making a further advance towards the attainment of the much-desired object of getting a bill introduced into Parliament for regulating the practice of pharmacy. But in neither of these directions was there any

present opening for a movement.   The Medical Defence
Association, which had formerly been a source of alarm, was
dying for want of occupation ; and the Legislature, after many
vain attempts to regulate the practice of medicine, was indis-
posed to meddle further with physic.   Both the medical and
pharmaceutical bodies were therefore reduced to a state of
constrained inaction as regarded legislation.   Attempts had
repeatedly been made to find some member of Parliament
who would undertake to bring a Pharmacy Bill before the
Legislature, but without success.   Mr. Warburton, who had
taken an interest in the subject, and was looked to as the
most likely person to become champion of the cause, was no
longer in Parliament, and nobody could be found to take his
place.   The medical profession had a member of their own
body, Mr. Wakley, to act as their advocate in the House, and
it was felt that if pharmacy had as zealous and able an
advocate inside as it undoubtedly had outside the House of
Commons, there would be some chance of accomplishing what
was required.   Who could be found, with means, talent, and
a chance of success, to seek a seat in Parliament as the champion of pharmacy ?   This was a question in many mouths,
but one not easily answered.

Among subjects which occupied the attention of the public,
and more or less prominently that of the pharmaceutical body,
in the years 1850–51, there were especially two that call for
notice here—one as showing the weakness, and the other as
indicating the means of strengthening, the bond of union
among chemists and druggists.   First, there was the design
for holding an International Exhibition in London; and
secondly, there was the alarm which had been created by
the occurrence of numerous cases of poisoning and especially
of poisoning with arsenic.   The Great Exhibition of 1851,
with its Crystal Palace, which sprang up like a vision in fairy-
land, and the crowds of visitors from every quarter of the
globe, which gave to London for a time an unusually cosmo-
politan character, together with the success of the undertaking in every respect, have become matters of history which
many look back to with interest, and some with a mixture of
satisfaction and partial regret, for it could not be said that
British pharmacy was well represented there.   This result
was principally caused by the difficulty experienced in getting

those who were able to contribute articles for exhibition to act in concert and to co-operate in carrying out a general plan for the display of such a collection of chemical and pharmaceutical products and drugs as might have been creditable to English pharmacy. The occasion afforded a favourable opportunity for showing to other nations what British commerce and manufacturing skill could produce in this department; but unfortunately it was not turned to the best account.

The questions relating to the sale of poisons more nearly affected the interests of pharmacy and more deeply engaged the attention of pharmacists than did the exhibition of pharmaceutical products. The subject was occupying the attention of the Government, of the medical profession, and the public generally. It appeared from the Registrar General's reports that a large number of deaths occurred annually from poisoning, and that more than one-third of these were caused by the use of arsenic. In 1849 the subject was brought under the notice of the Provincial Medical and Surgical Association by Dr. Tunstall, of Bath; and the Association petitioned Parliament to the following effect:—

1. That no druggist or shopkeeper be allowed to sell arsenic without a licence, under a penalty.

2. That no person be allowed to sell small quantities of arsenic unless combined with some material, the administration of which with food would be at once detected by the appearance or taste.

3. That no person be allowed to purchase arsenic unless accompanied by a witness.

4. And that the vendor do keep a book, in which he should make an entry of every sale of arsenic, to which the purchaser and his witness should affix their names and places of abode, and that this should be attested by the vendor.

Afterwards, the subject was submitted to the Pharmaceutical Society towards the end of 1849, and after being discussed at a meeting of the society, it was referred to the council, who immediately appointed a committee with a view to its further investigation. The committee drew up a series of questions, which were sent to every member of the society, together with the following circular:—

"LONDON, *November* 13*th*, 1849.

"SIR,—The accompanying questions are issued by a committee of the Pharmaceutical Society, appointed by the council to take into consideration the 'Sale of Poisons,' especially of arsenic, with a view of ascertaining whether any means could be adopted for preventing accidental and criminal poisonings.

" The questions are addressed to the members of the society generally; and the committee will feel obliged if you will favour them with answers to such of the questions as may come within the scope of your experience or knowledge. The committee will be glad also to receive information on any other points relating to this important subject.

" An early answer is particularly requested, as the committee will meet again before the expiration of this month.

"GEORGE WALTER SMITH, *Secretary.*

" QUESTIONS ON SALE OF POISONS.

" Do you sell arsenic ?

" Under what regulations do you sell it ?

" For what ostensible objects is it usually demanded?

" By what class of persons ?

" For what trades or manufactures is it required by your customers in small quantities ?

" Is it sold by oilmen, grocers, and general dealers in your town ?

" How many cases of poisoning by arsenic in your neighbourhood have come to your knowledge during the last twelve months, whether criminal or accidental ?

" In what manner do you send it out—in paper, bottles, or jars; and is it always labelled ' *Poison* ' ?

" Are you aware of any accidents attending the use of arsenic as sheepwash ?

" Are you aware of any accidents resulting from its use in steeping wheat ?

" Are poisons generally sold by oilmen, grocers, and general dealers in your neighbourhood ? "

At a meeting of council held on the 12th of December, 1849, Peter Squire, President, in the chair, the Committee on the Sale of Poisons presented the following " preliminary report " on the answers received in reply to the list of ques-

tions proposed by the committee, in reference to the SALE OF
POISONS, especially of ARSENIC.

"In the sale of small quantities of arsenic, the practice of
obtaining an indifferent witness is adopted by a large majority
of vendors. In many cases a written entry is made in a
register, and signed by all the parties. The word 'Arsenic' is
invariably put on the inner paper, and 'Poison' on the outer,
or *vice versâ;* and sometimes both words are placed on each
paper, either in writing or by printed labels. In many cases
the principal of the shop only supplies the demand, but does
not admit any of his own people as witnesses. It is sold
usually to well-known customers. It is often coloured, or
mixed with lard, soft soap, tar, etc. In some instances, where
strong grounds of suspicion have existed, cream of tartar has
been given with all the formality used in supplying arsenic,
by which substitution suicides have been prevented. Many
lives have also been saved by other precautions on the part of
chemists to whom application has been made for poison.

"The principal purchasers of arsenic are colour and chemical manufacturers, farmers, flock-masters, veterinary surgeons,
shipwrights, glass manufacturers, candle makers, and dyers.
These employ it largely; but the smaller or retail quantities
are demanded by braziers, white-smiths, bird-stuffers, game-
keepers, gardeners, grooms, whitewashers, painters, firework
makers, and by rat-catchers, housekeepers, and others of all
classes, for the destruction of vermin of all kinds.

"By many druggists in the country, arsenic is kept in one
pound and half-pound packets, weighed, wrapped, and labelled;
and it would be delivered to any shepherd or farmer's servant
in any quantity, on application by written order; or a pound
or more would be sold, with the usual precautions, to any
known customer connected either with farming or flocks, with
whose requirements the seller was fully acquainted. Arsenic
is used in dipping sheep, and it requires about forty pounds of
arsenic for every 1000 sheep. Some dippers number 40,000
sheep. Many druggists sell upwards of one ton of arsenic
per annum.

"The dippers are subject to serious affections of the hands.
The death of one is reported from Braintree. Deaths among
the sheep are frequent; but these are attributed to the care-
lessness of the operators.

"Arsenic is largely employed in steeping wheat. Persons in drilling the wheat so prepared have been seriously affected, although this is attributed by some to the lime necessarily used with it. Accidents have also occurred from the subsequent use of vessels in which the arsenic had been prepared. Many deaths have been known to occur amongst the stock from eating this prepared wheat, viz., horses, calves, pigs, and fowls; and also coveys of partridges, pheasants, and many small birds. With regard to calves thus poisoned, one lot can be shown to have been sent to the London market.

"In many districts sulphate of copper has superseded arsenic in the preparation of wheat. This process possesses the advantage of not requiring lime. In other parts the use of arsenic for this purpose seems to be unknown. Other substitutes for arsenic are proposed for washing sheep. Poisoning appears to have resulted, in some cases, from the purloining of arsenic by farm servants; in others from the facility with which it may be procured from the village shops. The care observed by the druggists in obtaining a witness and labelling the parcel is often of no avail, for the suicide and the murderer have respectively accomplished their determined purposes notwithstanding every precaution. Oxalic acid and laudanum are extensively used."

A supplementary digest of the correspondence on the sale of poisons was subsequently published by the committee, in which many interesting facts, too voluminous to be inserted here, relating to the sale of poisons, are mentioned.*

In March, 1850, a correspondence having taken place between the committee of the Provincial Medical and Surgical Association and the committee of the Pharmaceutical Society, a meeting of the two committees took place, at which the propositions which had been made for regulating the sale of poisons were discussed; and it was finally determined that a memorial should be forwarded to the Secretary of State, embodying the following propositions:—

"The sale of arsenic by retail should be restricted to medical men and chemists and druggists.

"Arsenic should only be sold to male adults, known to the vendor, personally, or on production of their written order.

---

* *Pharmaceutical Journal*, ix. 352.

"The vendor should enter the sale in a book, with the date, and the object for which it is required, to which the applicant and a witness (one or the other being known to the vendor) should sign their names, unless a written order is brought, in a handwriting known to the vendor, which order should be pasted in the book."

The Secretary of State soon afterwards gave notice in the House of Commons of his intention to introduce a bill for regulating the sale of arsenic; but the session was then so far advanced that its introduction was deferred until the next year, 1851, when it was passed without any serious opposition.

The passing of the Sale of Arsenic Act was an important step towards further legislation affecting the practice of pharmacy. It was found impossible in the then existing state of the law to limit the sale of arsenic to a class of men possessing a knowledge of its properties, because there was no legal definition of the terms chemist and druggist or pharmaceutical chemist; but in framing the Act and passing it through Parliament, it was felt that in this respect it was less efficient than it would have been if some such limitation as was recommended by the medical and pharmaceutical bodies could have been adopted. Something was gained, however, by the attention of the Legislature having been directed to this point in connection with the sale of poisons; and the opportunity was not allowed to pass without representing the importance of this feature of the case.

It was now felt that it was a favourable time for making further efforts to get a Pharmacy Bill introduced into Parliament. *The Pharmaceutical Journal*, taking a cheerful view of the prospects which pharmacists had before them, said, "The grand principle is now generally recognised, that the business of a chemist and druggist is something more than a mere trade, and that protection, respectability, and success are directly connected with professional qualification.

"Although we have no Lord Advocate espousing our cause in the House of Commons, although there is no parliamentary committee endeavouring to persuade us to improve our condition, yet our prospect is bright and cheering. Whether an Act of Parliament be obtained next session, or whether it be delayed for a few years, is a question which ought not to influence our proceedings or regulate our hopes. The society is gaining strength every year; it is acquiring a character which will reflect increasing credit and respectability on all its members; and when the paralysing effect of the late medical squabble has subsided, advocates will not be wanting in the houses of Parliament.

"In the meantime we must be our own advocates—every member and associate should put his shoulder to the wheel and do what he can, whether much or little, to promote the objects for which the Pharmaceutical Society was founded, recollecting that union is strength, and Heaven helps those who help themselves."

The writer of these sentences was one who not only had put his shoulder to the wheel, but had done more than any one else towards urging it forward; and now, for the further advancement of this object, he was prepared to enter a new arena and undertake new duties. Tired of seeking in vain for a member who, with an adequate knowledge of the subject, would undertake to pilot a Pharmacy Bill through Parliament, Mr. Bell signified his intention of trying to get a seat in the House of Commons, so that he might himself undertake that duty. It was not long before an opportunity presented itself. In November, 1850, a vacancy occurred in the representation of St. Albans, through the death of Mr. Raphael; and Mr. Bell offered himself as a candidate in the Liberal interest, while Alderman Sir Robert Carden was opposed to him as a Conservative candidate. The constituency of St. Albans was known in parliamentary circles to be not entirely above the influence of the sovereign; but this was a little weakness of which one who had never dabbled in politics might well be ignorant, as also of the right method of dealing with it. Mr. Bell left the management of the contest to his agents, who merely wanted to be supplied with the usual means, without which a contested election could not be conducted; and being supplied, he was returned by a good majority. It cannot be said that his brethren were enthusiastic on the occasion. There were, no doubt, very mixed feelings experienced by those who, having been accustomed to associate with the new member for St. Albans on terms of social equality, and, having never dreamt of his aspiring to or being peculiarly qualified for his present position, hardly

knew whether to view the step he had taken as a piece of
rash presumption or of spirited devotion to the cause with
which he had been so long identified.

He was now a member of the House of Commons, and it
remained for him to establish his character there. Unfortunately his title to his seat was almost immediately called
in question by a petition against the return on the ground of
bribery. The charge was fully established against the electors
and agents, but he himself was exonerated. The borough
was disfranchised, but the member retained his seat to the
end of that Parliament.

In 1850–51, new editions of two of the Pharmacopœias,
which constituted the official standards of authority with
reference to the composition of medicines in this country,
were published.

First appeared the Dublin Pharmacopœia, of which this
was the third edition, its long-lived predecessor having
maintained its position since 1826. The previous editions
had been issued in Latin; but this appeared in English, its
authors, the Dublin College of Physicians, following in this
respect the example which had been set by the Edinburgh
College in 1841. There was another important change made
in this edition of the work—a new system of weights having
been introduced which was a complete innovation. In place
of the long-established apothecaries' weights, a system was
adopted consisting of the troy grain, the avoirdupois ounce
and pound, and a new scruple and drachm differing in value
from any previously used.

Mr. Peter Squire, who had given a great deal of attention
to subjects connected with the Pharmacopœias, was the first
to appear as a commentator on the new work. In a paper
read before the Pharmaceutical Society he referred to the
changes which had been introduced in it, some of which
accorded with suggestions he had previously made; but he
regretted that other suggestions of his had not been adopted.

Mr. Squire had long been trying to induce an assimilation
in the strength and composition of all medicines ordered
under the same names in the three Pharmacopœias of the
English nation. He had also advocated the equalization in
neutralizing power of the diluted acids. The latter of these
suggestions had been adopted by the Dublin College; but, as

pointed out by Mr. Squire, discrepancies previously existing
between this and the other Pharmacopœias, had in several
instances been increased rather than diminished.   In the
discussion of Mr. Squire's paper, Professor Redwood showed
that the change which had been made by the Dublin College
in the weights directed to be used was unauthorized by the
law, and that the use of such weights would be illegal.

The new London Pharmacopœia was brought out in 1851.
It had been prepared by Mr. Richard Phillips, by whom an
authorized translation with copious notes was in course of
preparation when death put an end to his literary labours.

A brief notice of this distinguished chemist and pharmacist
will be appropriate here.

Richard Phillips was the son of a well-known printer in
Lombard Street, who, being a member of the Society of
Friends, placed his son with his near neighbour and associate
William Allen, of Plough Court.   Under the tuition of this
distinguished chemist and pharmacist young Phillips acquired
a taste for science and made some progress in its cultivation.
The family indeed appear to have had a tendency towards
scientific pursuits, for the elder brother, William, who succeeded his father as a printer, acquired a good reputation as
a mineralogist, and both brothers took part with others in
founding the Geological Society.

On leaving Plough Court Richard established himself in
business as a chemist and druggist at No. 29 in the Poultry.
In the pursuit of science he naturally devoted himself principally to the study of chemistry, and especially to that department of it which related to the preparation of medicines.

In 1811, while still carrying on the business of a pharmacist,
he published a small work entitled " An Experimental Examination of the Last Edition of the Pharmacopœia Londinensis,
with Remarks on Dr. Powell's Translation and Annotations,"
which brought him prominently into notice among medical
men.   In this work he showed by the results of a series of
experiments that the Pharmacopœia of 1809, which had been
brought out by a committee of members of the College, aided
by advice and assistance from Apothecaries' Hall, was in
many respects very defective and insufficient for the guidance
of those engaged in the preparation of medicines.   His
criticisms were found to be generally correct, and their effect

was greatly to damage the reputation of the Pharmacopœia to which they referred. The credit of the College of Physicians and Apothecaries' Hall was at stake, for they had undertaken, but had failed, to produce a Pharmacopœia that should satisfy the requirements of those for whom it was intended to be a ready guide and medium of communication. It was felt that something should be done to wipe off the stigma thus cast on the only two corporate bodies in England to whom the production of a Pharmacopœia could be referred. Accordingly arrangements were made for reprinting the work with corrections. But before doing this the operative department of Apothecaries' Hall was placed under the superintendence of an eminent Professor of Chemistry, William Thomas Brande, F.R.S., of the Royal Institution, whose assistance was thus obtained by the College in preparing the " Editio Altera " of 1815.

This edition, in which important changes had been made with the object of correcting previously existing defects, soon called forth another criticism from Mr. Phillips of even a more caustic nature than the previous one.

The pharmacist had thus proved that he was no mean chemist ; and he thus acquired sufficient reputation as such to enable him in the following year to obtain the appointment of Lecturer on Chemistry at the London Hospital. He had now become engrossed with scientific and literary occupations, to which he devoted the whole of his time, relinquishing his business engagements. Besides the appointment at the London Hospital he was at different times Chemical Lecturer at the Government Military College at Sandhurst, at Grainger's School of Medicine in Southwark, and at St. Thomas's Hospital.

In 1821 he conducted the *Annals of Philosophy ;* and when, at a subsequent period, this publication was merged into *The London, Edinburgh and Dublin Philosophical Magazine,* he became one of the editors, and remained so till his death.

In 1822 he was elected a Fellow of the Royal Society. He joined the Chemical Society from its commencement, and occupied the position of President during two years.

Although his criticisms on the Pharmacopœia gave offence to some members of the College of Physicians, they tended to gain for him a reputation even among medical men, as a sound chemist and good practical pharmacist. In fact, he was looked upon as an authority on pharmaceutical subjects; and when the next edition of the London Pharmacopœia was brought out, in 1824, he became the authorized translator of the work. Subsequently he assumed a more responsible position with reference to the work, as editor as well as translator and commentator, in which capacities his name is associated with the editions of 1836 and 1851.

In 1839 he was appointed Curator of the Museum of Practical Geology, which was then established, under the Government, in Craig's Court, Charing Cross, and subsequently removed to Jermyn Street.

Mr. Phillips had been actively engaged in preparing for the opening of the new premises in Jermyn Street, when, after a short illness, he died at his house in Camberwell, on the 11th of May, 1851, the day before that on which Prince Albert opened the new Museum. He had reached the 75th year of his age.

At the anniversary meeting of the Pharmaceutical Society which next followed after Mr. Bell's election for St. Albans, a resolution was passed that a petition from the society be presented to the House of Commons, to the following effect:—

" The humble Petition of the undersigned Members of the Pharmaceutical Society of Great Britain,

" Showeth,

" That in almost all civilized countries, those persons who prepare prescriptions and sell medicines are regularly educated in chemistry and other branches of knowledge and pass an examination.

" That in Great Britain no such provision is required by law, consequently uneducated and unqualified persons may, and frequently do, perform these responsible duties, by which means your petitioners have good ground for believing that the public sustain injury.

" That the Pharmaceutical Society was established in 1841 for the purpose of providing a remedy for this evil, by the introduction of a regular system of pharmaceutical education and an examination.

" That the arrangements adopted for this purpose have been attended with as much success as could be expected from such efforts on the part of a voluntary society; and your petitioners are persuaded from their experience, that the sanction of the Legislature is necessary in order to ensure the accomplishment of that reform which the safety of the public requires.

"Your petitioners, therefore, humbly pray that your honourable House will be pleased to pass an Act for regulating the qualifications of pharmaceutical chemists."

The petition was signed by fifty-six members who were present at the meeting, and it was presented by Mr. Bell on the same afternoon.

On the 12th of June, 1851, Mr. Bell moved in the House of Commons for leave to introduce a bill to regulate the qualifications of pharmaceutical chemists, and for other purposes in connection with the practice of pharmacy. Some opposition was offered to the motion by Mr. Henley; but leave was granted to bring in the bill, which was read the first time on the following day.

The purport of the bill, as introduced, may be gathered from the following concise outline of its clauses :—

Clause I. confirms the charter of the Pharmaceutical Society, except such parts as are altered or repealed in this Act.

Clause II. The Council to appoint a Registrar and other officers.

Clause III. The Registrar to prepare, from time to time, a list of all Pharmaceutical Chemists, their assistants, and apprentices, or students, respectively.

Clause IV. Registrar to keep books, etc.

Clause V. Certificate of Registrar to be good evidence in the absence of the contrary.

Clause VI. All members and associates of the Pharmaceutical Society to be registered, also every other person, within one year, on his producing evidence that he was exercising the business at the time of passing this Act.

Clause VII. Assistants, apprentices, and students to be registered.

Clause VIII. The Board of Examiners of the Pharmaceutical Society recognised.

Clause IX. The Council empowered to make and alter bye-laws, subject to the approval of one of her Majesty's principal Secretaries of State.

Clause X. Every person examined and having obtained a certificate to be registered.

Clause XI. Power to suspend or modify examination in the case of persons apprenticed before the date of the Act.

Clause XII. After one year from the passing of the Act it shall not be lawful for any person not duly registered to exercise the business, or to assume or use the name of Pharmaceutical Chemist, etc., or any name, sign, token, or emblem implying that he is registered under this Act, under a penalty not exceeding £20 nor less than £2. Penalties recoverable in the county courts, etc.

Clause XIII. No proceedings to be taken after the expiration of two months from the commission of the offence.

Clause XIV. Penalties to be forfeited to the Crown.

Clause XV. Registrar liable to penalty for the falsification of any register, etc.

Clause XVI. Penalty for procuring certificate of registry by fraudulent means.

Clause XVII. Act not to extend to or interfere with the rights, etc., of legally qualified medical practitioners.

Clause XVIII. Provided they do not take or use the name of Pharmaceutical Chemist, or Chemist and Druggist, etc.

Clause XIX. Exemption in favour of drysalters, vendors of patent medicines, horse and cattle medicines, or chemicals, etc., used for other than medicinal purposes, such parties not using any name, title, etc., implying that they are registered under this Act.

The second reading of the bill was moved by Mr. Bell on the 2nd of July, but it was not allowed to pass without opposition. Mr. Hume and Mr. Henley were among the opponents of the measure; and the Secretary of State, Sir George Grey, expressed a decided opinion that the bill, as introduced, was not likely to give general satisfaction, that it required much consideration, and ought to be before the public a considerable time before proceeding with it. He thought also that it was a measure that ought to accompany or follow, not to precede, one relating to the general practice of medicine. Finally, he suggested that the bill might be read a second time *pro formâ*, with an understanding that it should not be proceeded with any further that session.

Mr. Bell consented to adopt the suggestion of the Secretary

of State; and with that understanding the bill was read a second time.

Two days afterwards Mr. Wakley, speaking strongly in favour of the bill, tried to induce the House to alter the arrangement that had been previously made, and to proceed with the appointment of a select committee to which the bill might be referred, so as to admit of its being passed that session. This, however, was not complied with. The subject was brought forward again on two or three subsequent occasions. Mr. Bell was allowed to introduce some amendments with which the bill was printed, and it was then left to stand over till the following session.

While these proceedings were taking place in the House, 558 petitions, with 15,264 signatures, were presented in favour of the bill, and two petitions were presented against it, one from the Royal College of Surgeons of Edinburgh, and one from the Faculty of Physicians and Surgeons for Glasgow.

The amendments that had been introduced were for the purpose of ensuring the appointment of a Board of Examiners for Scotland, to meet in Edinburgh; of enabling members of the Pharmaceutical Society living in the country to vote by proxy or by post; of exempting assistants and apprentices already in the trade from the necessity of passing the examination; and of making registration permissive instead of compulsory with regard to those in business before the passing of the bill.

The result of this first attempt at legislation with reference to pharmacy was not considered to be discouraging. The objections raised in the House were, first, that the bill would interfere with free-trade principles by creating a monopoly; and, secondly, that it would tend to convert chemists and druggists into medical practitioners by giving them a professional education; but these were not felt to be serious objections, especially as the second had no foundation in fact. The point with reference to which objection had been anticipated and was most feared, namely, that it was intended to make the Pharmaceutical Society both an educating and examining body, was never alluded to. This was so far satisfactory.

On the 10th of June, 1851, the society sustained another

loss from death, by which it was deprived of its Treasurer,
Richard Hotham Pigeon, to whose valuable services in connection with the rise and early development of the association
we have repeatedly alluded.

Mr. Pigeon was a wholesale druggist in Throgmorton
Street. He had been apprenticed to Messrs. Fynmore and
Palmer, in the house in which he afterwards became a
principal, and in which he carried on a prosperous business.
He was one of the most respected members of the old Wholesale Druggists' Club, a commercial association established
for the purpose of discussing matters affecting the interests
of the wholesale trade, the members of which were in the
habit of meeting on 'Change, and occasionally of settling
knotty points over a city dinner. He had been Treasurer of
the Pharmaceutical Society from its commencement, and was
also Treasurer of Christ's Hospital, where he had conferred
great benefits through the tact and zeal he manifested in the
performance of his duties. Mr. Pigeon was a regular attendant at the meetings of the Pharmaceutical Society, and he
often contributed by his gentlemanly tone and conciliating
manners to maintain the regularity and dignity of the proceedings on such occasions. Mr. Pigeon died in the 63rd
year of his age.

During the official year, 1850–51, Mr. William Ince, the
representative of the old-established house of Godfrey and
Cooke, was President, and Mr. George Waugh, of Regent
Street, Vice-president of the society.

In June, 1851, when a further change took place, Mr.
Waugh having declined to take the office of President, it
was conferred on Mr. Thomas Herring, wholesale druggist
Mr. Henry Deane being at the same time appointed Vice-
president.

The son and namesake of the late Treasurer, Mr. Richard
Hotham Pigeon, succeeded his father in that appointment.

Comparing the position and prospects of pharmaceutica
chemists at this time with what they had been ten years
previously, there was no reason to be dissatisfied with the
aspect of affairs. The well-united band of zealous promoters
of pharmaceutical progress had worked steadily and successfully. Yet it was not all smooth sailing and sunshine. There
were dark clouds floating about, and sudden squalls arose

now and then. A few clever, active, but dissatisfied members
were ever trying to find out weak points in the management
of affairs. It had been made a subject of complaint, that the
government of the society was kept too exclusively in the
hands of the same set of men, who, with the officers, formed
a sort of happy family, in which differences seldom arose, but
in which a minority of the constituency, who differed in
opinion, was not represented. There is a tendency in societies
to get into such a condition as this, and there may have
been some justification for the complaint in this instance. The
ease and comfort of sliding in a groove are generally preferred
to rough jolting over the stones. But at least there was a
disposition among those in authority to do what was thought
to be most conducive to the welfare, and, if possible, the satisfaction, of the whole constituency; and therefore, when advocates of reform appeared openly in the field, instead of hiding
themselves behind anonymous circulars, some of these had no
difficulty in finding seats in the council. The usual effect
of putting grumblers into office, however, was not realized in
this instance, the result being that much unseemly contention
and obstruction to business were imported into the meetings
of the council, and continued as long as the new elements
remained there. The spirit that actuated these proceedings
extended even to the lecture room, where much annoyance was
caused to Dr. Pereira, by some members of his class supplying
garbled reports of his lectures to an opposition journal, which
had the bad taste to publish them in a form calculated to give
a very erroneous idea of their value. The Professor, to put a
stop to this offensive conduct, suspended his lectures and appealed to the council to protect him against such an unusual
and unlawful proceeding. The lectures were at that time
free to all members, associates, and apprentices of the society,
and it is due to the two latter classes to say that they presented a memorial to the Professor exonerating themselves
rom any participation in what had taken place, while members
not only of the society but of the council who were attending the lectures refused to join in this memorial. A suitable
assurance, however, was afforded to the Professor that there
would be no repetition of the practice he had complained of,
and the lectures were resumed, but not without a wound
having been inflicted, which no doubt contributed to cause

the resignation of his appointment by this distinguished Professor, who had the misfortune, in the eyes of an opposition party, to be a warm supporter of the society, its council, and its journal.

Soon after the conclusion of the session ending in July, 1851, Dr. Pereira having resigned his appointment, an arrangement was made with reference to materia medica and botany similar to that previously made in the case of chemistry and pharmacy, the two courses being united into one.

In accordance with this arrangement Mr. Bentley was appointed Professor of Materia Medica and Botany.

The council, under a pressure that was brought to bear upon them from without, were endeavouring to economize as far as possible the cost of keeping up the School of Pharmacy; but in doing this it was considered important to avoid the semblance of anything like a pecuniary advantage being derived by the society from that source, and therefore all persons connected with the society were admitted to the lectures without payment of fees.

We are now entering upon the year 1852, in which the first Pharmacy Act was passed. The state of political affairs seemed unfavourable to the prospects of pharmaceutical legislation. The year commenced with a change of ministry, and the prospect of a speedy dissolution of Parliament. At first it was considered doubtful whether an opportunity would be afforded in the then existing Parliament for renewing the attempt made in the previous session to get a Pharmacy Bill into the House. Sir George Grey, as Secretary of State, had been replaced by Mr. Walpole, of opposite politics; and although a Conservative Government might have been expected to be less tied to the maintenance of free-trade principles than its predecessor, the opinion of the new ministry, and the disposition of the House on the eve of a dissolution had yet to be ascertained.

It was thus under doubtful circumstances that Mr. Bell, on the 12th of February, moved for leave to introduce his bill, which was not granted without some opposition. The bill was essentially the same as that of the previous session, although a few further amendments had been introduced, to meet some of the objections urged against the measure.

The Master and Wardens of the Society of Apothecaries

strongly objected to the introduction of toxicology among the subjects of examination for the certificate of a pharmaceutical chemist, on the ground that a knowledge of that subject involved the medical treatment of cases of poisoning, which was out of the province of the pharmaceutical chemist. The terms used in the bill to denote the subjects in which candidates were to be examined were, " In the Latin language and classical knowledge, in botany, in materia medica, and in pharmaceutical and general chemistry, and toxicology." This last term was intended to represent a knowledge of the chemical nature and the appropriate antidotes of poisons, which it was considered every qualified chemist and druggist ought to possess; but as the former of these significations of the term was comprised under the head of general chemistry, and as objection was taken to the use of the term under the latter signification because it referred to a branch of medical practice, it was agreed that toxicology should be struck out of the bill.

The College of Surgeons of Edinburgh, and the Faculty of Physicians and Surgeons of Glasgow had opposed the bill under the impression that it would interfere with the rights and privileges of those bodies, the members of which were authorized to practise pharmacy; but amendments having been made that removed the objections previously existing in those quarters, the opposition was withdrawn.

The provision for establishing a separate board of examiners for Scotland also contributed to remove some objections to the bill, and to obtain for it several warm supporters in that part of the kingdom, among those who were previously indifferent or mistrustful.

Other amendments which were agreed to be made in the bill at this stage of its progress were of a trifling nature and need not be specified here, as much more important and radical changes were subsequently made, which gave a new character to the Act in the form in which it was passed.

On the 17th of March the bill was read a second time, and referred to a select committee, where a considerable amount of evidence was taken from physicians, surgeons, and general practitioners, connected with the several colleges and corporations in London and Edinburgh, and from representatives of the Pharmaceutical Society. Evidence was also taken on the laws relating to pharmacy in France, Germany, Sweden, Finland, Mauritius, etc.

The tendency of this evidence was to show that the cultivation of pharmaceutical knowledge had been much neglected in this country until it was promoted by the Pharmaceutical Society; that the success of medical practice depends to a great extent on the knowledge, skill, and judgment of those engaged in the selection and preparation of medicines; that the interests of the public are deeply involved in the adoption of such regulations as may best ensure a supply of qualified pharmaceutical chemists; that in Continental countries these regulations are made subject to legal enactment, but that in this country they have been disregarded by the Legislature.

It thus appeared that there was room and some need for legislation on the subject of pharmacy, and to this extent the committee was prepared to go with the promoters of the bill; but as a first measure of pharmaceutical legislation it was thought that something short of what was asked for would suffice; and in fact what was done was considerably short of what was asked for.

The bill, as submitted to the committee, gave a legal sanction and authority to the charter of the Pharmaceutical Society, and to the bye-laws made by the society. It provided for the appointment of a Registrar who was to make and maintain a register of all such persons as should apply for registration, and should furnish evidence of their having been engaged or employed as pharmaceutical chemists at the time of the passing of the bill, or should otherwise prove that they were entitled to be registered. It provided that all persons who, at the time of the passing of the Act, should be members or associates of the Pharmaceutical Society, and all other persons, not being members of the medical profession, who should, within one year after the passing of the Act, apply for registration and be able to prove that they were employed as pharmaceutical chemists in Great Britain at the time of the passing of the Act, should be entitled to be registered without the payment of any fee. It provided that all persons who, at the time of the passing of the Act, were engaged or employed as students, apprentices, or assistants to any pharmaceutical chemist in Great Britain, and who, within one year after the passing of the Act, should apply for registration, would be entitled to have their names entered in a list of students, apprentices, or assistants ; and the persons so registered would be entitled to be registered as pharmaceutical chemists on their commencing business on their own account.   It provided that the society should appoint a board of examiners for England, and also for Scotland, to conduct examinations "in the Latin language and classical knowledge, in botany, in materia medica, and in pharmaceutical and general chemistry," and to grant or refuse certificates of qualification to carry on the business of pharmaceutical chemist, or to be engaged or employed as students, apprentices, or assistants; and all persons obtaining such certificates would be entitled to be registered accordingly. Then it provided that after the passing of the Act it should be unlawful for any person, unless he were registered under the Act, or unless he had been in business before the passing of the Act, to exercise the business or calling of a pharmaceutical chemist in any part of Great Britain, or to assume any other name, title, sign, token, or emblem, implying that he was registered under this Act ; and that any infringement of this provision would cause a penalty to be incurred of not exceeding five pounds. Finally, it provided that "the term pharmaceutical chemist, used in this Act, should be construed to include chemist and druggist, dispensing chemist, and every other term denoting a dispenser of medical prescriptions and vendor of medicines, not being a member of the medical profession, or practising under a diploma or licence of a medical or surgical corporate body."

It soon became evident that the bill was not likely to pass the committee without considerable modification. The exclusive powers sought to be obtained, by which only qualified and examined persons would be allowed to dispense medicines and carry on business as chemists and druggists, were held to be incompatible with the principles of free-trade, and wholly at variance with the views which prevailed in the Legislature and had been recognised by Government in bills which had been introduced for regulating the practice of medicine.

At the same time the committee were not averse to giving the Pharmaceutical Society increased powers for the purpose of promoting its object of improving and extending the qualification of chemists and druggists. They were willing to afford the means of securing to qualified men who had passed the requisite examinations a title or titles by which they might be distinguished as such. But anything of a system of trade monopoly was strongly objected to; and those parts of the bill, therefore, which restricted the exercise of the duties of chemists and druggists to examined men were struck out leaving it a bill for confirming and extending the powers previously conferred on the Pharmaceutical Society by its charter of incorporation. The committee were also careful to guard against the liability of educated pharmacists doing what the apothecaries had formerly done, in gradually becoming a class of medical practitioners. Already toxicology had been struck out from the list of subjects on which examinations were to be conducted, and now it was further specified that such examinations should "not include the theory and practice of medicine, surgery, or midwifery."

With these and some other modifications, the bill, which was expected to have become a powerful lever in the hands of the Pharmaceutical Society for promoting the advancement of pharmacy and the interests of those engaged in its pursuit, became the well-known Act of 1852. Its promoters were disappointed; but still it was felt that something was gained, although much less than had been looked for.

The Act was passed on the 30th of June, 1852, and one of its provisions was that the then existing bye-laws should continue in force "until the next annual meeting of the society, to be held in the month of May, 1853." Meanwhile the Council of the Pharmaceutical Society were empowered to alter or amend the bye-laws and to make such new or additional bye-laws as they should deem necessary for the purposes contemplated by the charter of the society or by the Act; but all such original bye-laws, and all altered, amended, or additional bye-laws, were required to be confirmed and approved by a Special General Meeting of the members of the Pharmaceutical Society, and by one of her Majesty's principal Secretaries of State.

There were some important points to be determined with reference to the construction of the provisions of the Act and charter relating to the bye-laws, the settlement of which entailed a long course of litigation

In the first place, a question arose on the interpretation of the Act and the charter relating to the admission of chemists who commenced business on their own account after the date of the charter and before the passing of the Act. The council desired to admit into the society all such on production of satisfactory evidence that they were duly qualified, without obliging them to pass the ordeal of the board of examiners. This desire to put a liberal construction on the Act was in accordance with the opinion of members of the society very generally expressed at meetings specially convened in London and most of the large towns throughout the country.

At a Special General Meeting of the society held in Bloomsbury Square on the 4th of August, 1852, it was resolved,—

1. "That in order to bring the Pharmacy Act into more extensive and immediate operation, it is desirable that the Pharmaceutical Society should include among its members all duly qualified dispensing chemists throughout the United Kingdom."

2. "That this meeting recommends the council to adopt a liberal construction of the terms of the Act in regard to the admission of chemists in business on their own account before the passing of the Act."

3. "That the Pharmacy Act having been passed for the purpose of elevating the character and status of the pharmaceutical chemists of Great Britain by means of improved education, this meeting considers it of the highest importance that the members of the society should afford every encouragement and facility to their assistants and apprentices for preparing themselves to pass the examination."

4. "That the thanks of the society be given to Mr. Jacob Bell for his energetic exertions in promoting the passing of the Pharmacy Act through Parliament."

Meetings having a similar tendency were held at Liverpool, Manchester, Newcastle, Nottingham, Norwich, Bristol, Glasgow, Aberdeen, and Edinburgh.

At the Bristol meeting Mr. G. F. Schacht suggested the establishment of annual meetings for scientific objects connected with pharmacy, which should circulate through the chief towns in the provinces somewhat upon the model of those of the Provincial Medical Association. He thought such meetings would stimulate provincial members to a more active co-operation with the Pharmaceutical Society, and that they might be made highly instructive by selecting as the places of meeting towns which presented peculiar objects of manufacturing interest. This appears to have been the first publicly expressed idea from which originated the British Pharmaceutical Conference.

In Scotland the society had not hitherto made much progress, for although a Committee, with President, Vice-president, Treasurer, and Secretary, had from an early period existed in Edinburgh, the members in North Britain were not numerous, and the North British Branch would probably have hardly been kept together if it had not been for the zealous advocacy of the Honorary Secretary, Mr. Mackay. The granting of a separate Board of Examiners for Scotland did much to remove difficulties previously existing to progression there; but it was not until after the trade had been brought together at public meetings, which Mr. Bell attended, in Edinburgh, Glasgow, and Aberdeen, that the Pharmacy Act could be said to have been adopted in Scotland. A Society of Chemists and Druggists, for mutual improvement, had existed in Aberdeen since 1839, and this was now merged into the Pharmaceutical Society.

Strengthened by the general expression of opinion among members of the society as to the best mode of bringing the Pharmacy Act into operation, the council, with the view of giving effect to those opinions, prepared two new bye-laws, which were to the following effect:—

" Chemists and Druggists who commenced business on their own account after the date of the charter, and prior to the passing of the Act 15 and 16 Vict. c. 56, 30th June, 1852, and who shall, before the 1st of May, 1853, apply to be admitted as members by certificate of qualification according to the terms of the charter, shall, on production of certificates satisfactory to the council, be registered as ' Chemists and Druggists certified to be duly qualified for admission as members of the society.' The register on which the names of such chemists and druggists shall be entered, shall be closed on the day of the Annual Meeting of the said society in the month of May, 1853, when the existing bye-laws will cease to be in force, after which time the persons so registered shall be admitted as members of the society on payment of the entrance fee and the subscription for the current year. No person whose name is not included in the said register, unless an associate coming within the terms and meaning of the next following bye-laws, shall, after the period aforesaid, be admitted as a member of the society, except in the manner provided in the 10th section of the Act."

"Associates of the society who were admitted as such prior to the 1st day of July, 1842 (mentioned in the present bye-laws, section 1), shall be admitted as members of the society, on the production of certificates satisfactory to the council."

It was proposed, in accordance with the former of these bye-laws, that a certificate signed by two members of the society and countersigned by the local Secretary, to the effect that the applicant commenced business on his own account as a dispensing chemist before the passing of the Pharmacy Act, June 30th, 1852, and that he was a desirable person to be admitted as a member of the Pharmaceutical Society, accompanied by a statement of where he had served his apprenticeship or pupilage, might be taken as a satisfactory certificate to entitle him to be placed on the register of chemists and druggists.

It was also proposed that those not in business on their own account should be admitted for a limited time to a lenient examination on which they might receive a pass certificate.

A special general meeting of the society was held on the 8th of December, 1852, Mr. Joseph Gifford, President, in the chair, for the purpose of confirming or rejecting the foregoing bye-laws. Their adoption was moved by Mr. Bell, who explained the grounds on which they were required to enable the council to give effect to the resolutions passed at the previous meeting. Mr. Dickinson seconded the resolution, and it was carried unanimously.

The position taken by Mr. Dickinson on this occasion offered an agreeable contrast to that which he had usually occupied at meetings of the society. He now appeared as the advocate of an important proposition emanating from the council, and he warmly commended the liberal course they were adopting with reference to the admission of members. He expressed a hope that the society would ultimately comprise in its ranks all the respectable chemists and druggists in

the kingdom; but he would have been glad if the annual subscription could have been dispensed with, and he hinted that
the society had no legal power to enforce payment of the subscription by those who were once registered as pharmaceutical
chemists. He hoped, however, that the society would be supported, and that three important improvements would be introduced; first, the discontinuance of the annual subscription;
secondly, the retrenchment of all needless expenditure in the
School of Pharmacy; and thirdly, the publication of transactions by the society, under a publishing committee, with an
independent editor.

Had Mr. Dickinson continued temperately and consistently
to advocate these views, notwithstanding the fact that they
were in several respects opposed to those of the council, he
would probably have become the leader of a formidable opposition party; but he appears to have very soon changed his
opinion with reference to the admission of members into the
society, and the liberal course of proceeding which he commended at the meeting on the 8th of December, became the
subject of a long and bitter contention in which he repudiated
the validity of the bye-law the adoption of which he had
seconded.

The two new bye-laws having been confirmed by the
society, and also by the Secretary of State, afforded available
means for bringing a large number of chemists and druggists
and their assistants prospectively within the precincts of the
society; but their formal admission could not be effected until
after the meeting of the society in May, 1853.

Mr. George Walter Smith, the Secretary of the society,
had been appointed Registrar under the Act, and his duties
were now coming into operation.

Dr. Pereira, who had resigned his duties as Lecturer on
Materia Medica, was requested by the council to accept the
appointment of Honorary Professor of Materia Medica to the
society, which he acceded to. He had previously transferred
a large number of his materia medica specimens from the
London Hospital to the Museum of the Pharmaceutical Society,
and they were allowed to remain there for his and the
society's use.

Mr. Bell, having induced the late William Allen, F.R.S.,
while he was President of the society, to sit for his portrait

to Mr. H. P. Briggs, R.A., and a very successful likeness
having been produced, which was sent by Mr. Bell for exhibition in the society's rooms, he now presented this valuable
painting to the society, to be suspended in the council-room
with a view to its forming the first of a series representing
distinguished Presidents and officers of the society.

In the early part of this year, 1852, the council being
desirous of extending the usefulness of the collection of books
which had been gradually accumulating in the library of the
society, decided to allow them to circulate among the
members and associates, under certain regulations and restrictions.

The subject of the adulteration of food and drugs was
brought prominently under the notice of the public about this
time, through a series of articles which appeared in the *Lancet*
and the *Medical Times*.   The articles in the *Lancet* commenced in January, 1851, and purported to emanate from an
"Analytical Sanitary Commission;" but it subsequently
appeared that they were chiefly from the pen of Dr. Hassall,
and in substance they have since been reproduced in Dr.
Hassall's work on "Adulterations."   The articles in the
Medical Times commenced in January, 1852.

In these articles, unlike those published in the *Pharmaceutical Journal* in 1843 by Mr. Richard Phillips, the names are
given of the parties from whom the substances analysed were
obtained.

A good deal of dissatisfaction had arisen among chemists
and druggists at some of the seaports in connection with the
supply of medicines to emigrant vessels.   It had hitherto
been the general practice for medicines, together with other
stores required on board these vessels, to be supplied by
contract; and it was found that very inferior and sometimes
worthless medicines were thus often provided.   Her Majesty's
Land and Emigration Commissioners, who were responsible
for the carrying out of proper regulations, having received
numerous complaints of the bad quality of the medicines,
issued an order that they should in future be obtained from
Apothecaries' Hall.   Chemists and druggists were thus
excluded from a branch of trade which some of them had
been in the habit of carrying on in a creditable manner and
with satisfaction to those who had employed them.   The new

regulation was felt to be a stigma upon the body of chemists and druggists, and deputations from the trade waited on the Land and Emigration Commissioners to represent their view of the case, in which it was suggested that there should be inspectors appointed, capable of judging of the quality of the medicines supplied. The Commissioners however, could not undertake this responsibility; and the question having been referred to Professors Brande and Faraday for their opinion, it was decided that the best safeguard for the interests of the class of emigrants was to obtain the medicines from an accredited establishment such as Apothecaries' Hall.

In the early period of the year 1853, the Pharmaceutical Society sustained a great loss, and the medical and scientific world a shock, by the sudden and melancholy death of Dr. Pereira, who was carried off while still in the prime of life and the full vigour of his mental faculties. This sad event, although not immediately following, was indirectly caused by an accident which happened to the Professor while pursuing an investigation in his usual energetic way; and it may be added that the investigation was one arising from his connection with the Pharmaceutical Society and its journal. A substance had made its appearance in the drug market under the name of "isinglass from Para," which, as it differed entirely in its characters from any known varieties of true isinglass, excited some curiosity. A sample of it was sent to the Museum of the Pharmaceutical Society, and was described and figured in the *Pharmaceutical Journal*, vol. xii. p. 343. Pereira was endeavouring to ascertain the source of this remarkable substance, which appeared to consist of the dried ovaries of some large fish. Searching among specimens at the College of Surgeons, and having occasion to descend a winding stair to explore some of the treasures of the Hunterian Museum, he slipped when near the bottom, and falling on to his knees ruptured the *rectus femoris* muscles of both legs. This accident confined him to his room for some time, but did not appear to have affected his general health. He was still daily engaged in his usual literary occupations, and was just then preparing a new edition of his great work on materia medica. There was every prospect of his speedily recovering from the effects of the accident, but he was still confined to two rooms, and to locomotion in a wheel-chair.

In this comparatively helpless condition he was in the act of transferring himself from the chair to his bed, when the severe strain in doing so caused a rupture of one of the vessels connected with the heart. Three medical men were quickly in attendance; but he knew from the first what the fatal nature was of the mischief he had sustained, and declaring that nothing could be done for him, desired only to be allowed to draw his last breath in quietness. And thus within a few brief minutes the great Professor of Materia Medica passed from vigorous life to sudden death.

Jonathan Pereira, M.D., F.R.S., F.L.S., was born on May 22nd, 1804. His preliminary education was not in accordance with the position he was destined to occupy in after-life; his father, who was a London merchant, having been reduced from affluence to comparatively straitened circumstances. At fifteen years of age he was articled to Mr. Latham, a navy surgeon. He passed through his student's career with success, and obtained the vacancy which occurred in the office of Apothecary at the Aldersgate Street Dispensary. To gain this place he passed the examination for the licence of the Society of Apothecaries, and in the nineteenth year of his age was elected without opposition to the coveted post. Soon after, he established a class of pupils, to whom he gave private instruction preparatory to their examination. He was eminently successful; and in furtherance of his object he published a translation of the London Pharmacopœia of 1824, with a scientific description of the preparations, their reactions and decompositions. A little but invaluable work followed, called " Selecta e Præscriptis." Afterwards he published " A Manual for the Use of Students," and " A General Table of Atomic Numbers, with an Introduction to the Atomic Theory." On June 3rd, 1825, he became a member of the College of Surgeons, and being appointed Lecturer on Chemistry at the Aldersgate Dispensary, gave an introductory address on the rise and progress of the science, which comprised a notice of the latest discoveries.

In the winter of 1832 he became Professor of Materia Medica in the New Medical School in Aldersgate Street, and at the same period Lecturer on Chemistry at the London Hospital. At the persuasion of Dr. Cummin, who was the editor of the *Medical Gazette*, Pereira allowed his lectures to be published in that journal. They contributed greatly to raise his reputation abroad as well as in this country.

His class at the Aldersgate School became so numerous that he deemed it expedient to build a new theatre, which he did at an expense of about £700. His friends advised him to pause before sacrificing so large a proportion of his income (£1000 a year) in a building in which he could have only a temporary interest; but, without regard to minor considerations, he completed the theatre. He was invited to join St. Bartholomew's Hospital as Professor of Chemistry and Materia Medica; but the bye-laws requiring that all professorships in other institutions should be relinquished, Mr. Pereira could not accede to that arrangement.

Messrs. Longman were now desirous of launching the "Elements of Materia Medica," the first volume of which appeared in 1839; and the entire edition was sold before the appearance of the second volume, in 1840. The second edition of the work was published in 1842.

The prospect of a vacancy in the office of Assistant Physician to the London Hospital presented itself. In order to become a candidate, it was necessary that he should be a licentiate of the College of Physicians; and an examination was about to take place in a week or ten days from the time that the vacancy at the Hospital was made known. He waited on the President of the College, Sir Henry Halford, to ascertain the latest day on which he could be allowed to present himself, and an indulgence of two or three days was granted. He laboured night and day to refresh his memory on the details of the various subjects; and he passed with flying colours. His examiners declined to question him on the subject of materia medica. He applied for a degree at Erlangen, and received his diploma a few weeks after he had become licentiate of the College of Physicians.

On March 3rd, 1841, he was elected Assistant Physician at the London Hospital. He was appointed Examiner in Materia Medica at the London University in the year 1839.

Prior to the opening of the School of Pharmacy in Bloomsbury Square several Professors delivered introductory lectures with a view of promoting the undertaking. On March 30th, 1842, Dr. Pereira delivered one of these, and selected for his subject, "The Modern Discoveries in Materia

Medica." The completeness of the illustrations and the style of the delivery made a great impression, and it was recognised at once that the lecturer would be an invaluable acquisition to the school, and that every effort must be made to prevail on him to become one of its Professors. This plan could not be immediately adopted, but in the months of August and September he delivered two lectures, which afterwards were greatly amplified and published as a "Treatise on Food and Diet." Subsequently he gave several lectures on "The Polarization of Light," a subject in which he took a special interest.

In 1843 Dr. Pereira became Professor of Materia Medica to the Pharmaceutical Society, and delivered his introductory discourse in the month of September. His lectures were unrivalled for the amount of information conveyed, and the brilliance of the style in which they were delivered. His large correspondence, his powers of original research, his constant application of the microscope, and his unusual facility in explanation, invested the subject with the deepest interest. As a referee he was an inexhaustible source of knowledge, and he was always ready to give further information at the close of his lecture to any inquiring student. His time at this period was abundantly occupied in lecturing and in his professional duties. In 1845 he was elected a Fellow of the Royal College of Physicians, and almost immediately afterwards he became a member of the Pharmacopœia Committee of the College. As Curator of its Museum he discovered some curious manuscripts relating to materia medica. On resigning his office as Professor of Materia Medica at the London Hospital, he transferred the most important specimens of his museum, nearly 500 in number, to Bloomsbury Square. These specimens afterwards became the property of the society. He did not, however, cease to prosecute his researches; and fresh acquisitions continued to come in from foreign correspondents and other sources. The list of his separate communications was extraordinary, and he was a diligent contributor to the pages of the *Pharmaceutical Journal*.

Dr. Pereira died on January 20th, 1853, aged 49.

To perpetuate his memory, a marble bust was placed in the New College of the London Hospital, and a fund was raised by subscription, with which a prize was established in the form of a medal, called the Pereira medal, to be awarded annually by the Council of the Pharmaceutical Society to the candidate who should succeed at a competitive examination in the subject of materia medica. All candidates for this prize are required to have been associates of the society, and to have passed the major examination during the session in which the competition takes place.

On the 26th of March, 1853, another of the original members, a Councillor and late President, of the society, Mr. William Ince, was carried off by death. Mr. Ince had long occupied a prominent position as the representative of one of the oldest and most celebrated of the pharmaceutical establishments in London. He took an active part in the formation of the Pharmaceutical Society, had been a member of council from the commencement, was Vice-President of the society during the official year 1849–50, and President in 1850–51. In early life Mr. Ince had to contend with the difficulties which at that time stood in the way of the acquirement by students of even an elementary knowledge of the sciences appertaining to pharmacy. That he made some progress during his apprenticeship in a country town, in the acquirement of a knowledge of chemistry and other branches of science, was due to a strong innate desire to rise above mediocrity, and to the possession of a spirit of industry and determination.

On coming to London to seek his fortune, he soon succeeded in getting into the house of Godfrey & Cooke, in Southampton Street, Covent Garden, where he remained for the rest of his life, and where he acquired a high reputation for the qualities required in the successful management of a first-class pharmaceutical establishment. Mr. Ince had never been a man of strong health, and of late years he had become much enfeebled. He died at his residence in Kensington, in the 59th year of his age.

The Pharmacy Act, which passed in June, 1852, provided that during a period of nearly twelve months the then existing bye-laws of the Pharmaceutical Society should remain in force, together with any new bye-laws that might be formed and duly confirmed in the interim. Two new bye-laws had already been brought into operation, and as the time for holding the annual meeting in 1853 approached, it

was found that another was required for the purpose of
defining the method by which members residing more than
five miles from the General Post Office might vote for the
election of officers through the post. This was submitted
by the council to a special general meeting, held on the
6th of April, and having been confirmed there received final
confirmation by the Secretary of State.

The council were also, and had been for some time,
engaged in preparing the new code of bye-laws which was to
come into operation at the next anniversary meeting. While
performing this task it was found that Mr. Dickinson and his
friends were shifting their ground of opposition, or rather
that they were taking up new ground on which to oppose the
proceedings of the council. Hitherto the Dickinson party
had adopted the extreme liberal policy of desiring to bring
all existing chemists and druggists on to the register of
pharmaceutical chemists on easy terms, stating at the same
time that no person whose name had been once entered on the
register could be legally called upon to pay an annual subscription as the condition on which the name would be
retained there. It is obvious that if this had been sound
law, there would have been comparatively small inducement
for those who were registered to become members of the
society, and it would have been impossible to maintain the
institution in Bloomsbury Square in the form in which it had
hitherto existed; but when it was found that it was doubtful
law, and therefore an unsafe ground to proceed upon, another
was discovered which was thought to be more tenable,
although less liberal in its nature. It was now asserted that
it was illegal to place any person on the register of pharmaceutical chemists after the passing of the Act, unless they
had previously been members of the society, or had passed
an examination as specified in the 10th section of the Act.

As the new bye-laws recognised the legality of electing as
members, and therefore of placing on the register of pharmaceutical chemists, all those, about 800 in number, who had
been registered as "chemists and druggists certified to be
duly qualified for admission as members of the society," this
bye-law was opposed by the Dickinson party, first at a special
general meeting of the society held on the 11th of May for
the purpose of confirming it, when there were only four

dissentients to the confirmation, and afterwards before the Secretary of State, when the dissentients succeeded in inducing the Minister, Lord Palmerston, to give only a qualified confirmation in the following terms :—

"I hereby certify my confirmation and approval of the annexed bye-laws, confirmed and approved at a special general meeting of the Pharmaceutical Society of Great Britain, held on the 11th ult., for the space of one year from this date, and subject to the decision of a court of law upon the legal questions which have arisen or may arise in reference to any of them.   PALMERSTON."

"*Whitehall,* 17th *June,* 1853."

The process of electing members under the new bye-laws now proceeded rapidly, and among the names added to the register were those of John Abraham, William Murdock, and John Wright. But the legality of this proceeding was soon challenged by Mr. Dickinson.

On the 24th of November, 1853, in the Court of Queen's Bench, Sir Fitzroy Kelly (with whom was Mr. H. Lloyd) moved for a rule calling upon the Registrar of the Pharmaceutical Society to show cause why a *mandamus,* should not issue commanding him to remove the names of certain parties, namely, those above given, from the register of the society. This was the commencement of a long course of litigation, the details of which, being of a technical nature, would be uninteresting and difficult of comprehension. The whole gist of the case is admirably summarized by Lord Campbell, before whom it was heard, in the judgment he delivered on the 26th of January 1855, as follows :—

"The question raised by the special verdict is, whether the registrar did his duty in placing on the register of pharmaceutical chemists, made in November, 1853, the names of William Murdock and John Abraham ? The name of John Wright is also mentioned on the record; but as his title to be registered is the same as John Abraham's, he need not be further noticed. It is found that neither Murdoch nor Abraham were members of the Pharmaceutical Society on the 30th of June, 1853, when the Act of Parliament of the 15th and 16th of Victoria, chapter 56, passed, nor had either of them been examined under that Act; but each was in business on his own account as a chemist—Murdoch before the 18th of

January, 1843, the date of the charter of incorporation, and Abraham before the 30th of June, 1852, the date of the passing of the Act above mentioned. Each had obtained a certificate of this fact and of being qualified for admission as a member of the Pharmaceutical Society. Thereupon Murdoch's certificate was approved by the council, and he was elected a member of the society; and Abraham, having been registered as certified and qualified for admission according to certain bye-laws made in November, 1852, was afterwards elected a member of the Pharmaceutical Society, under bye-laws made in May, 1853. Both names were afterwards placed on the register of pharmaceutical chemists of November, 1853, above mentioned. Each was registered on the ground that he was a member of the society. The title of each to be a member is derived in part from the charter, and in part from the bye-laws, and the matter to be decided, is, whether the title of each was valid? By the charter, the society consisted of members of four classes :—first, those who were chemists on their own account at the date of the charter; secondly, those who should have been examined as the council should have deemed proper; thirdly, those who should have been certified to be duly qualified for admission; and, fourthly, those who should be elected as Superintendents by the council. Murdoch claimed to be in the first class, that is, a chemist on his own account at the date of the charter; Abraham claimed to be in the third class, that is, to have been certified to be duly qualified for admission; and as the charter is declared by the first section of the Act to be in full force, except such parts as are so varied and repealed thereby, and as the provisions of the charter relating to these two classes of members are not varied or repealed by the Act, that part of the title of each claimant which depends on the charter is made good. The Legislature intended an examination to be, in general, the condition on which the members were to be admitted ; but some other classes had been made admissible by the charter to prevent the displacement of existing interests, and the admissibility of the same classes was continued by the Act on the same principle, leaving the extent to which it should be carried to be regulated by bye-laws, to be made under proper precautions.   The remainder of the title of each of these claimants depended on the bye-laws, Murdoch claiming under

the bye-laws made under the charter before the statute, and
Abraham claiming under bye-laws made after the statute.
The bye-laws under which Murdoch claims, are clear from any
doubt. They were valid according to the charter, and their
validity was expressly continued by the second section of the
Act, and under them Murdoch was admitted as a member,
therefore his registration was right; the bye-laws under
which Abraham was admitted as a person certified to be duly
qualified for admission, were made after the passing of the
Act, that is, in November, 1852, and May, 1853, and their
validity depends on Section 2 of the Act, empowering the
council of the society to alter the bye-laws of the society
made under the charter, and to make new bye-laws for the
purposes contemplated by the charter or the Act, subject to
the proviso that the new bye-laws and the altered bye-laws
should be confirmed by a special general meeting and the
Secretary of State, and subject to the proviso that the existing
bye-laws should continue in force until the annual meeting
of May, 1853. As the bye-laws under which Abraham
claimed were new bye-laws, and not alterations of the
existing bye-laws, and as they were duly made and confirmed,
we think they were valid under the powers granted by the
Act, and were not restricted by the proviso continuing the
existing bye-laws until the annual meeting in 1853. Under
these Abraham is found to have been duly admitted. Thus
he also became a member of the society, and, if a member,
therefore entitled to be registered; for the Act makes no
distinction between different classes of members in respect of
registration, the registrar being bound by Section 5 from
time to time to make a complete register of all persons being
members of the society, that is, members at the time the
register is made. The meaning of the term 'Pharmaceutical
Chemist' was the subject of some discussion, and the Act does
not give any definition of it. The 6th section implies that a
pharmaceutical chemist is a generic term under which a
member of the society is comprised as a species. The 10th
section implies that a person who has passed his examination
without being elected a member is another species, and these
two species or classes are expressly declared by the Act to be
entitled to be on the register of pharmaceutical chemists, any
person not on that register being prohibited by the Act from

using the title either of pharmaceutical chemist or member of the society. To this extent the statute is clear, and this is sufficient for the decision of the present case. For these reasons we think that the registrar is shown by the verdict to have done his duty, and judgment therefore must be for the defendant."

It might be thought that this very lucid explanation of the case, together with the decisive judgment pronounced by so eminent a judge, would have been sufficient to satisfy the instigators of the proceedings and put a stop to further litigation and useless expense. Reasonable men were asking, what is the object of all this contention ? Is it a case in which a society of men who have acquired wealth and power, conferred upon them for public purposes, are trying to keep all the benefits of their position to themselves, and to exclude those of their brethren who are equally qualified with them from participating in benefits intended for the common good ? Is the Pharmaceutical Society a monopoly, and Dickinson the advocate of popular rights ? Or, is it a case in which the society is trying to perpetuate ignorance, while Dickinson appears as the promoter of education, and the advocate of rapid advancement in professional qualification ? Who are these men whose names are objected to; are they not men of equal standing in every respect with the best members of the society ? These were questions in the mouths of most of those who took an interest in the subject; and as the only possible answers appeared to leave no excuse for renewing the contest by carrying the case to a higher court, it was hoped that those whose attention had been for some time almost exclusively engrossed with the details of an unprofitable dispute, might now unite in furthering more worthy objects. But, alas for human nature ! There was one man who was dissatisfied with the decision of the Court of Queen's Bench, and who, having two or three avowed, and an unknown number of nameless abettors, signified his intention of carrying the case to a Court of Appeal.

All this harassing litigation produced, as might be supposed, a very prejudicial influence on the advancement of the society. It was repeatedly represented by the best friends of the association that a society divided against itself could not make satisfactory progress. All the opposition at this time experienced by the Pharmaceutical Society originated with and was supported by its own members, and the ill effects of this opposition were greatly enhanced by the mystery in which the names and numbers of the opposing parties were enshrined, and the difficulty experienced by most persons, who had not carefully studied the subject, in understanding the real merits of the questions in dispute.

While the case was being argued before Lord Campbell, on the 22nd of June, 1854, an interesting discussion arose with reference to the pronunciation of the word " pharmaceutical," which was reported as follows :—

Lord Campbell said there appeared to be a vexed question which he would like to have decided, namely, the proper pronunciation of the word "pharmaceutical," for some of the gentlemen pronounced the " c " in the word soft, while others pronounced it hard. He would ask the Attorney-General what he said it was.

The Attorney-General said, in his opinion it was soft. It no doubt came from the Greek ; but when it became English it was subject to the English rules. He had been cautioned by some of his learned friends as to the mode of pronouncing it.

Sir Fitzroy Kelly said, of course he should bow to the opinion of his learned friends, who were so much superior to him in learning as in everything else.

The Attorney-General said, that was rather too bad, as Sir Fitzroy Kelly had himself cautioned him.

Sir Fitzroy Kelly said, whatever his Lordship should say it was, that would be the mode to be adopted.

Lord Campbell.—Then let it be soft. Be it so.

Although suffering under the depression caused by internal dissension, the society continued to maintain its position, to promote the furtherance of its objects, and to grow in public estimation. It had already established a character for persistently confining its attention to its own proper business, that of advancing the study and improving the practice of pharmacy, and it was thus gaining confidence among members of the medical profession and others interested in the attainment of those objects. If any doubt or suspicion had at any time existed among members of the higher grade of medical men, that the cultivation of science by chemists and druggists might cause them to despise the shop and seek a professional character by following in the footsteps of the apothecaries of old, ten years' experience had tended to allay such apprehensions. It was seen that pharmacy afforded a sufficiently wide and honourable field for the exercise of talents and the application of much scientific knowledge; and as pharmacists continued to cultivate this field, medical men, who had previously occupied some of the ground, showed a disposition to resign merely pharmaceutical duties to those to whom they more legitimately belonged.

Hitherto pharmacists as such had never ostensibly taken part in the preparation of the *Pharmacopœia*. The editor of the last two editions of the *London Pharmacopœia*, it is true, had originally been a chemist and druggist, and his practical acquaintance with pharmacy was no doubt the principal cause of his having been selected for the appointment he so creditably filled; but Mr. Phillips, when he undertook the duty of editing the *Pharmacopœia*, had long ceased to be engaged in the practice of pharmacy; and he was perhaps better known for his general scientific and literary attainments than for special pharmaceutical knowledge. Since the death of Richard Phillips, in 1851, no one had appeared to take his place; but he had left, in the *Pharmacopœia* itself, a permanent record of the value of services which had been obtained from one who had been educated as a practical pharmacist.

The College of Physicians was now again looking forward to the preparation of a new edition of the *Pharmacopœia*; and with the view of obtaining the requisite assistance, application was made to the Pharmaceutical Society. After some correspondence on the subject, it was arranged that the society should appoint a committee of their members, from whom information on questions relating to the *Pharmacopœia* might be obtained by the Pharmacopœia Committee of the College of Physicians. It was suggested by the college that their communications should be addressed to the Chairman of the Pharmacopœia Committee of the Pharmaceutical Society, who also should be requested to attend at meetings of the Pharmacopœia Committee of the College of Physicians when they might require his assistance.

On the 2nd of August, 1854, the Council of the Pharmaceutical Society appointed as a Pharmacopœia Committee the whole of the members of their board; and at the same time it was resolved that there should be a working sub-committee consisting of not less than seven members, with power to request assistance from time to time from such members of the society as might be disposed to promote the object in view.

The sub-committee, which was appointed on the 17th of August, consisted of Henry Deane, Chairman, Jacob Bell, J. T. Davenport, T. N. R. Morson, Peter Squire, William Hooper, and Felix R. Garden. To this sub-committee Professor Redwood was appointed Secretary. Messrs. Sandford, Waugh, Herring, and Hills were afterwards, at different times, added to the committee.

It was resolved that it be the duty of the sub-committee to consider and report upon any proposed alterations referred to them by the Pharmacopœia Committee of the College of Physicians, and also to collect information respecting drugs and preparations not in the Pharmacopœia, which were in use in private practice, together with improved processes or formulæ to which it might be considered desirable to invite the attention of the college.

A printed list was prepared of all the materia medica and preparations contained in the London, Edinburgh, and Dublin Pharmacopæias, for circulation among the members of the society. This list was extracted, by permission, from the very useful book which had been published by Mr. Squire, entitled, "The Three Pharmacopœias," and 1500 copies of it were circulated. It was sent out accompanied with the following letter :—

"PHARMACEUTICAL SOCIETY OF GREAT BRITAIN,
"17, BLOOMSBURY SQUARE, *February*, 1855.

"The Pharmacopœia Committee of the Royal College of Physicians having been in communication with the Council of the Pharmaceutical Society on the subject of the Pharmacopæia, a committee of the society has been appointed to co-operate in the revision of the work.

"The following list has therefore been prepared for circulation, with a view of obtaining practical information.

"The Pharmacopœia Committee of the Pharmaceutical Society request your attention to the same, and will thank you to send at your earliest convenience answers to the following questions :—

" 1. Are there any preparations or articles of materia medica used in your neighbourhood that are not contained in the accompanying list ?   If so, please to add them.

" 2. Be so good as to prefix letters to each of the articles, indicating the frequency of their use, or otherwise, as follows :—

R.	Rarely.	F.	Frequently.
V. R.	Very rarely.	V. F.	Very frequently.
N.	Never,		

" 3. Do you find difficulty or confusion to arise from the nomenclature of the present Pharmacopœia?   If so, name the instances.   Signed,   " HENRY DEANE, *Chairman*."

The carrying out of the method thus adopted by the committee for obtaining information necessarily occupied a good deal of time.   A large number of the printed lists of materia medica, which had been sent to members of the society in every part of the country, were returned with marks attached to many of the articles in accordance with the desire which had been expressed; but, with this exception, very little information was elicited through the circulation of the lists.   The marked lists were collated, and it was found that many of the articles in the Pharmacopœia were so rarely used in medical practice that they might without any disadvantage be omitted.   The most important work, however, which had to be performed, namely that of suggesting alterations in the processes described in the Pharmacopœia, was left almost entirely in the hands of the working committee.

On the 2nd of April, 1856, the Pharmacopœia Committee of the Pharmaceutical Society presented their first report to the College of Physicians.   They described the steps they had taken for putting themselves in communication with practical pharmacists in various parts of the country, with the view of ascertaining what medicines were used in medical practice.   While this process was still in operation they had commenced a review of the alphabetical list of the articles described in the Pharmacopœia and had recorded their opinions on some of those contained in the early part of the list, which they proceeded to bring under notice.   They suggested the recognition in the Pharmacopœia of acetic acid in three different states with regard to strength, namely, those which were subsequently adopted and are still retained in the *British Pharmacopœia.* They suggested also that the diluted mineral acids, namely, hydrochloric, nitric, phosphoric, and sulphuric, should be of one uniform strength. It was at first thought that equal volumes of these diluted acids should contain the same quantity of the real or of the anhydrous acids; but this opinion was afterwards modified in favour of the suggestion of Mr. Peter Squire, that they should all have the same neutralizing power.   Several articles the names of which came into the early part of the alphabetical list were recommended to be introduced into the Pharmacopœia, among which were acetic ether, chloric ether, oxide of antimony, and oxide of silver.

The committee having thus given evidence that they were actively carrying out the wishes of the College of Physicians, continued to work assiduously in the same direction.   They issued another circular to members of the society throughout the country, asking for information and suggestions with reference to the following preparations, the introduction of which into the Pharmacopœia had been suggested; namely, benzoate of ammonia, phosphate of ammonia, iron alum, citrate of iron and quinine, jalapine, a blistering fluid, sedative solution of opium, and fluid extract of taraxacum.

Several of the members of the committee were active workers, who undertook the practical investigation of subjects that came under discussion, and some valuable results were thus obtained which deserved greater publicity than was accorded to them.   Of course differences of opinion frequently arose, and conclusions which had been arrived at were sometimes reversed when the subjects were reviewed and new light thrown upon them.   Those only who have had occasion to discuss the details of pharmaceutical processes with persons who profess to be familiar with them, can fully appreciate the difficulty of obtaining a concurrence of opinion even in a small committee.   The materials operated upon in such processes, and the products obtained, are often so variable and indefinite in composition and properties that it is difficult to form a judgment founded on any fixed and reliable principles.

The proceedings of this committee, of which there were

frequent meetings, extended over a period of six years, during part of which time official communication was kept up with the College of Physicians ; but on the passing of the Medical Act of 1858 the duty of preparing a British Pharmacopœia which should supersede the three Pharmacopœias previously in use and having authority in England, Scotland, and Ireland, having been conferred upon the Medical Council, the Pharmaceutical Society was requested to keep up its Pharmacopœia Committee in connection with the Pharmacopœia Committee of the Medical Council. This latter part of its proceedings will come under notice further on.

The Pharmaceutical Society was fortunate in having had so favourable an opportunity as the appointment and operations of the Pharmacopœia Committee afforded for proving to the outside world, as well as to its own members, that notwithstanding the weakening influence of internal dissension the society as a body continued to enjoy the confidence of the highest medical authorities.

It is satisfactory also to be able to record the rise and active operations, during this gloomy period of our history, of an association, mostly of associates and junior members of the society, who styled themselves the Phytological Club of the Pharmaceutical Society, and whose object was the extension of the study and application of the science of Botany. Professor Bentley was the president of this useful little association, which was founded in 1853 and was kept up until 1860.

Another association having a similar constitution, but the object of which was the encouragement of the study of chemistry and its allied sciences, was established in 1858 under the title of the Chemical Discussion Association of the Pharmaceutical Society. Professor Redwood was president of this association, which continued in active operation until 1866.

Having thus adverted to some of the favourable aspects which the progress of pharmacy at this time presented, we must return to the narrative of the law proceedings that were still pending.

The judgment delivered by Lord Campbell in the Court of Queen's Bench having been appealed against, as already intimated, the case came on for hearing before the Judges in the Exchequer Chamber on the 24th of April, 1855, when an application was made for an adjournment until the next sitting, and this was granted ; but while it was under consideration a discussion took place again on the pronunciation of the word pharmaceutical, when the following remarks were made :—

Lord Chief Justice Jervis.—Why do you call it the Pharma-*sutical* Society ?

Sir Fitzroy Kelly.—There was a discussion on that point in the Court of Queen's Bench, as to the question of philology. Their Lordships were unanimously of opinion that it was to be called Pharma*sutical*.

Lord Chief Justice Jervis.—I thought it was always known as *keu.*

Sir Fitzroy Kelly.—There was a great difference of opinion at the bar ; but the Bench as usual prevailed, and it is Phar-ma*sutical* now under authority.

Lord Chief Justice Jervis.—Then it is decided in the Court of Queen's Bench that it is *ceu.*

Mr. Baron Parke.—It is called *Cicero,* but in the Greek it is *Kikero.*

Sir Fitzroy Kelly.—That is not one of the points in error on which we ask your Lordship's judgment.

The case was then allowed to stand over until the 26th of May, when it was further adjourned to the 30th of May, 1855, on which day it was finally decided in a full court before the following judges :—

Lord Chief Justice Jervis, Lord Chief Baron Pollock, Mr. Baron Alderson, Mr. Justice Maule, Mr. Justice Cresswell, Mr. Baron Platt, Mr. Baron Martin, and Mr. Justice Crowder, each of whom delivered his judgment at length. It is suf-ficient here to say that the decision was unanimous, the eight judges affirming the judgment of the Court of Queen's Bench.*

After this decision the bye-laws of the society were con-firmed by Sir George Grey, Secretary of State, in the follow-ing terms, which were attached to a printed copy of the bye-laws :—

"I hereby certify my confirmation and approval of the annexed bye-laws of the Pharmaceutical Society of Great Britain.　　　　　　　　　　　　　　　　　G. GREY."

" *Whitehall,* June, 1855."

---

* For a full report of the judgments see *Pharm. Journ.,* vol. xv. p. 5.

There was very little anxiety or excitement manifested on the occasion of this concluding trial. So confident were those members who had watched the proceedings as to the final issue, that in anticipation of the result they were speculating on the best means of providing for an enlarged sphere of action of the society. At the anniversary meeting held on the 15th of May, the President, Mr. Henry Deane, suggested the purchase of a freehold building to comprise within its walls all the requisites for carrying on the educational and other business of the society in a manner consistent with the importance which the institution was assuming. He estimated the cost at not less than £15,000, of which he thought a portion, probably £5000, might be raised by a voluntary subscription, while the remaining £10,000 might be raised on the principle of a tontine in shares of £5 or £10, for which the society should guarantee four per cent. interest, equal to a rental of £400. This was obviously a question not calling for immediate action, and it was left for consideration.

One of the duties which the society, through its registrar, was required by the Pharmacy Act to perform, was that of preparing and maintaining a complete list of its members and as many who had been admitted into the society had ceased to comply with the terms of membership, it became necessary to ascertain whether and on what grounds the names of such were to be omitted from the list. In doing this about 600 letters were sent to defaulters, and the result of these applications afforded evidence of the vicissitudes occurring among this class of the population within a period of ten years. About two-thirds of those to whom application was thus made were found to have disappeared, some from death, some from emigration, retirement from the business, or other cause.

A corrected list of members and associates was ordered to be published in January, 1856, and another with further corrections in the month of July following, and also in the same month in each future year.

It was the duty of the society to protect the interests of registered pharmaceutical chemists by enforcing the provisions of the Act which prohibited the use of certain titles by unregistered persons, and they had occasion to exercise the power vested in them with respect to two chemists and

R

druggists who had issued labels on which was engraved a
copy, in miniature, of the certificate of membership, containing the words, " Members of the Pharmaceutical Society of
Great Britain." The parties had never been registered as
pharmaceutical chemists, and were not members of the society; they were therefore liable to a penal action; but ample
apology being offered, ulterior proceedings were allowed to
drop.

In 1855 and following year, a succession of cases of
criminal poisoning occurred which greatly agitated the public
mind, and forcibly called attention to the unguarded manner
in which poisons were supplied to those who desired to use
them, whether legitimately or otherwise.

In " the slow poisoning case at Burdon," the death of a
lady, Mrs. Wooler, appeared to have been caused by long-
continued administration of small doses of arsenic; but the
attempt to prove by whom or how the administration had
been effected, failed. The lady had been an invalid, and
under medical treatment, for some time before suspicions of
poisoning were entertained, and even then no decisive opinion
was formed until the death of the patient, which took place
about seven weeks after the suspicious symptoms first appeared. The medical evidence was distinctly that death was
caused by arsenic. This poison was found in the urine before
death, and in various parts of the body after death. It was
not in the medicines, nor could it be traced to the food.
Everything taken by the patient was administered by those
in attendance, and principally by the husband and a female
attendant. Suspicion finally fell on the husband, who was
put on his trial, but acquitted by direction of the judge. This
case occurred in June, 1855.

Another case of poisoning that caused considerable sensation occurred in February, 1856. The body of Mr. John
Sadlier, late M.P. for Sligo, was found on Hampstead Heath,
with evidence of death having been caused by poisoning with
essential oil of almonds. A bottle that had contained the
poison was found by the side of the deceased. There were
also papers found from which it was evident that this was a
case of suicide.

The trial and conviction of Palmer for poisoning his friend
Cook with strychnia followed soon after, and excited a much

greater amount of public interest than the preceding cases. Both Palmer and Cook had been largely engaged in betting transactions, and there were reasons why the former might have wished to get rid of his friend. He had previously, it appeared, got rid of his wife by similar means. The evidence went to show that Cook had been first treated with antimony, by which he was greatly debilitated, and that finally he was killed with strychnia. All the symptoms attending the death were those of poisoning with strychnia, but this poison was not found in the body. Antimony was found, but this could not be shown to have been the cause of death. The scientific evidence was clearly at fault, and this defect was turned to account by the witnesses for the defence. The prisoner was convicted on the medical and circumstantial evidence, the judge passing some severe strictures on the character of the scientific evidence, which he represented as partaking more of the nature of professional advocacy than of the impartiality that ought to characterize the evidence of witnesses in a court of justice.

The failure in this case to prove by chemical means the presence of strychnia, although it was obvious from collateral circumstances that repeated doses had been administered shortly before death, tended to shake the confidence of the public in chemical analysis.

A controversy afterwards arose as to whether strychnia disappeared as such when it exerted its poisonous action in a living body, or whether it remained after death, and could with certainty be detected by chemical reagents. The discussion which took place, although unduly acrimonious, cleared up much that was previously doubtful, and contributed to place the detection of strychnia among processes of extreme delicacy and practical certainty.

Rarely if ever has a case of poisoning excited so intense and wide-spread an interest as was manifested in connection with Palmer's trial.* Although at the time it conferred no honour upon the professors of chemistry, it was not without its influence upon the practice of their profession; and it probably tended also to exert an ulterior influence upon the practice of pharmacy.

* For details of the case see *Pharm. Journ.*, vol. xvi., p. 5.

The frequent occurrence of cases of poisoning drew serious attention to the subject. The crime had become not only common, but to a certain extent scientific. While science was increasing the facilities for the detection of poisons, the diffusion of such knowledge, and especially public discussions, such as had recently occurred, enabled the criminal to make choice of the means least easily discovered. The extension of this knowledge, moreover, imposed great responsibility upon those who dealt in poisonous substances.

Again another case. In July, 1856, William Dove, of Leeds, was put on his trial at York, and convicted of poisoning his wife with strychnia. The symptoms were marked and characteristic, leaving no doubt as to the cause of death, while it was equally evident by whom the poison had been administered. The evidence in Palmer's case appeared to have induced a belief by the culprit that strychnia could not be easily detected; but the chemists in this case were enabled to obtain satisfactory proof of the presence of the poison in the dead body.

A sense of alarm pervaded the public mind, which called for the application of some reassuring measure of protection against accidental or criminal poisoning.

On the 10th of July, 1856, Lord Campbell, in the House of Lords, said he rose to put a question to his noble and learned friend on the woolsack upon a subject of great importance. He would not then advert to the facts which had been disclosed during the trial of a recent case which had occupied the attention of all Europe; but he was shocked to say that for several years past the crime of poisoning had become remarkably common, and in his opinion some new law was imperatively required for the regulation of the sale of poisons. Many crimes of that kind had been caused by the institution of burial societies, the members of which had, in several instances, been proved to be accessory to the death of their own offspring. Another class of those cases arose out of the present system of life insurance. Persons caused insurances to be effected on the lives of others in whom they had really no interest whatever, with the premeditated intention of committing murder; and he knew from his own experience that murder was frequently committed in consummation of that intention. Until lately no restriction whatever had been placed upon the sale of poisons; it was possible to purchase arsenic as easily as Epsom salts, and the consequence was that cases of poisoning by arsenic became alarmingly common, especially in Essex and Norfolk. By a Bill introduced by the Lord-Lieutenant of Ireland, a check had been put upon the sale of arsenic. That poison was now therefore out of fashion, but another poison, nux vomica, had taken its place. Any one might go to any chemist in England, and buy a penny-worth of nux vomica by merely stating that he intended to use it for poisoning rats. Nux vomica, although not as powerful as strychnia, produced the same fatal effects; but even strychnia might easily be obtained. In some places people were not allowed to bathe except with a rope round their waists. That was carrying precaution to an extreme, but there certainly ought to be some restraint placed upon the sale of poisons.

The Lord Chancellor said the result of the investigation entered into by the Government five years ago was, that the measure then introduced was confined to arsenic. He understood that difficulties of a serious nature presented themselves in defining the different sorts of poisons; but he could not but think that a number of other poisons might be put in the same category as arsenic. He knew, however, it was the opinion of one of the most eminent medical men in London, that a great deal of mischief might be done by publishing the fact that there were seventeen or eighteen other articles quite as deadly as arsenic. He was informed that his right honourable friend Sir G. Grey had promised to give the subject his best consideration during the recess.

The question of legislation against poisoning became a chief topic of the press, and every imaginable shade of opinion was expressed. While this was being publicly discussed, there was another important matter in a more advanced state for legislation, which also affected the interests of pharmacy.

The means adopted by the *Lancet*, in 1851, for directing public attention to the adulteration of food and drugs through the publication of a series of reports in which the results of the analyses of various articles were given, together with the names of the tradesmen from whom they were obtained, led to the appointment of a committee of the House of Commons for the further investigation of the subject. This committee, of which Mr. Scholefield was chairman, commenced its sittings in July, 1855, and after examining a great number of witnesses, comprising men of various grades of scientific attainment, as well as men whose practical knowledge as dealers pointed them out as capable of giving valuable information, they reported the results of their inquiry to the House in July, 1856.

The evidence put before the committee was of a very mixed character, and as some of the witnesses appeared to speak from hearsay knowledge or from what they had picked up from books, which notoriously repeat each other and thus perpetuate statements which have long ceased to represent existing facts, there was a great tendency to exaggeration. There was also generally a want of the discriminating distinction which ought to be observed between impurities and adulterations, the former being often necessarily present in articles which are produced at prices which alone admit of their being used for certain purposes where the impurities are unobjectionable or of no material importance.

The council of the Pharmaceutical Society, in their report for 1856, observe with reference to the proceedings of this committee :—

" The appointment of a parliamentary committee to investigate the adulteration of food and drugs has brought prominently under the notice of the public many fraudulent practices, as well as various imperfections in the quality of commodities arising from accident or negligence. The attention of the society has always been directed to these abuses; and examples of impurity, with the means of detection when practicable, have been among the regular subjects of discussion at the Pharmaceutical meetings. A considerable improvement has taken place in the quality of drugs and chemicals in consequence of these efforts of the society, a circumstance overlooked by most of the witnesses before the parliamentary committee. The sweeping and indiscriminate charges which have been brought against the entire body of chemists, and extensively circulated by the press, have caused no less surprise than annoyance to those who have been for many years successfully using all their endeavours to bring about an improvement. The statements, which have been industriously circulated with a view of exciting alarm, are in most instances greatly exaggerated, and simply calculated to mislead the public."

At the time this statement was published the parliamentary committee had not presented their report, but they did so shortly afterwards. Looking at the composition of the committee it could hardly be expected that they should have been able to sift the evidence and rightly estimate the respective values of the contradictory statements contained in it. On the whole, however, the report was considered to give a tolerably fair view of the subject; and, with reference to the adulteration of drugs, it referred to what had been done by the Pharmaceutical Society in terms decidedly complimentary to the institution.

" It has been shown," it said, " that much good has arisen from the establishment of the Pharmaceutical Society, the members of which, being specially educated in the knowledge of drugs, are better able than heretofore to make proper selections and to detect adulterations."

The council of the Pharmaceutical Society thought this a suitable time to endeavour to counteract the effect of erroneous statements which had been circulated through the press reflecting on the manner in which chemists and drug-gists generally conducted their business. A paper was drawn up in the form of a circular, which was intended for general circulation and for insertion in the public papers. It was entitled " On the Education of Dispensers of Medicine and the Sale of Poisons." It recounted some of the prominent facts connected with the establishment of the Pharmaceutical Society, showing the efforts that had been made to introduce an efficient system of education, and an examination for the future members of the body. It referred to the incorporation of the society by Royal Charter, and to its being subsequently recognised by an Act of Parliament which conferred upon the members the title of Pharmaceutical Chemist, which title in the future would only be conferred on examined or qualified men. It represented the efforts which had been made by the society ever since its formation to improve the quality of medicines and prevent their adulteration, and the services it had rendered in collecting valuable statistical information relating to the sale of arsenic, which had facilitated the framing of the Arsenic Act. It pointed to the assistance the society could afford in promoting practicable and efficient legislation with reference to the sale of poisons; but at the same time it urged the importance of extending the means by which the scientific character and social position of chemists and druggists might be raised, as affording the best remedy for and security against the evils which had been complained of in connection with the preparation of medicines and the sale of poisons. The address concluded as follows : " The object of the above statement and remarks is, to direct attention to the fact that the reformation which recent events have shown to be required, and towards which the force of public opinion is tending was projected more than fifteen years ago by the Pharmaceutical Society, that great progress has already been made by its voluntary and unassisted agency, and that all that remains to be done may be effected by means of the society, if armed with more extended powers and assisted by the public."

There is reason to believe that the circulation of this document contributed largely to the removal of erroneous impressions which had been produced among a portion of the public, while at the same time it showed that there was still room for improvement in the regulations relating to the dispensing of medicines and the sale of poisons.

Various methods were suggested for guarding against accidents in dealing with poisonous substances, and among these the use of angular bottles and other vessels gave rise to much animadversion.

In a supplement to the Dublin Pharmacopœia, which was issued in September, 1856, it was—

" ORDERED,

" 1. That angular bottles or vessels, and none others, be employed in the dispensing of all medicines intended for external use.

" 2. That round bottles or vessels, and none others, be employed in the dispensing of all medicines intended for internal use.

" 3. That all the articles of the materia medica and preparations included in the list which is hereto appended, be kept in shops or warehouses in angular bottles or vessels ; and also that the same shaped bottles or vessels be employed in the case of such medicines and preparations being sold or delivered.

" 4. That all the articles of the materia medica and preparations not included in the list appended, be kept in shops
or warehouses in round bottles or vessels ; and also that the
same form of bottle or vessel be employed in the case of their
being sold or delivered.

" 5. That a similar rule be observed with reference to other
medicines, which, though not in the list of this Pharmacopœia,
may be kept by apothecaries or druggists, namely, that those
poseessed of dangerous qualities should be invariably kept
and sold or delivered in angular bottles or vessels."

The list comprised 33 articles of the materia medica and
130 preparations.

These regulations, which, it will be observed, applied only
to Ireland, were enunciated with the apparent authority of
an Imperial law, and in terms that would seem to indicate a
confident reliance in their efficacy. Those in that country to
whom they were addressed were struck with the boldness of
the appeal, but were not inspired with a belief in the practicability of carrying them into general effect, or the usefulness
of their imperfect application. Practical men were impressed
with the rashness manifested by the Dublin College of Physicians in issuing such important regulations, affecting all the
dispensers of and dealers in medicines throughout Ireland,
without consulting or generally advising with those most
seriously affected by them.

The appearance of the Irish poison regulations naturally
attracted a good deal of attention among English pharmacists,
and the subject was discussed at a meeting in Bloomsbury
Square, at which all the speakers concurred in disapproving
of the scheme, which was represented as visionary and impracticable.

A question arose about this time respecting the stamping
of grain weights used in dispensing. Several pharmacists,
residing within the city of Westminster, were summoned for
using grain weights that were not stamped, the law being
considered to apply to these, as troy or bullion weights,
although it did not apply to other apothecaries' weights.
As proceedings had never before been taken in similar
cases, and the weights in question were only used for dispensing and not for selling drugs, a defence was offered on
these grounds, and the Court having taken time to consider

the case, a decision was given on the 8th of May, 1856, at a Court of Burgesses at Westminster, in the following terms:—

"That it is the opinion of the Court that the weights used by chemists must be tested and stamped according to the standard of weights in use in Westminster, from one grain upwards: that as the question is now presented to the Court for the first time, it is their opinion that the fines already imposed on chemists should not be enforced: that the chemists are required to get their weights stamped within three months from this judgment, after which they will. be liable to have fines imposed on them, if found using unstamped weights."

A question also arose with reference to the dispensing of medicines in the army. Some serious accidents having occurred through mistakes made which were ascribed to the employment of incompetent dispensers, the subject was referred to a select committee of the House of Commons. It appeared that sergeants, and other men who had had no regular training for this duty, were often employed to dispense medicines. This practice was considered highly objectionable, and the committee recommended that no one should be considered eligible for employment until he had given proof before a Board in an examination, that he might, with safety to the sick soldiers, be permitted to dispense. The terms of this recommendation being indefinite, it was suggested that an examination, such as that of the Pharmaceutical Society, ought to be required, and this suggestion was to some extent adopted. At the time of the Crimean war it had been intimated that, in the appointment of dispensers, those holding certificates from the Pharmaceutical Society would have a preference given them; and subsequently, in 1857, when a large number of dispensers was required for service in India, the Director-General of the Army Medical Department refused to engage any candidate who could not produce the certificate of the Board of Examiners in Bloomsbury Square.

The Pharmaceutical Society had now been in existence for fifteen years, during which time most of the leading pharmacists in London, with one marked exception, had filled the office of President. The exceptional case was that of the man who of all others had taken the most prominent part in advancing the interests of the society. Mr. Bell had

hitherto refused to take office; but in 1856 he was induced
to allow himself to be placed at the head of the institution he
had so largely contributed to establish.   It is probable that a
feeling of declining health and strength, which rendered him
less capable of undertaking some of the numerous duties he
had hitherto performed for the society, may have led to his
accepting the office of President.   It cannot be said, however,
that Mr. Bell, as President, relinquished any of the work he
had been accustomed to do for the society.   He had made
two or three unsuccessful attempts to regain a seat in Parliament, and the anxiety and fatigue attendant on canvassing
and addressing large constituencies had brought on a disease
of the larynx which induced great debility, partly by preventing him from taking proper nourishment.

In July, 1857, Mr. Bell, as editor of the *Pharmaceutical
Journal*, wrote as follows :—" There is a manifest improvement and tendency to progress in the rising generation of
pharmacists at this time.   The School of Pharmacy was never
so well attended as it has been during the present session, and
the number of candidates for examination appears to be on
the increase.   The study of botany, which has hitherto been
too much neglected, is gradually acquiring that amount of
importance which it deserves, as a branch of the education
of the pharmaceutical chemist.   Upwards of eighty students
have entered the class during the present session, and the
regularity of the attendance indicates a growing interest in
the subject.   At this season of the year the study of botany
is an agreeable pursuit; and the lectures, being delivered in
the gardens of the Royal Botanic Society in the Regent's
Park, afford an opportunity for combining fresh air and
exercise with professional improvement.   The chemical class is
also well attended, and the number of pupils in the laboratory
has been greater than during any previous session.   In some
instances, however, the period of study has not been so long
as to ensure a competent knowledge of the principles and
practical details of the science; and it is a mistake to suppose
that this object can be attained by merely working in the
laboratory during two or three months.   This short time may
be sufficient to initiate the student in the elementary principles, and to awaken his interest in the science; but those
who desire to obtain a complete qualification for their pro-

fession, and to enjoy a favourable position for success in after life, must make themselves familiar with the entire range of the subject, including organic and inorganic chemistry, and especially the manipulations of the pharmaceutical laboratory.

" On taking a review of the last sixteen years, the gradual but steady progress of pharmacy in this country is very satisfactory, considering that the acquirement of this branch of education is entirely voluntary, and has enjoyed little or no encouragement on the part of the Legislature. In fact, the only inducement held out to the student as a stimulus to his industry has been the prospect of an honorary title.

" Recent events, and the notoriety of the deliberations which which have taken place respecting the sale of poisons, the dispensing of medicines, and the prevention of accidents, have led to a prevailing impression that some legislative enactment will shortly place pharmacy in a position which it has not hitherto occupied in this country. The natural tendency of such a prospect has been observable in the increasing activity among pharmaceutical students, the frequent inquiries respecting the books which should be read, the lectures to be attended, and the best course to be pursued by those who are dependent entirely on their own resources for improvement, and who, in country towns remote from the advantages of a school or college, are desirous of qualifying themselves for passing the examination. The voluntary system has effected a very marked improvement, but it is in the power of the Legislature to multiply these advantages tenfold."

The society was progressing, but at the same time it was losing some of its early supporters and friends. Among the number of these was Dr. Andrew Ure, F.R.S., who died on the 2nd of January, 1857. Dr. Ure was born in Glasgow in 1778, and he pursued his studies in the Universities of that city and of Edinburgh, where he took the degrees of Master of Arts and Doctor of Medicine. In 1830 Dr. Ure came to live in London, and in 1834 he was appointed Chemist to the Board of Customs. He had previously, in 1821, published his Dictionary of Chemistry, and subsequently, in 1837, he brought out his most important work, " The Dictionary of Arts, Manufactures, and Mines." He was largely consulted as one of the chemical authorities of the day, and especially by manufacturers and those requiring analyses in relation to technical subjects.

During the last thirty years of his life he was in the habit of performing most of his analyses by means of standard solutions of most of the reagents, according to a system on which he based his method of alkalimetry.   Dr. Ure was a man of indefatigable industry, and he pursued with enthusiasm the laborious researches in which he was professionally engaged.   For the last three or four years of his life he was obliged from the state of his health to retire from the more active professional exertions in which he had for many years been engaged.   He died at the age of seventy-eight.

An event that calls for special notice here, was the illness of Mr. George Walter Smith, the Secretary of the Pharmaceutical Society, which necessitated the resignation of his appointment by this important officer, who had performed so much good service to the Society.   Equally deserving of very special notice was the appointment of Mr. Elias Bremridge as the new Secretary, by whom the affairs of the society have been and still are so ably conducted.   Mr. Bremridge was elected in March, 1857.

Attempts were still made, and had been so almost continuously, to frame a medical Bill that should satisfy the bulk of the medical profession ; but as yet reformers in this direction appeared to be as far as ever from the attainment of their object.   Two Bills were before Parliament, namely, those with which the names of Mr. Headlam and Lord Elcho were respectively identified, but there was strong opposition to both, and no likelihood that either would pass.

In May of this year (1857), a Bill was brought into Parliament, " to restrict and regulate the sale of poisons," which called forth a vigorous opposition from the pharmaceutical body.   This Bill provided that no poison should be sold unless the sale was made to a person of full age and in the presence of a witness of full age who was known to the person selling the poison and to whom the purchaser was known, and unless there was produced and delivered to the seller a written certificate signed by the clergyman of the parish, or a legally qualified medical practitioner, or a justice of the peace, justifying the use for which the poison was required.   Provision was made for keeping a record of all the circumstances attending the sale.   Provision was also made that all colourless poisons should be coloured with soot, or indigo, or archil, and if contained in paper that there should be an outside wrapper of tin foil with a label of "POISON" in conspicuous letters. Dealers in poisons and medical men who used them were required to keep all poisonous substances in a closet set apart for that purpose under lock and key. Then with reference to the dispensing of medicines it was provided that all liquid medicines intended for external use, and all medicines containing any poison, should be supplied in quadrangular blue glass bottles, labelled in conspicuous capital letters, white on a black ground, "POISON," or "FOR EXTERNAL USE," the word "POISON," or the words "FOR EXTERNAL USE," being also cast or moulded in raised letters in the glass on the four sides of the bottle.

Mr. Bell, in an article in the *Pharmaceutical Journal*, said with reference to this Bill, "Although it cannot be supposed for a moment that the Bill is at all likely to be passed in its present form, yet the principle displayed in it may be taken as an indication of the direction in which legislation is tending; and the experience of those who are practically conversant with the subject must be brought into requisition to expose the absurdities of the measure, and to point out the boundary line between the sublime and the ridiculous."

Immediate steps were taken by the Council of the Pharmaceutical Society to elicit an expression of opinion on this measure. A public meeting was appointed to be held in Bloomsbury Square, which all those interested in the subject were invited to attend. This was held on the 3rd of June, and resolutions were unanimously passed representing the effects of imposing unnecessary restrictions, which would defeat the object contemplated, and augment rather than remove the evils which had led to this injudicious attempt at legislation.

On the 6th of June a deputation from the society waited on Lord Granville at the Council Office in Whitehall, and strongly urged upon him the necessity of greatly modifying the provisions of the Bill. The subject was fully discussed, but without any very apparent result.

On the 8th of June a communication was received from the House of Lords, requesting the attendance of two members of the deputation to give evidence before a committee to which the Poison Bill had been referred. This was complied with : several meetings of the committee took place, evidence was given by London and also provincial pharmacists, and suggestions were made for modifying the Bill so as to render it practicable and capable of effecting the objects in view. The committee made several important alterations in the measure, the general tendency of which may be inferred from the following observations by Mr. Bell on the amended Bill when it reappeared in the House. " To those," says Mr. Bell, " who are practically conversant with the subject, it will be obvious, after a few moments' consideration of the alterations, that the last state of the Bill is worse than the first. The Bill, as originally drawn, would have been simply impracticable, and therefore inoperative. It would, in the first instance, have caused some inconvenience ; but by degrees it would have become,—like the Ecclesiastical Titles Act,—a dead letter, defied and disregarded by those whom it was intended to restrain, and merely serving to expose the impotence of legislators when they get out of their depth. In the Bill as altered, the intended precautionary provisions are considerably impaired ; and while there is a pretence of adopting the suggestions offered to the committee in regard to the qualifications of persons dealing in poisons, it is proposed to attain this object by annihilating the legitimate source of pharmaceutical improvement, and substituting a superficial examination, to be performed by a mixed Board, consisting of six persons, under four independent jurisdictions, remunerated according to the number of candidates, and invested with irresponsible and inquisitorial powers."

The provision, in the amended Bill, for granting licences to persons who were to be allowed to sell poisons, was as follows :—

" After the —— day of —— no person other than a legally qualified medical practitioner shall sell any poison without a licence to vend drugs granted under this Act.

" For the granting of licences and the examination of persons desirous of obtaining licences under this Act, six examiners shall be appointed from time to time, three of whom shall be appointed by Her Majesty under her sign manual, and the College of Physicians of London, the Society of Apothecaries of London, and the Pharmaceutical

Society of Great Britain shall severally appoint one of the remaining examiners; and every examiner appointed by her Majesty shall hold office during her Majesty's pleasure, and every other examiner shall hold office for such term as the body by whom he is appointed shall think fit and direct."

In November, 1857, the Council of the Pharmaceutical Society drew up and circulated among the members a series of questions with the object of obtaining statistical information as to the real or principal sources of danger in the sale of poisons. This elicited some valuable information which the committee embodied in a report,* a copy of which was sent to Lord Granville with a request for an interview. On the day before this was to have taken place, however, the ministry resigned, and further proceedings with reference to their Sale of Poisons Bill were suspended.

While the foregoing events relating to the sale of poisons were transpiring, another subject affecting the interests of pharmacy was brought prominently under notice. The Government had been induced, on the recommendation of a commission appointed at the instigation of the Board of Inland Revenue, and consisting of Professors Graham, Hoffmann, and Redwood, to authorize the use of duty-free spirit for certain purposes in the arts, if mixed with ten per cent. of purified wood spirit, or methylic alcohol. The addition thus made to spirit of wine was found to render it unfit for human consumption as a beverage, without materially impairing it for the greater number of the more valuable purposes in the arts to which spirit is usually applied. The mixed spirit was called methylated spirit, and it was made and supplied under excise regulations and inspection. It had not, however, been contemplated, nor was it intended, that it should be used in the preparation of medicines, except in cases in which none of it would remain in the product; as, for instance, in the extraction of alkaloids for the preparation of their salts. The objects which had been contemplated in the introduction of methylated spirit were to benefit the manufacturing arts in which spirit might with advantage be used, and to lessen the temptation to produce spirit by illicit distillation. It had well fulfilled those objects; but it had recently been found

---

* *Pharm. Journ.* vol. xvii. pp. 300, 346, 445.

that in some instances it had been used in pharmacy for the preparation of tinctures, with the view of cheapening their production. This unauthorized use of methylated spirit was brought under the notice of the Pharmaceutical Society, at their meetings in October and November, 1857. It appeared that a sort of implied sanction had been given to its use in pharmacy in consequence of orders having been sent to Apothecaries' Hall from the Army Medical Board for soap liniment, and some other preparations intended for external application, to be made with methylated spirit. The instructions to adopt this method of preparation being imperative, authority was obtained from the Inland Revenue Board to comply therewith, and this authority was afterwards extended to other pharmaceutical preparations. As soon as this became known to the Council of the Pharmaceutical Society, the President communicated with the College of Physicians on the subject, and the licence, which had been unadvisedly given, and which, if not promptly objected to, would have opened the door to a great abuse, was speedily withdrawn.

The two following minutes were prepared by the President and Censors of the College of Physicians, the former for publication in the *Gazette* and in the medical journals, and the latter for transmission to the Board of Inland Revenue.

" ROYAL COLLEGE OF PHYSICIANS,
" *Nov.* 25*th*, 1857.

" The Censors of the Royal College of Physicians, having learned that in the manufacture of tinctures and some other preparations of the Pharmacopœia, it has latterly become the practice of certain druggists and manufacturers to use methylated in the place of pure spirit, hereby declare their disapproval of such an unauthorized departure from the instructions laid down in the Pharmacopœia."

" ROYAL COLLEGE OF PHYSICIANS,
" *Nov.* 25*th*, 1857.

" The President and Censors of the Royal College of Physicians, having had their attention called to an unauthorized departure from the instructions of the Pharmacopœia in the manufacture of tinctures and other preparations, by the use of methylated instead of pure spirit, have

s

found it necessary publicly to express their disapproval of such departure, and beg to call the attention of the Board of Inland Revenue to the fact that an assumed authority for this deviation from the rules of the Pharmacopœia is said to have been derived from an order or minute of the Board of Inland Revenue, giving a general permission to use methylated spirit in the preparation of medicinal tinctures and extracts."

These proceedings were followed shortly afterwards by a communication from the Board of Inland Revenue, addressed to the Secretary of the Pharmaceutical Society, enclosing a copy of the minutes they had received from the College of Physicians, and stating:—

" INLAND REVENUE OFFICE, LONDON, W.C.

"*February,* 1858.

" SIR,—

" I am directed by the Commissioners of Inland Revenue to send you the accompanying minute of the Censors' Board of the Royal College of Physicians of London, and to state that the Commissioners have ascertained that the Colleges of Edinburgh and Dublin concur in the desire of the London College to dissipate the impression that a departure from the rules of their Pharmacopœia has been countenanced by the legalization of methylated spirits.

"Such an impression can only have arisen from very erroneous views of the powers and intentions of this Department; but, since it appears to prevail, it is necessary that the Commissioners should distinctly warn all persons using the methylated spirits in medicinal preparations, that the permission granted by this Department conveys no authority to apply the spirits in any manner not sanctioned by the Colleges of Physicians.

"I am, Sir, your obedient servant,

"THOMAS DOBSON, *Assistant Secretary.*"

The action thus taken by the College of Physicians and the Board of Inland Revenue, checked the further progress of the objectionable practice which had commenced with reference to the pharmaceutical use of methylated spirit.

A good deal of discussion took place at this time with reference to the use of paper-hangings which had been coloured with arsenical pigments. Statements were published, which appeared to be supported by strong evidence, to the effect that serious injury to health frequently occurred to persons who occupied rooms in which arsenical papers were used. But on the other hand chemists failed to detect in the atmosphere of such rooms the slightest trace of arsenic, except in some instances where the pigment, or the coloured surface of flock paper, had been mechanically removed and remained suspended in the air. The balance of evidence, however, went to show that the injury caused was not confined to cases of the latter kind.

The dentists had lately been in a state of excitement, which to some extent affected chemists and druggists, for among the occupations in which the latter occasionally engaged, were those of extracting teeth and performing some other operations of dentistry. In this country dentists had hitherto occupied a position similar to that of the chemists and druggists prior to the year 1840. They were not recognised by the medical profession ; and, having no distinct separate existence, it was difficult to define what their occupation and qualifications consisted or ought to consist in. There were men among them who possessed the requisite qualifications, surgical, medical, and mechanical, to enable them to deal with the teeth under all the conditions in which the services of a dentist are required ; but there were some with little or no qualification. Recently attempts had been made to introduce some organization in this heterogeneous body, to sift the good from the bad, to establish a regular system of education and examination, and to indicate qualification by a title. The dentists were fifteen years behind the chemists and druggists in commencing this movement, but the spirit of reform was now actively fermenting. Some of the leading and best qualified men among those engaged in the practice of dentistry formed an association called the Odontological Society, while another more numerous class established the College of Dentists on principles less exclusive than those of the other association. Both societies were aiming at the same object, namely that of securing for the public the services of men, recognisable by certain titles, who should be qualified to perform the various operations connected with the treatment, extraction, and supply of teeth. The leaders among them could not agree upon any proposed method of amalgamating the two institutions, and therefore both continued to work independently, and not without good effect.

Chemists and druggists, although not wholly a united body, were not divided in the same way as the dentists were. There was but one organization formed for the purpose of educating and bringing into fellowship a class of men to whom the duties of pharmacy might be safely entrusted. The organized pharmacists were a comparatively small section of the whole body of chemists and druggists, and they had not of late years been increasing in numbers; but the important work committed to them was being steadily and effectively carried out. The various departments of the establishment in Bloomsbury Square were gradually expanding and their operations were becoming more important, so that it was evident that more accommodation than the premises hitherto occupied could afford, would soon be required. As already intimated, a proposition had been made to obtain, by purchase or otherwise, a freehold building for the use of the society; but the address in Bloomsbury Square had become so identified with the Pharmaceutical Society that the council were easily induced to extend the accommodation there in preference to seeking premises elsewhere. An opportunity for doing so had now occurred, the lease of two adjoining houses, 72 and 73 Great Russell Street, being offered, together with an extension of that of 17, Bloomsbury Square. These together formed a block of buildings which had originally been united as a nobleman's mansion; and the whole was now secured by the society for a period of ninety years. The newly-acquired part of the premises was at present occupied by tenants, but it could be appropriated for the use of the society when required.

Whilst the society was thus extending the means by which it was carrying out its objects, it was at the same time sustaining the loss of some of the wise heads which had contributed so much to its establishment on a sound foundation and which had subsequently directed its councils during a period of distraction and difficulty. The year 1857 did not close without adding to the list of the early Councillors and past Presidents who were now numbered with the dead. Mr. Joseph Gifford, of the Strand, was one of these. The position he occupied among his brethren, as an old member of the trade, may be gathered from the fact that at the meeting of chemists and druggists held at the Crown and Anchor on the 15th of February, 1841, for the purpose of considering Mr. Hawes's Bill, he was called to the chair. He was an active member of the committee appointed on that occasion to watch and oppose the progress of the Bill, and from the foundation of the Pharmaceutical Society until the year in which he died he had been a member of the council. During the official year 1852-3 he filled the presidential chair. He died on the 7th of September, 1857, in the 77th year of his age.

The position of British pharmacists and of chemists and druggists at this time could not be said to be all that might have been desired. The Pharmaceutical Society had its charter and an Act of Parliament, giving to its members certain privileges and imposing certain duties upon them as a body; but the advantages resulting from all they had gained in these respects were not generally felt to be of a substantial nature. Pharmacists were carrying out objects for the benefit of the public, but in what way were the originators and supporters of the costly arrangements by which a better-qualified class of pharmacists was supplied to the public, themselves benefited? Was it by raising up competitors in trade with qualifications of a more demonstrable nature than their own? Questions such as these could not fail to occur to the minds of many; and although they were often answered to the satisfaction of the conscience, and although many also felt that in promoting the education of others they were advancing their own education, still there was an anxious looking for a more profitable investment than had hitherto been made in the Pharmaceutical Society. Nor was it merely the retrospective view that failed to satisfy. Prospectively there was a dark mist and obscure vision of medical legislation and a Poison Bill with threatened innovations which were calculated to undermine what had already been done by the Pharmaceutical Society and to destroy the hope of further beneficial legislation for the body of chemists and druggists. It was well that good men were still found in the council chamber, and that these were supported by a yearly increasing phalanx of men of the rising generation who owed to the society and the cause with which it was identified the proud position they occupied as educated and examined men.

We are entering now on the year 1858. Jacob Bell was

President of the Pharmaceutical Society, with W. L. Bird as Vice-President, Daniel Bell Hanbury as Treasurer, and Elias Bremridge as Secretary and Registrar. The parliamentary session opened with the prospect of ample work for the officials of the society.

Attempts at medical legislation had so frequently proved abortive and yet were so constantly renewed, that agitation on the subject began to be looked upon as a chronic disease for which there was no remedy. Year after year Bills had appeared in Parliament, been discussed, opposed, and finally withdrawn. Still it was admitted by all those who inquired into the subject that there was much need for medical reform. Lord Elcho, Mr. Headlam, and Mr. T. Duncombe had respectively tried their hands at it, and now gave it up in despair, but not without an implied promise from the Government that they would once more try to settle this difficult question.

Lord Palmerston's ministry, with the' resignation of which the progress of the Poison Bill had been suspended, having been succeeded by that of the Earl of Derby with Mr. Walpole as Home Secretary, the two subjects of medical reform and the regulation of the sale of poisons were undertaken by them. The report of the committee of the Pharmaceutical Society, which, as already stated, had been submitted to Lord Granville, was now laid before Mr. Walpole, and an intimation was received that the society would be made acquainted with the purport of any measure the Government purposed introducing. The council drew up a Bill, based on that of the previous session, but modified so as to meet the views of pharmacists generally, which was submitted to the Government and by them to the College of Physicians. Practically, however, the Bill taken up by the new ministry was that of their predecessors, and it still contained some very objectionable provisions to which it was incumbent on the society to offer a strenuous opposition. It had been introduced in the House of Lords, and now Lord Derby had charge of it. Suggestions were made by the council for removing the grounds of the strong objection they had to parts of the measure, and hopes were at one time entertained that these would be acceded to. Some modifications were made, but there was one point on which the Government and the society were still at issue, as the following correspondence will show :—

"15, LANGHAM PLACE,
"*June* 7, 1858.

"My Lord,—

"I regret the necessity of troubling your Lordship on the subject of the Sale of Poisons Bill, but I think it better at this early stage to point out any provisions that appear to be objectionable, instead of deferring it to a later period. The provision to which I chiefly refer is the proposal to supersede the Pharmaceutical Society by the appointment of a new Board of Examiners, to examine candidates for the distinction of "Licensed Druggist." For about eighteen years the Pharmaceutical Society has been endeavouring to introduce a regular education and examination of all chemists and druggists. During nearly the whole of this time, very little encouragement has been obtained from the Legislature or the Government ; the efforts of the society having been met either with indifference or opposition, and the necessity for education and examination having been scarcely admitted to exist. It is now generally acknowledged that some qualification in those who dispense medicines, including poisons, is necessary for the safety of the public, and it is also acknowledged that the Pharmaceutical Society has done service to the public in promoting this object, for which its establishment is expressly designed. Yet in carrying the principle into practice, it is now proposed to appoint another Board of Examiners, the tendency of which would be to divert candidates from the channel of education and examination provided by the society, substituting a qualification which must of necessity be inferior to that of a pharmaceutical chemist, and frustrating the endeavours of the society to raise the standard of education. The distinction between a pharmaceutical chemist and a licensed druggist would scarcely be recognised by the public ; and as the examination for a licensed druggist would be attended with the smallest amount of trouble and expense, the Pharmaceutical Society would be superseded. I have seen the President of the College of Physicians, and some other influential members of the college, who, I have reason to believe, are favourable to the views of the Pharmaceutical Society on this subject. I therefore most respectfully and earnestly request that the further progress of the Bill may be deferred until an opportunity has been afforded for a conference

with the representatives of the College of Physicians and of
the Pharmaceutical Society.   I may also observe that the
opinion which was received by your Lordship as that of the
Royal College of Physicians, was in fact the opinion of a
deputation consisting of physicians and others.   I should be
able, if favoured with an interview, to explain more fully the
facts of the case, and also to point out other objections to the
constitution of the proposed Board of Examiners.

" I have the honour to remain, my Lord,

"Your Lordship's obedient servant,

"JACOB BELL."

" To the Right Hon. the Earl of Derby."

The following reply was received the same day :—

"DOWNING STREET, 7th June, 1858.

" Sir,—

" I am directed by Lord Derby to acknowledge the receipt
of your letter of this day's date, relative to the Sale of Poisons Bill, and to acquaint you that the Bill in question is to
be committed pro formâ to-night, to allow of amendments
being printed. His Lordship will send you a copy ; but he
cannot admit the validity of your objections to the proposed
Board of Examiners.

"I have the honour to be, Sir,

"Your most obedient servant,

"MAURICE DRUMMOND."

" To Jacob Bell, Esq."

This was immediately acknowledged as follows :—

" My Lord,—

"I have the honour to acknowledge the receipt of your
Lordship's favour of this day. I regret that your Lordship
does not admit the validity of the objections to the proposed Board of Examiners, as upon that question the
Pharmaceutical Society will stand or fall. I am obliged to
leave town on business for three days, on my return I look
forward to receiving a copy of the Bill as amended.

" I have the honour to be, etc., etc.

"JACOB BELL."

"To the Right Hon. the Earl of Derby."

An interview was to have taken place between Lord Derby and a deputation from the society ; but this was prevented by his lordship's indisposition. The deputation had a satisfactory interview with the College of Physicians, and communicated the result of this to the Government. Another attempt was made to get an interview with Lord Derby, but without avail; and the third reading of the Bill in the House of Lords was appointed for the 8th of July. On this day the Poison Committee met, and arranged to attend at the House of Lords to hear the fate of the Bill. A reporter was retained, with instructions to furnish a verbatim report of the debate. Several noble lords went down to the House, prepared to support amendments which it was expected would be proposed. While the parties interested in the question were waiting for the debate to commence, the words, " Read a third time," and " Bill do pass," pronounced at the table, were indistinctly heard. A noble lord said, " That was the Poison Bill which passed." Another said, " No ; it has not come on yet." But upon inquiry it was ascertained that the Poison Bill had actually passed, *sub silentio*, and without any of the amendments which the Committee had hoped to have succeeded in getting introduced.

What was now to be done ? The committee, greatly annoyed and somewhat bewildered, retired from the House, beaten but not disheartened. Trusting to the strength of their cause, they had hitherto hoped to be able to convince the Government of the reasonableness of their proposed amendments. Up to the present time,—six o'clock p.m. on the 8th of July,— no attempt had been made to stir up an active opposition to the Bill among the members of the trade generally. For nearly a month, however, copies of the Bill had been circulated through the country, and much correspondence had taken place between the council and the members, which showed that a strong feeling of opposition to the measure existed among the entire body of chemists and druggists. It had now become necessary to turn this to account as a means of influencing the House of Commons, where the ultimate fate of the Bill rested.

Within two hours from the time at which the third reading of the Bill had been so quietly carried by the Lords, circulars were in the printer's hands, convening a meeting of members of the society in London. Circulars were also prepared, informing the local secretaries of the failure of the efforts of the council, with a short statement describing the provisions of the Bill as passed by the Lords, and suggesting means for opposing it in the Commons. In twenty-four hours the symptoms of a coming storm were manifest. Petitions began to come in, Members of Parliament received earnest letters from their constituents, and in the course of two or three days the entire House of Commons was sensibly influenced by the pressure brought to bear upon it. Deputations from the country and members of the council clustered in the lobby of the House, to meet their representatives and to convey their sentiments, directly or indirectly, to Mr. Walpole, who invited them to form a deputation to attend at the Home Office to discuss the question. This interview was arranged to take place ; but on the previous evening Mr. Walpole stated in the House, that communications had been sent to him from every quarter, almost from every village, stating that the chemists had serious objections to the Poisons Bill; and although he did not quite agree with all of them, yet, as he thought the Bill required great amendment, he proposed not to proceed with it that session. The Bill was therefore withdrawn.

This was looked upon as a great victory gained by the society, for the Government had evidently, at one time, determined to carry this measure notwithstanding the opposition offered to it by the council. They had not then learnt to estimate the power which the society was capable of exerting by means of its organization throughout the country.

But although the Government had failed in their attempts at legislation respecting the sale of poisons, they succeeded in carrying their Medical Bill, and this result was a matter of even greater general surprise than the other.

The Medical Act of 1858 was the means of bringing about important changes in the medical profession, and at least one important change in relation to pharmacy.

The duty was assigned to the General Council of Medical Education and Registration, of causing "to be published under their direction a book containing a list of medicines and compounds and the manner of preparing them, together with the true weights and measures by which they are to be prepared and mixed, and containing such other matter and things relating thereto as the General Council shall think fit, to be called 'British Pharmacopœia;' and the General Council shall cause to be altered and republished, such Pharmacopœia as often as they shall deem it necessary." And by a subsequent Act it was provided that the British Pharmacopœia should supersede the Pharmacopœias of London, Edinburgh, and Dublin. The Colleges of Physicians were thus relieved from the responsibility of preparing new Pharmacopœias, this duty being transferred to the representatives of those and other medical corporations in the Medical Council.

The London college, as we have previously noticed, had for several years been making preparations for a new edition of their Pharmacopœia, and in doing so had requested the assistance of the Pharmaceutical Society. Some valuable information had been collected through the combined action of the pharmacopœia committees of the college and the society; and it was anticipated, although no specific arrangement had yet been made for the production of the British Pharmacopœia, that the matter which had been thus prepared world be made available for use in the new work. The committees, therefore continued their labours.

In the North there was evidence of increased activity. The Edinburgh College of Physicians now followed the example which had been set by the Pharmaceutical Society some years before, as the following circular, addressed to medical practitioners and chemists in Scotland will show :—

"Royal College of Physicians, Edinburgh,
"11th August, 1858.

" Sir,—

" A committee of this college is at present engaged in collecting such information as it is presumed the new Medical Council will expect from the royal colleges, before a national Pharmacopœia is published under their auspices.

" I am instructed by the committee to request from you any information which you can supply on the following heads :—

" 1. Articles of materia medica frequently prescribed, but not included in the last edition of the Edinburgh Pharmacopœia.

" 2. Changes in any of the processes of the Edinburgh Pharmacopœia which you consider desirable.

" 3. New processes which you follow, or are inclined to suggest, for the preparation of any article in the Pharmacopœia.

" Any communication on the above subjects, if made to me, will be highly valued, and duly acknowledged by the committee.

" I am, sir, your obedient servant,

" WILLIAM ROBERTSON, M.D.,

" <i>Secretary of Pharmacopœia Committee.</i>"

As chemists in Scotland had previously received a circular similar in purport to the foregoing, from the Pharmacopœia Committee in London, some doubt existed as to whether they were expected to communicate with the Edinburgh or the London committee, or with both. This question was raised at a meeting of the committee in London, and drew forth the following letter :—

" Sir,—

" At a meeting of the Pharmacopœia Committee, held Oct. 26th, a letter having been read from Mr. Deane, Chairman of the Pharmacopœia Committee of the Pharmaceutical Society of Great Britain, enclosing a circular issued by the College of Physicians of Edinburgh to the pharmaceutical chemists of that city, and inquiring with which college the members of the Pharmaceutical Society in Edinburgh should in future communicate on the subjects mentioned in that circular, Mr. Redwood being also present by invitation on the part of Mr. Deane, who was unable to attend,—

" <i>It was resolved,</i>—That, in the opinion of this committee, it is desirable that the members of the Pharmaceutical Society of Edinburgh should be left at liberty to reply individually, according to their own experience, to the inquiries of the College of Physicians of Edinburgh ; but in order that the London and Edinburgh colleges may receive the same recommendations, and to further the production of a national Pharmacopœia, it is desirable that the members of the Pharmaceutical Society in Edinburgh should, as a body, communicate with the Pharmaceutical Society in London, and that the London society should communicate their final conclusions and recommendations to both colleges.

"I have the honour to be, Sir, your obedient Servant,

"FRED. J. FARRE, M.D.,

"*Chairman of the Pharmacopœia Committee.*"

"To the Chairman of the Pharmacopœia Committee of the Pharmaceutical Society of Great Britain."

Evidence having been thus afforded that the Colleges of Physicians and the pharmaceutical chemists were disposed and prepared to render all the assistance they could in the production of the new Pharmacopœia, it remained for the Medical Council to organize the necessary arrangements for carrying this important object into effect, nor were they long in doing so. Pharmacopœia committees were appointed in England, Scotland, and Ireland.

At a meeting of the Council of the Pharmaceutical Society specially convened on the 15th of December, the following letter was read:—

"84, HARLEY STREET, CAVENDISH SQUARE,

"*10th Dec.*, 1858.

"Sir,—

"The British Pharmacopœia Committee is desirous that the Council of the Pharmaceutical Society should appoint a member to co-operate with the London sub-committee in the preparation of the British (national) Pharmacopœia, and the committee is desirous that such appointment should be made with as little delay as possible.

"I am, Sir, your obedient servant,

"A. B. GARROD, M.D., *Secretary.*

"To the President of the Pharmaceutical Society."

After some discussion, it was resolved,—

"That Mr. Squire be appointed a member to co-operate with the London sub-committee in the preparation of the British Pharmacopœia."

A further correspondence relating to the Pharmacopœia took place a few days later, as follows—

"ROYAL COLLEGE OF PHYSICIANS,

"*Dec.* 16th, 1858.

"Sir,—

"I have the honour to enclose you a copy of resolution

passed at the *Comitia Majora* held at the Royal College of
Physicians on Saturday the 11th instant.

"I have the honour to be, Sir, your obedient servant,

"HENRY A. PITMAN, M.D., *Registrar.*"

"To the President of the Pharmaceutical Society."

"*Resolved*, That the thanks of the College be given to the
Society of Apothecaries and to the Pharmaceutical Society,
for the valuable assistance afforded by them to the Pharmacopœia Committee of the College."

This communication having been duly acknowledged, the
correspondence and co-operation which had been maintained
since 1854 between the London College of Physicians and
the Pharmaceutical Society respecting the Pharmacopœia was
terminated. It soon appeared, however, that the services of the
Pharmacopœia Committee of the Pharmaceutical Society were
not yet to be dispensed with, as the following correspondence
will show :—

"HARLEY STREET, CAVENDISH SQUARE,

"18*th Dec.*, 1858.

"My dear Sir,—

"The Pharmacopœia Committee requests the Pharmaceutical Society to continue their committee and to communicate through their delegate, Mr. Squire, any information
on subjects relating to the British Pharmacopœia.   One
point upon which they are now desirous of obtaining information, is the extent to which the drugs and preparations
are employed, as this concerns the list of materia medica
which will form the first portion of the work.

"Believe me, dear Sir, yours very truly,

"A. B. GARROD,

"*Secretary to the Pharmacopœia Committee
of the Medical Council.*"

"To Jacob Bell, Esq."

Proceedings similar to the foregoing were taking place at
the same time in Edinburgh.   At a meeting of the Council of
the North British Branch of the Pharmaceutical Society in
Edinburgh, the Secretary read a letter which he had received
from Professor Christison, as convener of the sub-committee
of the committee to which the General Medical Council of
Education and Registration had entrusted the preparation and

publication of a national Pharmacopœia, requesting that the Edinburgh Branch of the Pharmaceutical Society would have the goodness to appoint two of its members to be associated with the existing Pharmacopœia sub-committee, and lend their valuable services in assisting to prepare the new Pharmacopœia.

After some deliberation it was resolved, "That J. F. Macfarlan, of 17, North Bridge Street, and James Robertson, present President of the society here, be appointed representatives of the Pharmaceutical Society at the board of said committee; and it was also further resolved that the Council should strongly recommend to the sub-committee to admit Dr. Douglas Maclagan as representing the honorary members of the society in Scotland."

These proceedings on the part of the Pharmacopœia Committee of the Medical Council were justified by resolutions which had been passed at the first meeting of the General Council of Medical Education and Registration held in the hall of the Royal College of Physicians, London, on the 23rd of November, 1858, which were to the following effect :—

" 1. That the following gentlemen be appointed a committee to prepare and publish the national Pharmacopœia with all convenient speed :—Dr. Christison, Dr. Thomas Watson, Sir James Clark, Bart., Mr. Green, Dr. Apjohn, Mr. Syme, Dr. Williams, Dr. Andrew Wood, Mr. Nussey, Dr. Leet, with power to add to their number; Dr. Christison to be convener.

" 2. That this Committee shall have full power to communicate with the three Colleges of Physicians, and to request their co-operation in preparing the Pharmacopœia, and to beg them for that purpose to appoint Fellows of the several Colleges to be associated with the committee of the General Medical Council.

"3. That the committee shall have power to communicate with the Pharmaceutical Society for the same purpose.

"4. That the committee shall have power to appoint a chemist or chemists, to carry on such chemical and pharmaceutical researches as may be found necessary, and to pay those gentlemen such remuneration as the committee of the General Council may think advisable.

" 5. That a sum of £500 be voted by the General Council, from the registration fees of existing practitioners, in order to defray the cost of preparing the Pharmacopœia for printing."

It was also resolved,—

" That it be an instruction to the Pharmacopœia Committee that the Pharmacopœia be published in the English language, with the list of the materia medica and compounds in the Latin language."

It could not have been otherwise than gratifying to the Pharmaceutical Society to find that it was thus placed in so prominent and honourable a position by the Medical Council in relation to the one subject on which it claimed to possess an amount of practical knowledge superior to that of medical men who were not engaged in pharmacy. It was the highest public recognition that could have been given, by the most competent authority in the kingdom, that the subject of pharmacy was being and had for a series of years been, cultivated, advanced, and practised, legitimately, consistently, and with effect, by those who were now invited to assist in the compilation of a national Pharmacopœia. The compliment was gracefully paid to those who were thought to have deserved it. But it was felt that no small amount of responsibility was thus thrown on to the representatives of British pharmacy; and the President of the society was foremost in expressing an anxious solicitude for the credit of his brethren. Mr. Bell knew that for four or [five years the society had been invited by the College of Physicians to perform a similar service; and, with the exception of what had been done by some three or four members of the London committee, little if anything had been contributed. It was indeed hardly to be expected that very much should have been elicited under the circumstances. If the appeal was intended to be made to members of the society generally, or to the body of chemists and druggists, the subject, or at any rate the mode of dealing with it, was so perfectly new to them, that a sense of diffidence would in most cases have deterred those who may have had a knowledge of facts worth communicating from putting them forward. Then the circumstance that there was a committee of pharmacists, and also other committees, engaged on the work, would be considered by the members generally to have relieved them of responsibility on the subject. The several committees in London and elsewhere were asked to confine their attention to certain specified subjects, and their reports were to be submitted to a subsequent revision by the general committee. This division of labour and responsibility could not be considered favourable to a successful result of the undertaking, and yet on this occasion it could not well have been avoided. The British Pharmacopœia work, however, was in active operation.

In carrying out this important work, one of the questions that appeared to present considerable difficulty in the way of its being satisfactorily settled, was that of the system of weights and measures to be recognised in the Pharmacopœia, for use in prescribing and dispensing as well as preparing medicines. This subject had already been discussed at meetings of the Pharmaceutical Society, and considerable difference of opinion was found to exist, not only among members of the society, but among scientific and practical men outside the society, who had devoted much attention to the subject. Prior to the year 1850, the three Colleges of Physicians in the United Kingdom had agreed in adopting the same weights, namely apothecaries' weights, in their Pharmacopœias; but in that year the Dublin College, in bringing out a new Pharmacopœia, adopted a new system of weights, previously unknown, and still unrecognised by law, in which the avoirdupois pound and ounce were used with the troy grain, but with a new drachm and scruple. In this system the avoirdupois ounce was divided into 8 drachms, each representing 54·68 troy grains ; and the drachm was divided into 3 scruples, each representing 18·22 troy grains. The principal object in adopting this system was, to do away with the inconvenience and source of error arising from the use of two sorts of weights, one for buying and selling drugs, and the other for prescribing and dispensing them. But the Irish system had the grave defect that two of the weights, the drachm and scruple, were illegal, and that the grain was not an integral part of either the ounce, drachm, or scruple. The system did not meet with approval in this country.

Several propositions were made for removing the difficulties which stood in the way of having one common system of weights and measures alike applicable and suitable for buying and selling, prescribing and dispensing medicines ; or at least of having weights suitable for prescribing and dispensing medicines, that were integral parts of those used in ordinary commercial transactions.

T

There were many persons, especially among those whose pursuits had taken a scientific turn, who were favourable to the adoption of the French metrical system; but public opinion was not yet prepared for so great a change as this would have involved. Others, although doubting the feasibility of introducing the metrical system in this country, yet approving of a decimal arrangement of weights, suggested certain modifications of one or other of our existing systems, with the view of giving them a decimal character.

Mr. Warder, at a meeting of the Pharmaceutical Society held in December, 1858, suggested a decimal division of the avoirdupois pound, into 10 ounces, 100 drachms, 1000 scruples, and 10,000 grains. This was a radical change, which was scarcely considered worth a consideration.

Mr. Abraham, of Liverpool, at an earlier date, in 1855, in discussing the subject of weights and measures, maintained that a decimal system was much to be desired; and that, although the time was probably far distant when the Legislature would compel the general use of a decimal system of weights, he thought something might be done to lessen the inconvenience experienced in the use of existing systems in this country. He suggested that in all pharmacopœial formulæ only two denominations of weight should be specified, namely the troy grain and the avoirdupois pound of 7000 grains; that quantities less than a pound or some aliquot part, should be expressed in grains, and that sets of grain weights should be kept, consisting of 6000, 3000, 2000, 1000, 600, 300, 200, 100 grains, and the small weights commonly used in dispensing.

Mr. Griffin, at a meeting of the Pharmaceutical Society in March, 1855, proposed a decimal system of weights and measures which at least possessed the merit of completeness. This system cannot be more concisely or better described than in the terms used by Mr Griffin on the occasion referred to. "He considered that the change might be effected without much difficulty, because a decimal relation already existed between the avoirdupois pound, our standard for weights, and the gallon, our standard for measures. Ten avoirdupois pounds of water, at 60° Fahr., make an imperial gallon. One pound of water is sixteen fluid ounces, or four-fifths of a pint. Its volume is a decigallon, or the tenth part of a gallon. If the avoirdupois pound were divided into 1000 units of weight, and the decigallon into 1000 units of measure, we should have a decimal system as perfect as that of France, a system in which there would be a strict correspondence between the weights and measures, and yet without interference with the existing legal standards. The unit of weight in the proposed system would be equal to 7 imperial grains. The corresponding unit of measure would be of the bulk of 7 grains of water. It would be necessary to give different names to these units, in order to distinguish the weight from the measure. The weight might be called a *Baro*, and the measure a *Barim*. 1000 baros would be equal to a pound, and 1000 barims would be equal to a decigallon. Weights intermediate between the pound and baro would be obtained by taking the ounce at the tenth part of the pound, and the drachm at the tenth part of the ounce. The measures would be subdivided correspondingly. The formula 1·525 pound would then represent 1 pound, 5 ounces, 2 drachms, and 5 baros. The French decimal system is exactly similar to this, for 1·525 k. is read 1 kilogramme, 5 hectogrammes, 2 decagrammes, and 5 grammes. It has, however, been found in France that the denominations existing between the kilogramme and the gramme are too cumbrous for popular use, so that the formula 1·525 k. is commonly read 1 kilogramme, and 525 grammes, omitting the intermediate denominations. The same result would, no doubt, to some extent occur with us, and the formula 1·525 lb. would be read as 1 pound and 525 baros. The weights and denominations of ounce and drachm would nevertheless be highly useful, for the formula ·525 would be $5\frac{1}{4}$ ounces, and ·025 would be $2\frac{1}{2}$ drachms." " The proposed decimal ounce would contain 700 of our present grains, and would bear to the avoirdupois ounce the relation of 70 to $43\frac{3}{4}$ or 16 to 10, and to the troy ounce the relation of 70 to 48, or nearly of 3 to 2. Being divisible into 10 drachms, and into 100 barims, and also, if required, into halves and quarters, it offers as many subdivisions as are likely to be required for any purpose of science or commerce.

" The term *grain* could disappear, unless it were thought fit to retain it for the unit instead of adopting the word baro. The term *pint* would also disappear, unless retained to denote the decigallon, instead of denoting, as it now does, the octogallon. Such terms as *fluid* ounce and *fluid* drachm are too clumsy to be worth retaining. It is expedient to have terms that will at once distinguish between a measure and a weight."

" The barim = 7 grains of water, is a very convenient unit volume for liquid measures. The French centimetre cube = 1 gramme of water, contains 2·2 barims; but in practice this unit has been found to be inconveniently large, and in consequence nearly all scientific instruments are graduated to half *centimetre cubes*, a division that bears to the barim the relation of 1·1 to 1·0."

When the Pharmacopœia Committees in connection with the Medical Council had entered on their work, and it became necessary to decide what weights and measures should be used in describing the processes, some further suggestions were made bearing on the subject.

Dr. Charles Wilson, of Edinburgh, submitted a proposition to the Edinburgh Committee which was favourably received there in the first instance. It was to the following effect :— that the troy grain should be reduced to 0·91145 of its recognised weight, in which case the grain weight would correspond with the weight of a minim measure of distilled water. Then, 20 such grains representing the scruple, 60 such grains representing the drachm, 480 representing the ounce, which would coincide with the avoirdupois ounce, and 7680 representing the pound, coinciding with the avoirdupois pound, would form a system in which the pound and ounce would correspond with the standard imperial weights of those denominations established by law, while the subdivisions of the ounce into drachms, scruples, and grains would bear the same relations to the ounce that the apothecaries' drachm, scruple, and grain bear to the troy ounce. This proposition was freely discussed both in Edinburgh and London, but the prevailing opinions were unfavourable to its adoption.

Propositions were also made by Mr. Peter Squire and by Mr. Robert Warington.

Mr. Squire objected to the introduction of the avoirdupois weight for use in the Pharmacopœia, and strongly urged the retention of the apothecaries' weight. He recommended that in all formulæ in which weights are used, in addition to giving the apothecaries' weight there should be a separate column in which the quantities should be represented according to the metric system, the latter being expressed in approximate equivalents, which, as he pointed out, could be easily done in whole numbers.

Mr. Warington's proposition was in the same direction as Mr. Griffin's, but not worked out to the same extent. He suggested that the pound avoirdupois of 7000 grains should be taken as the unit, and decimated for the lower denominations down to 70 grains, the extreme of the scale being one grain.

There were thus ample materials put before the General Committee of the Medical Council, from which to choose a system of weights and measures; but the great diversity of the propositions made, and the differences of opinion expressed with reference to them, probably tended as much to perplex as to convince the committee, and the result was that no one of the propositions was adopted.

Mr. Bell, although suffering in health from the effects of a chronic affection of the larynx, which rendered the use of his voice and even the swallowing of food painful and difficult operations, was unremitting in his endeavours to stimulate his fellow-members to a creditable display of what pharmacists, after eighteen years' training, could do towards the production of a Pharmacopœia. He wrote a paper which was read at a Pharmaceutical meeting on the 3rd of February, 1859, on some of the processes of the Pharmacopœia which he thought required revision. But although he could thus use his pen, he was at this time unable to read his paper, or even to be present at the meeting.

Two subjects which had previously occupied the attention of the Legislature and called forth a good deal of discussion among pharmacists, were now again brought prominently into notice by the introduction of Bills into Parliament "for preventing the adulteration of articles of food and drink," and "for regulating the keeping and sale poisons." A recent accident which had proved fatal to the lives of many persons, had contributed to keep up the excitement which had existed for several years in the public mind with reference to the latter of these subjects.

A manufacturer of cheap peppermint lozenges at Bradford, had, through the mistake of a druggist's assistant, put white arsenic instead of sulphate of lime into his lozenges, and these had been sold at a stall in the public market. The result was that twenty persons who ate some of these lozenges died, and about two hundred others suffered more or less severely from the effects of the poison.

This happened in the latter end of October, 1858. The case served to illustrate the effects of adulteration as often practised, and of the careless and unrestricted way in which poisons were kept and sold. It appeared that the lozenge-maker, in the production of his cheap lozenges, was in the habit of substituting sulphate of lime (gypsum) for part of the sugar, and to prevent those employed in the manufacture from knowing what the adulterant was, it was called " daff," under which name it was kept and sold by druggists.

Having occasion to prepare a batch of lozenges in readiness for market day, the lozenge-maker sent to a druggist for twelve pounds of " daff." The druggist was ill in bed, and his assistant, who had been with him only a few weeks on trial with a view to his being apprenticed, having no previous knowledge of the business, and not knowing where the "daff" was kept or what it was, went to his master's room to inquire. He was told it was a white powder in a cask in a corner of the attic; but was not informed that close by the cask containing the " daff" there was another cask containing white arsenic, and that there was no visible label on either of them. The lad, finding a cask as described with a white powder in it, which proved to be arsenic, took the quantity required, and having supplied it to the customer, it was made into lozenges with sugar and oil of peppermint. These were supplied in the market next day at less than a penny an ounce. Each lozenge contained about ten grains of arsenic.

The parties implicated in this transaction were put on their trial for manslaughter, and acquitted, the druggist being merely censured for not having the arsenic cask properly labelled.

It was no matter of surprise to find, after the occurrence of this dreadful accident, that the Government were again prepared to introduce their Poison Bill. The council, in anticipation of this result, had prepared the draft of a Bill such as they could assent to, and this was submitted to the Home Secretary, Mr. Walpole, who, on the 3rd of February, 1859, introduced the Government Bill. The most objectionable provisions of the Bill of the previous session were omitted in this; but still it could not be allowed to pass without modification or opposition. A deputation from the council waited on the Home Secretary and urged their views; further concessions were made by the Government; and the Bill was ultimately so far emasculated that it was not thought to be worth any further attempts to carry it, and it was accordingly withdrawn.

The Bill for preventing the adulteration of food and drink also failed to pass, although, after the discussions and criticisms it had undergone, it began to assume a more practicable character. In one respect, however, a great step was now taken towards the prevention of the adulteration of drink, by the adoption by the Government of a method of diverting the sewage of London from parts of the Thames from which water was drawn for domestic use. Powers for carrying ou t the Main Drainage of London were given to the Metropolitan Board of Works, which had been constituted in 1855, the year in which Professor Faraday, by dropping his card from a steamer into the muddy river and representing the rapidity with which it became invisible, so forcibly drew attention in the *Times* newspaper to the highly polluted state of this great sewer.

Several communications were made through the Pharmaceutical Society which appeared to have originated in a desire to assist those who were engaged in preparing the British Pharmacopoeia. Mr. Henry Deane had been experimenting on the preparation of soap liniment, and contributed some valuable suggestions for preventing its gelatinization in cold weather. Mr. Giles, of Clifton, originated a lengthy discussion on spermaceti ointment, in which he took exception to the frequently occurring practice of using bleached olive oil in its preparation. Numerous short notes on pharmacopoeial processes were contributed by Mr. B. S. Proctor, of Newcastle; Mr. Thomas Southall, of Birmingham; Mr. Boucher, of Bristol; Mr. C. R. C. Tichborne, and Mr. Muskett, of Dublin. Mr. Haselden and Mr. Bell furnished papers on concentrated infusions and fluid extracts; Mr. T. H. Hills on the preparation of lard, and on extract and fluid extract of taraxacum; and Professor Bentley, on the best time for collecting and on the constituents of taraxacum root. These and other contributions served to show that there was not only the disposition but the power to render valuable assistance in compiling the important work with the production of which the Medical Council was entrusted.

In some respects the position of pharmacy and of those who were making its cultivation and improvement the objects of their exclusive professional pursuit, may be said to have been susceptible at this time of a very favourable comparison with what they had been in times past. There was now a well-organized body of what might be called pharmacists proper—of men whose special pursuit was that of pharmacy. They were recognised by law, appealed to and consulted by the highest medical authorities in the country on purely pharmaceutical subjects, and, through the influence of a well-sustained system of professional education, were acquiring the power of efficiently fulfilling what was required in this department of medical practice. There was room for congratulation in reviewing the past, room for satisfaction in many respects in the contemplation of the present, but ground for some uneasiness even now, and still more for apprehension in regard to the immediate future. Great as were the benefits conferred upon the cause of pharmaceutical progress by the almost exclusive devotion to its interests of the energies of a man of superior abilities, who had enlisted all the means at his command in the furtherance of this cause, there was reason to fear that so much had been left to be carried out by those individual exertions, that should they unfortunately fail, the advancement of the cause must sustain a severe check.

With loss of health Mr. Bell's effective exertions were now failing. For many months he had been losing strength, while the disease which preyed on his physical powers, having resisted all efforts to subdue its ravages, assumed a chronic form and threatened the speedy destruction of its victim. Those who were brought into personal communication with Mr. Bell were not unprepared for the fatal issue now impending, nor was the sufferer himself less sensible than his friends were of the serious nature of his malady. In concluding the eighteenth volume of the *Pharmaceutical Journal*, after briefly reviewing the objects and results of his editorial labours, he concluded by saying, "The Editor, having been for a considerable time suffering from a pulmonary disorder, attended with debility and loss of voice, feels that it will be necessary for him at no distant period to relinquish the responsibility of the management of the *Journal*. Should his anticipation in this respect be realized, it is his intention to place the *Journal* more directly under the control of the Council, and arrangements have been made with this object."

This sentence was written at the end of May, and published ostensibly on the 1st of June, 1859. It contains the last editorial words contributed to the *Pharmaceutical Journal* by the man who for eighteen years had been its editor and proprietor.

Practically the printing and issuing of the *Journal* bearing date the 1st of June, took place some days before that date; and on the 1st of June there was a meeting of council, at which Mr. Bell presided. On this occasion the President expressed his intention of presenting the copyright of the *Journal* to the Society, coupling this statement with an explanation of his views and desires as to its future management.

Before another number of the *Journal* appeared, the remains of Jacob Bell had been consigned to their last resting-place. After trying the effects of change of air at Hastings and other places, the atmosphere of Tunbridge Wells was found to suit him best, and here he had been staying for a short time before his death, which took place on the 12th of June, 1859.

The announcement of this sad event was a source of unfeigned grief to a wide circle, not only of personal friends but of those who merely knew Mr. Bell by name and were accustomed to consider him an almost essential advocate and supporter of the good work in which the Pharmaceutical Society was engaged. His short life had been devoted to the one chief object of his ambition, the union of the whole body of chemists and druggists in association, for the establishment of a sound and comprehensive system of pharmaceutical education, for the attainment of parliamentary recognition and support in securing to a body of qualified pharmacists the privileges to which they were entitled, for elevating the professional status of such a body, and for generally advancing the interests of pharmacy. He had seen the fulfilment of

much of his object, and died in the faith that others who had
hitherto co-operated with him would live to see the more
complete accomplishment of the work.

Jacob Bell was the eldest surviving son of John Bell, and
was born at 838, Oxford Street, in the parish of St. James,
Westminster, on the 5th of March, 1810. His early education
was provided at home. At twelve years of age he was sent
to the school of his uncle, Frederick Smith, at Darlington,
where he remained four years, and received a good general
and classical education, such as was considered suitable for the
business occupation for which he was intended. Frederick
Smith's school had been established for supplying a superior
education to the children of wealthy members of the Society
of Friends. It acquired a good reputation as a classical
school. The progress that young Bell made there was considered satisfactory. In some respects he took a prominent
part among the scholars, and was especially distinguished for
the facility with which he wrote essays, composed facetious
dialogues in Hudibrastic style, and illustrated them with very
clever pen-and-ink sketches. In connection with a school-
fellow he contributed to the maintenance for some time of
a humorous manuscript periodical which was devoted to
school news and chit-chat.

On leaving school Jacob Bell took the position of an
apprentice in his father's business. His father at that time
had two partners, one of whom, Thomas Zachary, resided on
the premises; and the young apprentice was put under the
immediate control of this partner and was made to submit
to all the regulations to which apprentices and junior assistants were subjected. The early closing movement had not
then come into operation. A senior assistant, with one or
two juniors, commenced their duties at eight o'clock in the
morning, and were actively engaged in the shop until eleven
o'clock at night, when the door was finally closed, the shutters
having been put up, when practicable, at nine o'clock. Other
assistants were in attendance in the evening on half-duty,
ready to be called upon if necessary. None were allowed
to leave the premises in the evening without special permission; but those off duty were free to go out in the morning before breakfast. The evening hours of those not on
duty were either spent in the counting-house at the back of

the shop or in the bed-rooms, where each assistant had a desk
and a few shelves on which to keep such books as he was
enabled to provide for himself, and where the studious occupied themselves to their great benefit.   At breakfast and
tea time conversation was not allowed, as all were engaged
in reading.   There was a book-case in the room containing a
few books, mostly religious, with "Thomson's Dispensatory,"
"Thomas's Practice of Physic," and a few other works of that
sort.   But most of the reading done was in general literature,
and the books either belonged to the readers or were obtained
from public libraries.   No light literature was admitted, and
systematic scientific study was but rarely pursued by chemists'
assistants at that time.   The writer of this notice having been
associated with Jacob Bell during his apprenticeship, and
being in fact his most intimate associate, the reading and
studies of these two were carried on to a great extent in
unison, and took after a time a distinctly scientific turn.   In
an establishment in which there were, as here, several assistants, all kept under strict discipline and all occupying their
leisure time with studies of one sort or another, but without
any definite curriculum being imposed, there was naturally
some diversity in the studies adopted.   There was poetical
Watson, logical Jones, classical Hodgson, commercial Nelson,
and especially Alsop, who made chemistry and chemical
analysis chief subjects of his study, and the influence of whose
example was not unimportant.

The writer has often looked back with satisfaction to the
great benefit he derived from the regular half-hourly readings
at breakfast and tea time every day during seven years of his
early life spent at 338, Oxford Street.   It was the practice to
take books of substantial information and read them through
in this way.   No better system of study by reading could be
devised.   The mind was never wearied, nor was the continuity
of the subject too much broken up.   Fortunately there were
no cheap serial publications then, and newspaper reading
was not allowed to engender a taste for idle gossip or frivolous
excitement.

The young apprentice, Bell, now began to take a better
position in the house.   He attended lectures on chemistry
at the Royal Institution, and on the practice of physic at
King's College.   He was relieved from the shop-duties of an

apprentice, and allowed to take out-door exercise on horse-
back. This was his favourite recreation, and he became an
accomplished horseman. Nor were his studies confined to
subjects appertaining to pharmacy. He had always manifested
a taste for the fine arts, and especially for drawing. He
attended the morning classes at Sass's drawing-school, and
took lessons in oil-painting from his friend Mr. H. P. Briggs,
R.A. During his apprentice days he recorded in a journal
the incidents of his business life, in which he introduced a
large number of pen-and-ink sketches, some of which possessed
considerable merit. Various members of the household, including even some of those in authority, if their exercise of
discipline clashed with the laxer ideas of the young master,
figured in some caricature representations, in which, however,
the supremacy of law was always maintained. He became
after a time the occupant of a larger bedroom than that which
in the first instance sufficed for him, and this was soon made
into bedroom, sitting room, and laboratory. A chemical
furnace was fixed in it, and many of the experiments were
imported here from the lectures at the Royal Institution.
Even the roof of the house was converted into a laboratory,
and there also processes of dissection in connection with comparative anatomy were conducted.

It will be readily conceived that a young master endowed
with these exuberant tendencies for the cultivation of art and
science, would be calculated at times to disturb the equanimity
of the ruling authority in a quiet quaker family. But Jacob
Bell, although possessed of a lively imagination, sensitive to
the pleasures derived from the study of objects of art, and
ever active and enthusiastic in all he undertook, had judgment
and discretion enough to enable him to distinguish between
what was admissible in connection with business occupations
and what might be legitimately indulged in by those who
were relieved from such responsibilities. His love and appreciation of art had enabled him to form numerous acquaint-
ances among artists and the patrons of art, and he was thus
led into a kind of society widely different from that of the
families among whom he had been educated. He threw off
all appearance of quakerism, and entered with much spirit
into the enjoyments of fashionable society. Being a good
rider and accustomed to ride good horses, he became fond of

hunting, but had the discretion to avoid bringing his hunting attire into the house of business. He relinquished this occupation, when he found that his father took it greatly to heart, and was grieved to think that his son could engage in such cruel sport. But Jacob was no hypocrite, and never tried to pass for anything better than he was. He entertained to the last a strong belief in some of the leading principles fo quakerism, but did not include among these the necessity or desirableness of adopting what are called the quaker peculiarities of dress or language. Nor did he consider the higher influences of music sensual in any objectionable sense, or the cultivation of high art calculated to degrade or corrupt rational and well-educated human beings. At the period at which the Pharmaceutical Society was founded, John Bell's partners had left the business and Jacob was taking their place. He had now assumed the position of master in the establishment, and having an ample income, he shortly afterwards took a house for his private residence in Langham Place. Reference has already been made to the pharmaceutical meetings held at the house of business in Oxford Street. That was before the house in Langham Place had been taken. Among the acquaintance which Jacob Bell had formed at this time were the Landseers, especially Edwin, afterwards Sir Edwin, Briggs, Frith, Ward, Cooper, Stone, Hunt, and other eminent artists of the day; Charles Dickens, Thackeray, Talfourd, and other literary celebrities; numerous musical performers, and a host of medical and other scientific men. There were brilliant parties in Langham Place, to which Mr. Bell was accustomed to invite several of his pharmaceutical friends; but these were not pharmaceutical meetings such as had previously been held at 338, Oxford Street. Those meetings had been transferred to Bloomsbury Square, where the Pharmaceutical Society was now in full operation.

Frequent reference has been made throughout the latter part of this Historical Sketch to the active part which Mr. Bell took in all the proceedings of the society. None of his labours, however, were more serviceable to the society than those which were expended on the *Pharmaceutical Journal*. After the hours of business were ended journal work usually commenced, and from eight or nine o'clock in the evening until often past midnight, two or three times a week, or sometimes oftener, the editor and sub-editor were associated in editorial work, or in conference on questions affecting the interests of the cause to the furtherance of which the Pharmaceutical Society and its *Journal* were devoted. Not unfrequently these conferences were relieved or enlivened by an adjournment to her Majesty's Theatre, where Mr. Bell usually had a box throughout the opera season, or to some other place of amusement. Very soon after the appointment of Dr. Pereira as Professor to the Society, he was induced to render valuable service in the selection of articles on Materia Medica for the *Journal*, and to superintend the translation of such as were taken from foreign journals. Once a month the editor and sub-editor spent an evening at Dr. Pereira's house in Finsbury Square, to arrange the matter for a forthcoming number, and provide for the future. Those meetings continued up to the time of Dr. Pereira's death, after which a new arrangement was made, by which assistance was obtained from Professor Bentley, Mr. Daniel Hanbury, and Mr. Joseph Ince. It might be confidently said that none of those who were thus associated with Mr. Bell in editorial work were otherwise than impressed with the feeling that they had a leader who was worthy of the position, who never gave them the slightest ground for thinking that their services were under-valued, or who was accustomed to over-estimate his own powers. Mr. Bell was not above asking advice from those he thought most capable of assisting him in judiciously treating the subjects referred to in leading articles in the *Journal*. A vast deal of time was thus often occupied in consulting members of council and others, and trying, at least, to reconcile the opinions offered with those he might consider it his duty to express.

For some years before Mr. Bell's death, Mr. John Barnard had acted as his private secretary, and in that capacity had rendered great service in connection with journal work.

It was no easy matter at times to satisfy members of the society that all was being done that ought to be done towards obtaining for the society and its members the much desired legislative recognition, together with the concession of some exclusive privileges. There was an ever-recurring murmur of complaint that without an Act of Parliament the Pharmaceutical Society could not be of any great service to those

who were contributing to its support. Mr. Bell had been in
frequent communication with those members of the House
of Commons who were thought to be most likely to take up
the subject of pharmaceutical legislation, with a view of introducing a Bill into Parliament. Warburton, Wakley, Duncombe, and others were tried, but they were either indifferent
or lukewarm, or not prepared to advocate the required
principles. There was much ignorance among members of
Parliament generally of the qualifications required for the
practice of pharmacy, and it was felt that it would be a
dangerous experiment to introduce a Bill into Parliament
unless it were in charge of a member fully conversant with
all the circumstances under which legislation was required.
In connection with medical legislation, advantage had been
experienced by the general practitioners in having a man
like Mr. Wakley in the House, who, when the subject was
discussed, had a knowledge of all its bearings, and could
advocate the cause of that section of the medical profession to which he was attached. It had been repeatedly
asked, "Why cannot pharmacy have its representative and
advocate in the House of Commons?" No man was known,
more likely than Mr. Bell, to be induced to undertake, if it
were possible for him to obtain, so important a position.
Although sensible of the difficulty of attaining to it, Mr. Bell
was not unwilling to undertake the duties of the position.
The project had not been much discussed, except among a
few of Mr. Bell's friends, who favoured the proposition, when
an opening presented itself at St. Albans, caused by the death
of Mr. Raphael, in November, 1850. Mr. Bell determined to
offer himself as a candidate for the vacant seat. He was now
entering the arena of politics, and so little had he been accustomed to take part in political questions, that at first he
hardly knew which party he belonged to, but he soon found
that the tendency of his early associations had been to give
him a bias in favour of Liberal principles. He was, therefore,
the Liberal candidate for St. Albans, and after a sharp contest
with Alderman Carden, the Conservative candidate, was
returned by a good majority. His proceedings in Parliament,
the partial success of his endeavour to carry his Pharmacy
Bill, his disappointment with the result in that respect, and
his still further disappointment and mortification at finding

that, through the unprincipled conduct of the agents employed
at his election, the borough of St. Albans was disfranchised,
and he was practically deprived of a constituency, although
allowed to retain his seat to the end of the Parliament—all
this has already been noticed.

Mr. Bell's object in seeking a seat in Parliament was simply
that of promoting the passing of a law for regulating the
practice of pharmacy. He succeeded in getting a law passed,
but not the law that was desired, and further legislation was
therefore still wanted. He had not yet accomplished his
object, and as the Parliament to the end of which he retained
his seat was dissolved on the 1st of July, 1852, the day after
that on which the Pharmacy Act received the royal assent,
he had to seek a new constituency or leave to others the
accomplishment of the task he had undertaken. He had
not been implicated in the unlawful proceedings by which
his agents brought discredit on his election for St. Albans,
but the notoriety which the transaction had acquired, left a
sort of stigma, which was never entirely removed, and this
no doubt stood in the way of his getting another seat. He
contested Great Marlow at the election which took place in
the autumn of 1852, but was unsuccessful. At a later period,
in 1854, a vacancy having occurred in Marylebone, the
borough in which he resided, he became a candidate in
opposition to Viscount Ebrington, and although again unsuccessful, he polled a greater number of votes than the successful candidate had obtained at the previous election. In
this contest Mr. Bell received the cordial support of those of
his pharmaceutical brethren who resided in the borough,
showing that a prophet may have honour among his own
kinsmen. It was at this election he appears to have laid the
foundation of the disease which ultimately proved fatal to
him. Having occasion to address large assemblages in different parts of the extensive borough, and being at the same
time unmindful of the requirements of nature in the way of
sustenance, he overtaxed his physical powers, and by unduly
straining his voice, contracted an ulceration of the larynx,
from which he never recovered. That his devotion to the
interests of pharmacy continued undiminished has been
shown by the frequent reference we have had occasion to
make to his services in that direction up to the time of his

death. His friend and partner, Mr. T. H. Hills, and his friend and frequent adviser in cases of doubt or difficulty, Mr. T. N. R. Morson, were his last visitors at Tunbridge Wells, where he died on Sunday, the 12th of June, 1859. He had selected a spot for his interment in the Tunbridge Wells Cemetery, close to the grave of his former friend, Dr. Golding Bird. The instructions he left for his funeral were consistent with his unostentatious deportment through life; but although the arrangements for the ceremony were directed to be confined to his immediate relations, the Council and officers of the Pharmaceutical Society could not be restrained from following the last earthly track of him with whom they had so long laboured harmoniously, and to whom they were accustomed to look, as to one capable of fulfilling the parts both of counsellor and leader.

The loss of one who had filled so important a position as that which Jacob Bell occupied among the members of the pharmaceutical body, was felt to be a serious blow to the interests of the cause with which he had been so intimately associated, but at the same time it was hoped that this misfortune might stimulate others who, although perhaps equally zealous, had hitherto been less energetic, to increased activity. It was obviously important, at any rate, that the depressing influence of the loss of a leader should not be allowed to paralyse the exertions of those whose duty it was now to fill up the ranks. Meetings of the Council were held on the 14th and 16th of June, and again on the 6th and 20th of July. Mr. T. N. R. Morson was elected President, and Mr. Peter Squire, Vice-President. Mr. Adolphus F. Haselden was also elected to fill the vacancy in the Council.

At the meeting of Council on the 6th of July, the following minute and resolutions were passed :—

" The Council of the Pharmaceutical Society, on this its first meeting after the death of its President, Mr. Jacob Bell, desires to record its grateful sense of the invaluable services rendered by him to this society, from its earliest commencement to the day of his death, and of the total self-abnegation in which those services were ever given.

" In order to give permanence to this expression of gratitude :—

" *Resolved*,—That a committee be appointed to take the

requisite steps for forming a Capital Fund, out of which one or more scholarships, bearing the name of Jacob Bell, may be established in connection with the society.

" *Resolved,*—That the following be appointed a committee for carrying out the preliminary arrangements connected with the above resolution:—President, Vice-President, and Treasurer; Messrs. Deane, G. Edwards, Lescher, Sandford, and Waugh, with power to add to their number; and that they report to a special meeting of the Council."

At this meeting of Council the following communication was received:—

"25, CAVENDISH SQUARE, W., 20*th June*, 1859.

" GENTLEMEN,

" By the direction of Mr. James Bell and Mr. Thomas Hyde Hills, the executors of the late Mr. Jacob Bell, I forward to you an extract of his will, whereby the sum of £2,000 is bequeathed to the trustees of the Pharmaceutical Society.

"I have the honour to be, gentlemen,
"Your very obedient servant,
" To the Council of the Pharmaceutical   " GEO. BRACE.
Society of Great Britain."

" *Extract of the Will of Jacob Bell, deceased, late of No.* 15, *Langham Place, and No.* 338, *Oxford Street.*

" I give and bequeath the sum of two thousand pounds to the trustees for the time being of the Pharmaceutical Society of Great Britain, which two thousand pounds are to be paid exclusively and in priority to other legacies out of such part of my personal estate as is by law applicable to such payment, and to be expended in establishing or otherwise increasing the efficiency of a School of Pharmacy, or in promoting pharmaceutical education, in such manner as the Council of the said society may deem expedient, but so that the receipts of the trustees shall be good discharges to my executors."

It was thereupon resolved,

" That the Council gratefully acknowledge the announcement of the bequest of £2,000 by their late highly respected President, Mr. Jacob Bell, to the Pharmaceutical Society, and pledge themselves faithfully to carry out his expressed wishes in the disposition thereof, to the best of their ability."

The President, Mr. Morson, informed the Council that Mr. Bell had, in his presence, executed the transfer of the copyright of the *Pharmaceutical Journal* to the society, and that the document was in the hands of the executors.

At a subsequent meeting of the Council, a communication was received from the solicitor, Mr. Brace, to the effect that, acting under instructions, he had made the requisite entry of the *Pharmaceutical Journal and Transactions* in the Registry book of the Stationers' Company, on behalf of the Pharmaceutical Society.

At a special meeting of the Council, held on the 20th of July, the following report was received and adopted:—

The committee appointed to consider the preliminary steps to be taken for carrying out the proposed establishment of Pharmaceutical Scholarships as a memorial of the late Mr. Jacob Bell, report:—

1. That they deem it desirable, if the amount subscribed be sufficient, to establish two or more scholarships, to be in the gift of the Council of the Pharmaceutical Society for the time being.

2. That they recommend that one or more of these scholarships be open to registered apprentices, and associates of the society who are under 21 years of age, and who shall be considered to have established their claim thereto by capability, industry, and general good conduct: and that in addition to these there be others of a higher grade to be offered, with the view of encouraging the further prosecution of scientific study, to associates under 24 years of age who have passed the major examination.

3. That they propose the following form of circular to be sent to the members, associates, and registered apprentices of the society:—

" Many members of the Pharmaceutical Society and friends of the late Mr. Jacob Bell, having expressed a desire that some monument or testimonial should be erected to the memory of their late President and friend, as a proof of their high estimation of his disinterested exertions in promoting the advancement of pharmaceutical knowledge, thereby elevating those engaged in the practice of pharmacy to the social position occupied by their brethren in other countries, and also his activity in defending them from injurious legislation, the Council have resolved that no more appropriate mode of accomplishing this object, nor one more in accordance with the expressed opinions and wishes of the man they desire to honour, could be adopted than the establishment, by a general subscription, of scholarships, to be called 'The Bell Memorial Pharmaceutical Scholarships,' which shall be awarded, under suitable regulations, to industrious, well-conducted, and competent registered apprentices and associates of the Pharmaceutical Society.

" The details, including the extent of the proposed scholarships, and the conditions on which they shall be awarded, must necessarily depend on the amount of subscriptions obtained; but the Council feel assured that such a sum will be subscribed, as will enable them to establish not only minor scholarships for young men less favoured by fortune than by industry, but also one at least for the advancement of high scientific attainments, so that there may thus be two classes of scholarships tending to advance the reputation and dignity of the Pharmaceutical Society."

The response to this address was both general and liberal. Within a few months subscriptions were received amounting to nearly two thousand pounds, which was invested in the names of trustees, and this sum enabled the Council to found two scholarships of the value of thirty pounds a year each. These scholarships, which are held for one year, are awarded to students in the society's school.

While this memorial was being founded, the Council were considering the most suitable application to make of Mr. Bell's bequest of two thousand pounds; for although it could only be used for the promotion of pharmaceutical education, the precise mode of applying it had not been defined. Those who had control over the fund knew pretty well what Mr. Bell's desire would have been with reference to it, and they were anxious, as far as possible, to act in that direction. They knew that nothing would have been farther from Mr. Bell's desire than the disconnection of the school and the society. There was, however, a proposition for the removal of the laboratory from 17, Bloomsbury Square, to other premises; and as this seemed to present a means by which the school might be enlarged, and much additional accommodation at the same time obtained for other purposes for which

the society required more house-room, the Council favoured
the plan, and gave instructions that inquiries should be made
for premises in the neighbourhood.   Contiguous premises in
the rear of the society's house had been vacant some time
previously, which would have answered the purpose, but they
were not now to be had, nor could any others that were eligible
be found.   The difficulty thus experienced arose partly from
the fact that all the property in the neighbourhood, with the
exception of that which the society occupied and had a lease
of, belonged to the Duke of Bedford, and the Duke's agent
was unwilling to allow a chemical laboratory to be established
on the Bedford estate.   The society had obtained a long lease
of the block of building forming the corner of Bloomsbury
Square and Great Russell Street, which had formerly been a
nobleman's mansion, but had subsequently been divided into
three houses.   The house, 17, Bloomsbury Square, which was
first taken by the society, was one of these.   The whole
block formed an exceptional instance of an isolated building,
belonging to another ground landlord, in the midst of the
Bedford property.

But even this building in its then existing state, although
capable of affording all the accommodation otherwise required for the use of the society, seemed to offer no facility
for the construction of a laboratory.   After it had been decided that the society should occupy the whole of the building, and a suggestion was made that a suite of laboratories
might be erected at the top of the house, extending over the
whole area, which would afford the required accommodation,
this was thought to be a feasible arrangement, and the
opinion of an architect was obtained, which fully justified
the suggestion.   Plans were then prepared for extensive
alterations of the premises, and these were carried into effect
at a cost of several thousand pounds.

Another important matter which occupied the attention of
the Council was the adoption of suitable arrangements connected with the editing of the *Pharmaceutical Journal*.   As
the work had now become the property of the society, it
became necessary to consider what position it should occupy
with regard to the opinions expressed in it editorially.   It
was difficult to lay down any precise rule for the guidance of
those entrusted with its management; but it seemed obvious

that, under the altered condition of proprietorship, it would be desirable to impose a greater amount of restraint upon the expression of opinion than had previously been exercised or required. Three editors were appointed, each taking a special department; namely, Professor Redwood, for Chemistry and Pharmacy; Professor Bentley, for Botany and Materia Medica; and Mr. John Barnard, for Commerce. There was also a committee appointed by the Council, consisting of the President of the society for the time being, Mr. T. N. R. Morson, and Mr. Daniel Hanbury, who conferred with the editors once a month.

We have now entered upon the year 1860, which was characterized by the absence of any great excitement or activity in the pharmaceutical world. Within there was no hot contention or open discord on matters social or political, and without there was no attempt to interfere by legislation with the interests of pharmacy. Several papers were published on pharmaceutical subjects, but they were mostly brief notices of experiences in the preparation or use of medicines either ordered in, or proposed to be introduced into, the Pharmacopœia, and originating in a desire to assist the Pharmacopœia Committee in the work they had in hand. There was, however, one marked exception to the general character of the papers published, in the case of a series of papers which were commenced at this time by Mr. Daniel Hanbury, on "Chinese Materia Medica." These papers, although of slight practical importance, possessed considerable literary and pharmacological interest. Among works of a more substantial character may also be mentioned, Professor Bentley's "Manual of Botany," a book worthy to take its place by the side of Fownes's "Manual of Chemistry." The *Chemical News* (with which was incorporated the *Chemical Gazette*) commenced its career at this time.

In Bloomsbury Square, the house of the society was surrounded by scaffold-poles, and the arrangements of the establishment were in a state of disorder and reorganization. Students were working at chemical and pharmaceutical operations, not in their accustomed places, but wherever unoccupied space could be found for them, and especially in the room that has since become the library. It might be said that the Pharmaceutical Society was moving under the influence of a subdued tone—at low tension—and gathering up its strength for future operations.

That a renewal of strength was necessary was made evident by the breaches which death was repeatedly making in the ranks of those who had been foremost in the fight. The leader had gone, and with him, before him or after him, had departed many of his able coadjutors, whose places were not yet filled up.

Mr. George Walter Smith, the first Secretary and Registrar of the Pharmaceutical Society, died on· the 24th of May, 1860. We have had occasion to allude to the active part Mr. Smith took in the formation of the society in 1841, and subsequently. As Secretary, and afterwards as Registrar, he continued to discharge his duties with untiring energy and great ability, until the end of the year 1856, when declining health obliged him to give up all active pursuits. His latter years were spent in retirement at Brighton, where he died.

In the short space of little more than a month afterwards, one who had been most closely associated with Mr. Smith in the work of establishing the Pharmaceutical Society was called to follow him.

Mr. Robert Adolph Farmar died at his residence in Mount Street, Lambeth, on the 29th of June, 1860. We have already so fully referred to the valuable services rendered by Mr. Farmar in conjunction with Mr. Smith, when the society was first started, that it is only necessary here to say, that he continued to take a warm interest in the society's proceedings up to the time of his death.

Scarcely had this same year expired when another very able, active, and influential member of the society and of its Council followed in the same inevitable track, leaving a gap not easily filled. Mr. J. F. Macfarlan, of Edinburgh, died on the 20th of February, 1861. In early life, Mr. Macfarlan had obtained the diploma of the Royal College of Surgeons of Edinburgh, and for a short time he practised medicine, but he afterwards devoted himself exclusively to the business of a chemist and druggist and manufacturing chemist, in which he was highly successful. He took great interest in public affairs, whether political, religious, social, moral, or economic. When the Municipal Reform Bill first became law in 1833, his fellow-citizens marked their appreciation of the value of his services by placing him at the head of the poll. He was also elected one of the magistrates, and he worthily administered judgment from the bench of the police court. On the formation of the Pharmaceutical Society he became one of the members, and for many years was the representative of the North British Branch at the London Council Board. The early adhesion to the society of a man of so much influence as Mr. Macfarlan had acquired, was of considerable importance to the interests of the cause in Scotland. The Pharmaceutical Society did not in the first instance make much progress there. So much was this the case, that when the Pharmacy Bill was first drafted, its operation was confined to England; and even in 1858, Mr. Bell, in writing on the subject of the North British Branch, said: "The Pharmaceutical Society is not yet fully established in Scotland. Some of the leading chemists of Edinburgh joined it at or near the commencement, and have been steadfast in their endeavours to extend its influence, and commend it to the favourable notice of their neighbours; but it was difficult to overcome the prevailing impression, that it was a London society, and could confer but little benefit on members at a distance. Consequently it made slow progress in the North, and for several years it was doubtful whether any success would attend the endeavour to establish an effective branch in Scotland." A committee in connection with the Bloomsbury Society had been in existence in Edinburgh for several years, but it was not until shortly before the passing of the Pharmacy Act, in 1852, that a separate board of examiners was appointed there. In 1858 an attempt was made to get increased support for the Pharmaceutical Society in North Britain, and a meeting was held in Dundee, at which Mr. Mackay, the active Secretary to the society at Edinburgh, read a paper on "The past and present state of pharmacy; with a special reference to the origin and progress of the Pharmaceutical Society."

It is to the steady, persistent exertions of Mr. Mackay that we must chiefly ascribe the successful establishment and active operations of the North British Branch of the Pharmaceutical Society. After the death of Mr. Macfarlan, Mr. Mackay was elected a member of the London Council Board.

Notwithstanding what was done by the Chemical and Pharmaceutical Societies, it appeared that there was need for a further diffusion of the knowledge of chemistry, for at this time (1860), in and about the City of London, there were intelligent men, merchants, clergymen, and men of position, who could be induced to believe in some of the wildest assumptions of alchemy. Evidence of this was afforded by the short public career in London of a Hungarian refugee, named Nicholas Papaffy, who represented that he had an invention by which he could convert base metals into standard silver. He did not aspire to gold. But he was anxious to join with some men of capital who might be satisfied with making silver by his invention for his and their common benefit. He wanted some bismuth, aluminium, and a few other ingredients; a crucible, a furnace, and men willing to advance capital. All these were placed at his disposal, and he proceeded to manipulate in the presence of Barnett, Cox, Cole, and Company. From the crucible a mass of silver of some ten pounds weight was produced, and confidence was established. Capitalists were induced to join in the undertaking. The members of the new company took offices at 104, Leadenhall Street, and began trading. The inventor was to receive £12 a week as his share of the profits, and having drawn about £600 in advance, and raised, it was said, about £10,000 on bills drawn in the name of the company, he quietly decamped, leaving the furnace and crucible to liquidate the debts, while he pursued his travels in search of new victims, and further discoveries in alchemy.

The year 1860 must not be passed over without noticing a law which came into operation in this year, " For preventing the adulteration of articles of food or drink." This was the first Adulteration Act, which was passed on the 6th of August, 1860, as the result of a lengthened inquiry which took place on the subject before parliamentary committees, and originating with the investigations made chiefly by Dr. Hassall, and published in the *Lancet* in 1851, and subsequently. The Act applied exclusively to the adulteration of food and drink, and did not therefore affect pharmacy. Even with regard to food and drink, its action was not very stringent or likely to be effective. It enacted that, " Every person who shall sell any article of food or drink with which, *to the knowledge of such person*, any ingredient or material *injurious to the health* of persons eating or drinking such

article, has been mixed; and every person who shall sell
expressly warranted as pure and unadulterated any article of
food or drink which is adulterated or not pure, shall, for
every such offence, forfeit and pay a penalty not exceeding
five pounds, nor less than five shillings, together with the
costs of conviction." For carrying the law into effect, local
authorities were empowered to appoint analysts for their
respective districts, but this appointment was left optional
with them. Then the analysts were to possess "competent
medical, chemical, and microscopical knowledge," which was
generally so construed as to require a medical qualification.
Practically, the law remained a dead letter.

A question had more than once arisen with reference to the
sale of an article called "Dandelion Coffee," which had come
into use in some districts, and consisted either of the torrefied
root without admixture, or of the simply ground dry root
mixed with a certain proportion of coffee. This latter preparation seemed to fall within the provisions of the excise law,
which required a licence to be taken out for the sale of coffee,
and at the same time sanctioned no other mixture than that
of chicory. In 1852, Mr. Bell had asked the chairman of
the Board of Inland Revenue whether this preparation was
included among the prohibited mixtures of coffee, and if it
were, how chemists should act when medical men prescribed
dandelion coffee for their patients. In reply, it was stated
that the Board would not interfere if the dandelion coffee
were used as medicine. As this was not considered a satisfactory settlement of the question, Mr. Brady, of Newcastle,
in 1860, on behalf of himself and others, induced the Council
to make a further application, the reply to which was that
the sale would not be interfered with provided the articles
were found free from any admixture of coffee. In order to
legalise the sale of a mixture of dandelion with coffee, three
conditions were to be fulfilled :—1. The dealer must have a
licence. 2. The mixture must be sanctioned by the Board
of Inland Revenue. 3. It must be stated on the label, *This is
sold as a mixture of coffee and dandelion.*

A suggestion having been thrown out that the difficulty
might be overcome by substituting cocoa for coffee, it being
supposed that no licence was required for the sale of cocoa,
the following letter was received bearing upon that point :—

" INLAND REVENUE OFFICE, LONDON,
Jan. 14*th*, 1860.
" SIR,—

" The excise licence under which cocoa is saleable, is for
the sale of tea, coffee, cocoa, chocolate, and pepper.   A
licence is not required for the sale of vinegar.   It is clear
that the Board could not authorize the mixture of dandelion
with cocoa, or the sale of an article called dandelion cocoa,
for the law imposes a penalty of £100 and a forfeiture of
the goods upon any cocoa dealer keeping any vegetable substance as an imitation of, or substitute for cocoa, or calling
any such substance by ' any name of cocoa.'   The law in
this respect is exactly the same as with respect to coffee, the
difference being that the mixture of chicory with coffee,
under certain restrictions, has been allowed by authority of
the Treasury, while no similar authority exists regarding
cocoa.

" THOS. DOBSON, *Assistant Secretary.*"

A rather important regulation was adopted by the Royal
College of Physicians in April, 1860, which seemed likely to
operate beneficially for the interests of the pharmaceutical
body.   It was decided to create a third class of medical men
connected with the college, who, in regard to the nature of
their practice, would occupy a similar position to that of the
apothecaries or general practitioners, but with a restriction
that they should dispense medicines only for their own
patients.   The two previously existing grades recognised by
the college, under the designations of Fellows and Members,
were restricted from dispensing medicines, and they only,
under the new regulation, would be recognised as physicians.
The members of the new grade were to be designated Licen-
tiates of the College of Physicians.   They would not be
entitled to the appellation of Doctor, but would virtually be
general practitioners, holding a licence from the College of
Physicians, and having authority to dispense medicines to
their own patients, but not being allowed in any other way to
engage in the sale of medicines.

It might have been inferred at this time, from some
surrounding circumstances, that the interests of members of
the Pharmaceutical Society, as well as of the whole body of
those engaged in the practice of pharmacy, were in a satis-

factory state of progression towards substantial improvement. But the appearance of quiet prosperity, caused by the absence of threatened interference from without, and of active opposition within, which had prevailed for nearly two years, was rather delusive than real.　The spirit of opposition to the proceedings of the society in Bloomsbury Square had never died out, and only required some active agent, capable of instilling life into the elements and of inducing their organization, to cause them to become again a source of trouble.　Nor was it long before a movement was made in that direction.

In 1861 a society was formed called "The United Society of Chemists and Druggists," the objects of which were thus represented :—

"The society is based upon the principle of co-operation, as essential to the strength. and progress of chemists and druggists as a trading community, with the following objects :—

" 1. The establishment of a Benevolent Fund for the assistance of members in sickness, destitution and death.

" 2. To carry out, by district meetings and combined action, any improvement that may be deemed necessary for the welfare of the trade.

" 3. To promote early and Sunday closing.

" 4. To watch the progress of, and support or oppose any legislative enactment that may affect the interests of chemists and druggists as a trading community.

" 5. To answer any legal questions relating to the trade rights of members, free of cost.

" 6. To keep a register of the transfer of businesses, required partnerships, and situations for assistants, and to be the general excipient and exponent of any other trade requirement."

The committee in their first report stated that they wished to place the society upon a broad numerical basis, and to enable them to do so successfully they determined that the admission fee should be within the means of the poorest member.　It was fixed accordingly at five shillings, and the payment of this fee constituted the only condition of membership.

It could hardly be said, as regarded the Pharmaceutical Society, that the new association was either an opposing or a competing body. The objects of the two societies were to a great extent different, and the parts of the trade to which they respectively appealed were also different; but as they had some objects in common, and as the same members of the trade were not likely to subscribe to both, there was naturally a little jealousy between them. At a later date, however, the United Society took up a position of direct antagonism to the Pharmaceutical Society.

In some respects the appearance in the field of an association having even the semblance of a competitvie character was calculated to produce a beneficial effect on the older society, by stimulating those at the head of affairs to more active exertions, and possibly, also, by inducing them to consider how far their proceedings, and the institution itself with which they were connected, were based upon sound principles, and afforded adequate security for a continuance of the prosperity they had hitherto enjoyed.

In the early part of the year 1861, Mr. Haselden, a member of the Bloomsbury Council, and a frequent contributor to the *Pharmaceutical Journal*, started the question, " Are we progressing ? " which raised a lengthy discussion on several matters of deep import to the welfare of the society and the cause in which it was engaged. The question opened several distinct considerations, but that which assumed the most serious aspect related to the financial prospects of the Pharmaceutical Society. It appears that to some extent this view of the subject originated the discussion, and it is due to the Secretary of the society to say that he was mainly responsible not only for the suggestion, but for the practical form which the subject officially assumed. In the report of the Council presented at the anniversary meeting in May, 1861, reference was made to the bye-laws in the following terms :—" Upon a careful examination of the provisions of the bye-laws, and a reference to the practical working of the existing regulations, relating to the encome of the society, your Council have come to the conclusion that some alteration should be made in the terms of contribution as applied to those hereafter to be admitted into the society, in order to ensure a permanent income adequate to the maintenance of the institution in a fully efficient state."

The data on which this statement was founded had been

previously given in a leading article in the *Pharmaceutical Journal,* in which reference was made to the present and prospective sources of income to the society. Referring to the financial statements which were annually presented at the anniversary meetings, including that which had been then prepared, it was asked, "Does the financial statement afford a correct indication of the strength of the Pharmaceutical Society with regard to numbers? And the answer to this question will be in the negative. Those who now enter the society by *examination are not called upon by the bye-laws to pay an annual subscription, as the fee of five guineas, paid on admission, entitles them to the privileges of membership for life; and according to the existing regulations they continue to receive the Journal of the Society without any further payment.* These members, as well as associates and registered apprentices by examination, do not, with the exception of those admitted during the current year, in any way appear in the financial statement. We cannot, therefore, estimate the numerical strength of the society from this document. The members and associates may be classed under several different heads. Thus we have :—

" 1. Members who have paid a composition fee of twenty guineas, under the original bye-laws.

"2. Members who have paid a composition fee of ten guineas, under the existing bye-laws (1861).

" 3. Members paying an annual subscription of one guinea, admitted before 1853.

" 4. Members who have paid a composition fee of five guineas, admitted by examination since 1852.

" 5. Associates paying an annual subscription of half a guinea, admitted before 1853.

" 6. Associates who have paid the examination fee of three guineas if previously registered, or of five guineas if not registered, admitted since 1852.

"7. Registered apprentices paying an annual subscription of half a guinea, admitted before 1853.

" 8. Registered apprentices who have paid the registration fee of two guineas, admitted since 1852.

"Of these several classes, only 3, 5, and 7 appear from year to year in the financial statement, and the numbers representing them are necessarily decreasing, as no fresh additions can now be made, and their ranks are annually thinned by death and other causes."

It was obvious from this view of the subject, that under the then existing regulations the income of the society must continue to fall off year by year, and that the society would at no distant period die a natural death, unless its current expenses were reduced to the very limited amount derivable from the interest on capital, together with the small number of fees paid on admission by examination, if these should be included. That an alteration was required in the terms on which members, associates, and apprentices, who became such for the future, should be enabled to partake of the benefits conferred by the society, was admitted by all. But in considering what these changes should be, it was suggested by some persons that a further attempt should be made to enlarge the boundaries of the society by admitting old established chemists and druggists into membership, if they produced satisfactory certificates of qualification, and were willing to pay an entrance fee and annual subscription. This was the point on which the discussion principally turned, and with reference to which much difference of opinion was found to exist. Strong objections were urged against relaxing the terms of admission in favour even of old established chemists who had failed to take advantage of the opportunities presented to them at and before the passing of the Pharmacy Act. Pains were taken to ascertain the opinions of members throughout the country on this point, and they were found to be so far adverse to the proposal that it was entirely relinquished. Other changes, however, were adopted almost unanimously, the most important of which consisted in the substitution of annual subscriptions for the fees previously paid by members, associates, and apprentices on their admission into the society. Members were required to pay an annual subscription of a guinea, and associates and apprentices of half a guinea each.

The new bye-laws by which these and other slight changes were effected were passed at a specially convened meeting of the society held on the 15th of January, 1862, subject to some slight alterations which the Council agreed to make for the purpose of more clearly specifying that the door should not again be opened for the admission of members without examination. Another meeting was held on the 16th of April, to receive the final amendments introduced by the Council, and it was then moved by Mr. Sandford, Vice-President, seconded by Mr. Breton, of Brighton, and carried unanimously, " that the said code of bye-laws, as amended, be confirmed and approved as the bye-laws of the society, and take effect from the date of confirmation thereof by one of Her Majesty's principal Secretaries of State, and that all other bye-laws of the society be abrogated." The sanction of Her Majesty's Secretary of State to these bye-laws was given on the 23rd of June, 1862.

The arrangements for the International Exhibition were now occupying much public attention, and several leading pharmacists were conferring together for the purpose of ensuring a creditable exhibition of the materials, both raw and manufactured, that were employed in medicine in this country. A committee was formed consisting of the whole of the Council of the Pharmaceutical Society, the professors of the society, and Messrs. Allchin, Barnes, Bastick, Brewer Cracknell, Darby, Hanbury, Horner, R. Howard, S. Howard, T. Morson, jun., and R. Warington, with T. H. Hills, Treasurer, John Garle, Honorary Curator, and Elias Bremridge, Honorary Secretary. It was resolved,—

" 1. That it is desirable to ensure, as far as possible, at the International Exhibition of 1862, such an exhibition of substances used in medicine as shall fairly represent the existing state of pharmacy in this country.

" 2. That the formation of a collection of drugs and pharmaceutical preparations, contributed by different exhibitors, but arranged systematically in one large group, comprising, if possible, all the substances used in medicine in this country would tend to fulfil the object contemplated in the foregoing resolution."

It was considered desirable to adopt, as far as possible, one uniform method of displaying the articles exhibited in this joint pharmaceutical collection; also that the articles should not be enclosed in glass cases, but arranged on shelves, so that they might be examined by the public under the supervision of an attendant. A subscription was started for defraying the expenses incurred in carrying out these arrangements.

The Council, in their annual report, presented at the meeting of the society in May, 1862, referring to this exhibition stated,—

" The Pharmaceutical Society having been called on to illustrate the present state of pharmacy in the International Exhibition, the Council endeavoured, by the formation of a committee, to enlist the assistance of the members generally and others, that it might appear worthily on so important an occasion.

" The result has been that an extensive collection of drugs and preparations used in medicine has been formed, and placed under the care of an attendant. It has been a principal object in making this collection to obtain specimens from a great number of sources, so that a fair representation may be afforded of the materia medica of this country, arranged in one group, and exhibited in such a way that those who take an interest in this subject may have the means of thoroughly examining the specimens and comparing them with similar substances exhibited in the foreign department."

The collection was considered very creditable to those who united in getting up this joint exhibition of British drugs and medicines ; and not only this part, but the whole of the Exhibition of 1862 proved a success, notwithstanding the adverse influence produced by the death of the Prince Consort, with whom the undertaking had originated.

It had been intended, if the British Pharmacopœia had been published in time, to have included a collection of all the articles described in it as a separate department within the joint pharmaceutical collection at the Exhibition ; but unlooked-for delay in the preparation of the work completely frustrated that object. The prospect had been held out by the Pharmacopœia Committee that the work would probably be issued during the winter of 1861 ; and a meeting of the English, Irish, and Scotch committees took place in September of that year, at which it was expected that final arrangements for publication would be made ; but new difficulties arose and more work had to be done.

In the years 1856–7 a new regulation was introduced by the Director-General of the Army Medical Department with reference to the evidence of qualification required in the persons appointed to dispense medicines for the army. In some instances candidates for the appointment had been required to produce certificates of having passed the examination of the Pharmaceutical Society; but the regulation was not then acted upon uniformly. In 1862 it assumed a more definite character, as indicated by the following letter:—

"ARMY MEDICAL DEPARTMENT, 9th January, 1862.

"SIR,—

"In acknowledging the receipt of your letter of the 2nd instant, I have the honour to inform you that no gentleman can be appointed to a Dispensorship in the army whose age is more than twenty-six or less than twenty-one years; and no name can be placed on the list of candidates until the applicant produces evidence of bearing a good moral character, of having passed the examinations of the Pharmaceutical Society of London, and of having been duly registered as a pharmaceutical chemist.

"I have the honour, etc.,

"J. H. GIBSON, Director-General."

The improvements which had been for some time in progress at the house of the Pharmaceutical Society had provided greatly increased accommodation for the operations connected with the various departments of the establishment. The library and museums, the rooms for examinations, the Secretary's offices, and council and committee rooms, were all re-arranged and extended. A tolerably good lecture theatre was provided, and above all, forming the uppermost story of the enlarged premises, there was a suite of well-lighted and ventilated laboratories, capable of accommodating a large number of students. All this extension of facilities for carrying out the objects of the society had not been effected without the expenditure of a large sum of money, and the members naturally looked for some return in the way of an extension of the amount of work accomplished. In one respect, however, the provisions made were defective. Enlarged museums and library called for more exclusive and efficient services of a curator for the one and a librarian for the other. It had become the practice for many years past, with a view to economy, to heap many duties on to the shoulders of a few officers, and this was especially the case with regard to the departments alluded to, and to the laboratory, lectures, and scientific committees. Formerly the laboratory had been almost always full to overflowing; but now that its accommodation was more than doubled, it was found that in order to keep it in the same satisfactory condition, more undivided attention was required from the professor, and it was therefore decided to appoint a teacher for this special duty.

In 1862 Mr. John Attfield was appointed, under the title of Director and Demonstrator of Chemistry and Pharmacy, to take the entire management of the practical classes in the laboratory, with the understanding that he was to devote himself entirely to the work. At a subsequent period the title of the office was changed to that of Professor of Practical Chemistry; and the professor, in addition to this title, took the degree of Ph.D. The *Pharmaceutical Journal* of October, 1862, remarked: "The laboratory and the lectures were established and are maintained for the benefit of pharmaceutical students, whose special requirements have been studied in the educational arrangements which have been made. These arrangements have been recently revised and improved by the Council, and a new programme is issued, which may be obtained from the Secretary. If the efforts thus made to render the school of pharmacy fully efficient should be responded to by pharmaceutical students as they ought to be, and as we trust they will be, the present session may prove the commencement of a new era, in which the provisions for education so liberally made and maintained for many years, will be not only received, but sought after, and not only recognised, but appreciated and duly acknowledged by young men who, in their turn, will become creditable members of the pharmaceutical body, and active promoters of pharmaceutical education."

During the session of the School of Pharmacy which had just passed, a number of former and present students of the school presented a handsome testimonial to Professor Bentley, consisting of a silver tea service and an illuminated address on vellum.

In July, 1862, the first "Act for the Safe Keeping of Petroleum" was passed. Subsequent Acts relating to the same subject have been passed in 1868, 1871, and 1879.

A very important subject, affecting the interests of the

Pharmaceutical Society and of its members individually, came
before the notice of Parliament in 1862, in connection with a
Bill relating to the mode of summoning juries. Hitherto the
only privilege which the Legislature had conferred on members
of the Pharmaceutical Society was the exclusive right to use
a title which might be understood to imply a professional
qualification. This, although a privilege of some value to
those who had a sound justification for its use, was by many
thought but little of, and something of a more substantial
nature was looked for which might act as a stimulus to the
work by which alone the title could be fully justified. An
opportunity presented itself, in connection with the Juries Bill,
for obtaining a concession to pharmaceutical chemists which
was acknowledged to be a material benefit. Professional men
had long been exempted from the duty of serving on juries.
This was conceded to medical men on the ground that their
professional services were required by the public who employed
them, and that to take them away from the performance of
such duties might be the means of inflicting serious injury on
their patients. It was considered that a somewhat similar
ground for exemption existed in the case of chemists and
druggists, and advantage was taken of the passage of the
Juries Bill through Parliament to make a claim on their
behalf. There were, however, two difficulties in the way of
promoting the claim on behalf of the whole body of chemists
and druggists,—first, that there was no sufficient means of
defining who was a chemist and druggist, and secondly, that
if all who assumed the name were exempted, it would seriously
diminish the jury lists and increase the difficulty already
experienced in getting the duty of juryman efficiently performed. An exaggerated statement which had been put
forth by the United Society of Chemists and Druggists, to
the effect that there were about forty thousand chemists and
druggists in the country, strengthened the influence of the
latter objection and rendered the claim of the whole body
quite untenable. The difficulty was overcome by confining
the claim to registered pharmaceutical chemists ; and a clause
was prepared, to the effect that " All persons duly registered
as pharmaceutical chemists according to the provisions of an
Act intituled, an Act for Regulating the Qualifications of
Pharmaceutical Chemists, shall be and are hereby absolutely

freed and exempted from being returned and from serving
upon any juries or inquests whatsoever, and shall not be
inserted in the lists to be prepared by virtue of the principal
Act or of this Act." This clause was proposed to be introduced into the Bill while passing the committee in the House
of Commons; but although from the promises of support given
there was every prospect of its being accepted without opposition, it was at last opposed by Sir George Grey, on the
ground that, as the Bill related ostensibly to the *mode* of
summoning juries, this was not the proper occasion for exempting persons from serving on juries, and that if pharmaceutical
chemists ought to be exempted, this should be effected by a
Bill introduced for that purpose. In the face of this opposition
the motion was not pressed to a division, and the Bill therefore passed the Commons without the proposed clause. It
was discovered afterwards, however, that although the House
of Commons had rejected the clause for exempting pharmaceutical chemists, they had at the same time introduced a
clause for exempting the "managing clerks to attorneys,
solicitors, and proctors," which seemed inconsistent with the
statement made by Sir George Grey. The result of the
efforts which had thus been made on behalf of pharmaceutical
chemists was entirely unexpected, and appeared to have
originated either in a misapprehension or in the exercise of
some unseen influence.

When the Bill went into the House of Lords a petition was
presented from the Council of the Pharmaceutical Society
praying their lordships to extend to pharmaceutical chemists
the privilege for which they had in vain asked the Commons.
The justice of the claim having been admitted by several
noble lords, including Lord Chelmsford and Lord Portman,
who had charge of the Bill in the upper House, a clause
similar in effect to that previously proposed in the House of
Commons was introduced in the Lords' Committee, and this
was passed through the House without any opposition. The
exemption, however, was now made to comprise veterinary
surgeons as well as pharmaceutical chemists.

As no opposition to these exemptions was in the slightest
degree hinted at during the progress of the Bill through the
House of Lords, it was hoped the Commons would accept the
Bill in the form in which it was returned to them, especially

as they had already sanctioned the introduction of exemptions by exempting lawyers' clerks.

A petition was presented to the House of Commons as had previously been done to the House of Lords, and interest was made with members of the House through local secretaries and others throughout the country. But unfortunately the objection of the Secretary of State was not removed, and the ground of his objection had, in one respect, been strengthened by the addition of a new class of men, namely, veterinary surgeons, for whom exemption was now asked. Sir George Grey therefore again appeared in opposition to the clause introduced by the Lords, and having moved its non-confirmation, the numbers on a division were equal, namely fifty-three on each side. The Speaker had therefore to give the casting vote, which he did in favour of Sir George Grey's motion.

The Commons having thus rejected an amendment which had been introduced by the unanimous decision of the House of Lords, it became necessary to return the Bill to the Upper House for their reconsideration. This took place on the 28th of July, when Lord Wensleydale, after reading the second clause of the Bill, said their Lordships had amended it by adding words which exempted the registered pharmaceutical chemists from serving on juries, and he thought it a wise alteration of the law. Physicians and surgeons had, in consequence of their being often required in cases of great emergency, been exempted from these duties; and he could not see any reason why the members of the Pharmaceutical Society, which consisted of only about 2000 members, should not be placed in the same category. These gentlemen were employed in very responsible and delicate duties, in making up prescriptions, and it was desirable that they should not be called away from those duties to attend at distant places as jurymen. There were, he said, about 40,000 persons * employed as chemists and druggists, who no doubt made up prescriptions, but those gentlemen did not undergo any examination, nor were they members of a registered society. It was not intended to apply the exemption to them. He then moved

---

* This statement was obviously founded on the erroneous assertion emanating from the United Society of Chemists and Druggists, to which allusion has been previously made.

that the alterations made in the Bill by the Commons, so far
as they affected or concerned the registered pharmaceutical
chemists, be not agreed to, but that the amendments made in
that respect by their Lordships be insisted upon.

The question was then put, "That all the words which
related to the pharmaceutical chemists be retained in the
Bill," and it was declared that the "contents" had it.

Lord Denman then begged to move that the amendments
made by the Lords in favour of exempting veterinary surgeons, who were much fewer in number than pharmaceutical
chemists, and who often rendered service in saving the lives
of animals, should be insisted upon. On this question being
put, the "non-contents" had it.

This result was considered favourable to the prospect of
obtaining the consent of the House of Commons to the exemption of pharmacists, for, as veterinary surgeons were now
excluded, the Commons could with better grace give way.

The question came again before the Commons on the 31st
of July; and as Sir George Grey had intimated his intention
of not offering any further opposition to the Lords' amendment in its altered form, it was hoped the difficulty had been
overcome. But although the Home Secretary appeared to
have been appeased, opposition arose from another quarter.
Mr. Edward Craufurd moved, " That this House doth insist
upon its disagreement to so much of the Lords' amendment
in page 1 line 13, as their Lordships insist upon." On the
question being thus again raised, Sir George Grey and Sir
G. C. Lewis expressed their intention to support the motion.
This was an exciting moment. The Lords were with us, but
ministers in the Lower House were against us. On a previous
occasion the Commons had been equally divided. How will
the division be now? Motion put, that the Lords' amendment be rejected. Ayes 12—Noes 45.

The Secretary and a few members of the Council, who had
been anxiously watching the proceedings and waiting the
result, retired, and went on their homeward way rejoicing.

It must not be supposed that this very satisfactory result
was obtained without great exertions being made to secure
it. The Council, with the Secretary in London and the local
secretaries and members throughout the country, were
actively engaged in urging upon Members of Parliament the

importance of the question and the true merits of the claim
made on behalf of the pharmaceutical body. It is very certain,
that without the vigilance, promptness, and energy displayed
at head-quarters, and chiefly by the Secretary, without the influence brought to bear when and where it was most required,
and without the support derived from the soundness of the
principles upon which the claim was urged, the battle would
not have been won, and the Council in Bloomsbury Square
would, at least for that year, have been deprived of the satisfaction of congratulating themselves and their constituents
upon the triumph achieved through the influence of *organization, registration*, and *qualification*.

The importance of the attainment of this result was admitted by all who were capable of discerning the influence it
would exert on the position and prospects of the Pharmaceutical Society. The *Lancet*, in an article headed " The Druggists' Franchise," did full justice to the claims of those who
by a course of training had acquired a character to which, as
well as to the nature of their occupation, they were indebted
for this acquisition of privilege.

The year 1862 forms one of the epochs of our history. Two
decades had elapsed since the starting of the society in
Bloomsbury Square, the commencement and ending of each
of which was signalized by an important event; the granting
of the Charter in 1842, the passing of the Pharmacy Act in
1852, and the attainment of enfranchisement, or freedom from
service on juries, in 1862. These may be represented respectively as the epochs of *recognition*, of *designation*, and of *enfranchisement*.

To the question " Are we progressing ? " a satisfactory
answer might now have been given. The laws and bye-laws
the passing of which had tended to confirm the stability and
promote the success of the Pharmaceutical Society, served at
the same time to represent the progress of pharmaceutical
knowledge and the advancement of pharmacy, for it was only
as these results occurred and could be traced as practical out-
comes of the society's operations, that recognition and aid
could be obtained from the Government and Legislature.

Evidences of the state of pharmaceutical knowledge among
pharmacists have been afforded in the references we have had
occasion to make to work done and duties undertaken and

efficiently performed. That much of this work was not of a
highly scientific character is not surprising. Scientific training was required for scientific work, and it would have been
unreasonable to look for the latter before the former had
produced its required effect. Those who contributed to the
advancement of pharmacy in the early stages of the operations
in Bloomsbury Square, wisely, if not necessarily, confined their
attention principally to the practical details of pharmaceutical
processes and operations. In this direction a good deal of
useful work had been done. Processes for the preparation of
tinctures, infusions, extracts, pills, ointments, and other forms
of medicine had been submitted to experimental investigation
or commented upon and freely discussed. This in fact
formed the most useful kind of matter that could have been
furnished at the pharmaceutical meetings at that time ; and
indeed at all times it must form much of what is available for
such occasions. Among the class of pre-existing pharmacists
who chiefly contributed to keep up a supply of papers for the
meetings and Journal, may be mentioned Deane, Morson,
Squire, Bell, Savory, Barry, Ince, Southall, Haselden, Alsop,
Bastick, Barnes, Greenish, Sandford, Smith, Donovan, Mackay,
Hooper, Bland, Whipple, etc. To these may be added the
professors in the Bloomsbury school who were outside the class
of pharmacists, and the professors who had sprung from that
stock and might therefore be included in the class. Then
there was a class of younger men who were becoming every
year more prominent and the record of whose work was to be
found in the transactions of local associations in various parts
of the country, as well as in that of the parent Society. These
were mostly the offspring of the system of education which
had originated with the Pharmaceutical society. Some of
them had been for several years guiding spirits to whose influence the good work done in promoting the cultivation of
scientific as well as practical pharmacy was due, especially
in provincial districts. Thus we have John Baker Edwards
and Henry Sugden Evans at Liverpool, Richard Reynolds at
Leeds, Henry B. Brady and Barnard S. Proctor at Newcastle,
G. F. Schacht and R. W. Giles at Bristol, Charles Ekin at
Bath, T. B. Groves at Weymouth, Edward C. C. Stanford
at Worthing and afterwards at Glasgow, Daniel Hanbury,
Benjamin H. Paul, Joseph Ince, Michael Carteighe, Samuel

Gale, Charles Umney and others in London and elsewhere, who were exercising important influences upon the present and future condition of British pharmacy.

The unauthorized use of methylated spirit in pharmacy was brought again prominently under notice in 1862, by Mr. Richard Reynolds, of Leeds, Mr. H. B. Brady, of Newcastle, and others. The attention, not only of the Pharmaceutical Society, but also of the College of Physicians, had been directed to this subject several years previously, in 1857, and it was then thought that the practice complained of had been suppressed; but it now appeared that a much more extensive use than was then made of methylated spirit for medical and other illegal purposes, had subsequently arisen. The spirit was purified and used for making tinctures and other preparations, and in some instances it was sold as an intoxicating beverage. Such a result might have been anticipated as a natural consequence of the leniency adopted by the Excise authorities as indicated by the following communication :—

"INLAND REVENUE OFFICE, LONDON, *July 29th*, 1862.

"SIR,—In reply to your inquiry of the 22nd instant, I am desired to acquaint you that the Board do not object to the manufacture and sale of any strictly pharmaceutical preparation made with methylated spirit, so long as it appears that such preparations are used for medical purposes, and not made a cover for such spirit being used as a beverage. I am to add, that a licence is not required for the sale of any medicinal preparations made with methylated spirit.

"THOMAS DOBSON, *Secretary.*"

It was felt that under these circumstances it became an imperative duty on the part of the Pharmaceutical Society, to adopt the most efficient means they could to check a practice which, if continued, would be highly injurious to the interests of pharmacy, by causing a depreciation and debasement of drugs, and a loss of character among druggists. At a meeting of the Council held on the 4th of February, 1863, the following protest was entered in the minutes, and ordered to be published in the transactions of the society :—

" The attention of the Council having been directed for some time past to the use in pharmacy of methylated spirit, in the place of pure spirit of wine, they think it incumbent

upon them, as the representatives of a society founded for the
promotion of pharmaceutical science in this country, to declare
their opinion that such substitution is highly undesirable.

" Methylated spirit is a compound of pure spirit of wine, to
which one-tenth of its volume of imperfectly purified wood-
naphtha has been added, the object of such addition being
that of rendering the mixture *unpotable* through its offensive
odour and taste.   This spirit, being sold duty free, can be
employed by the chemical manufacturer as a solvent in many
processes, for which, from its greater cost, duty-paid spirit
would be commercially inapplicable.   But, in the preparation
of those medicines which contain spirit as the vehicle or
menstruum by which more active substances are administered,
the employment of a compound so uncertain and offensive as
methylated spirit, is, in the opinion of the Council, highly improper, and by no means to be justified upon the plea of its
lower cost.

" The Council desire to draw the attention of pharmaceutical chemists to these facts, and earnestly request their co-
operation in discountenancing such a substitution."

This was all that appeared to be practicable for the furtherance of the proposed object while the law remained as it was.
In process of time, however, changes were effected in the law,
and also in the regulations which the Board of Inland Revenue
was authorized to impose on those who used methylated spirit.
Laws were passed in 1865 and 1866, by the former of which
methylated spirit, if purified, was made subject to the same
duty as ordinary spirits, and by the second the use of methylated spirit was prohibited, under a severe penalty, from being
used in the preparation of any medicine for internal use, except
sulphuric ether and chloroform.   In accordance with the
altered state of the law, the Board of Inland Revenue, on the
9th of August, 1866, issued a " General Order " to the effect
that " The use of methylated spirit or any derivative thereof in
the manufacture or preparation of tinctures, medicated spirits,
hyponitrous ether, or other pharmaceutical preparations, or in
the manufacture or preparation of any other article or substance capable of being used as a beverage, or internally as a
medicine, is now illegal, and the sale or possession thereof by
any person is also illegal.

" Should any chemist desire to use methylated spirit in any

process necessary for the production of substances used in medicine, and in which no spirit or derivative thereof shall remain after the completion of such process, special application must be made to the Commissioners for leave to use the methylated spirit for such purpose."

A subsequent order in 1870, stated "that chemists be allowed to use methylated spirit in the production of a new medicine termed hydrate of chloral, as being an article within the scope of the 5th paragraph of the General Order of the 9th of August, 1866, viz., one in which no methylated spirit or derivative thereof, remains after completion of the process of manufacture."

In the year 1863 an important fresh development of British pharmacy took place, which resulted in the formation of a new association, the chief object of which was the encouragement of scientific inquiry and research among those engaged in the practice of pharmacy. At an earlier period, in 1852, Mr. Schacht, of Clifton,—at a meeting of chemists and druggists held for the purpose of considering the provisions of the Pharmacy Act,—had suggested the establishment of annual meetings for scientific objects connected with pharmacy, which should circulate through the chief towns in the provinces, somewhat upon the model of the Provincial Medical Association. He thought that meetings of this character, held annually in different localities, would have the effect of stimulating the provincial members to a more active co-operation, and that they might often be made highly instructive by selecting, as the places of meeting, towns which presented peculiar objects of manufacturing interest. Mr. Schacht contemplated making these peripatetic meetings a department of the Pharmaceutical Society. The idea, however, was not further worked out at that time, and the state of the society was not then such as to favour its being carried into effect. After ten years of incubation it began to show symptoms of active vitality. Mr. Reynolds, of Leeds, resuscitated the scheme in a slightly modified form, proposing to establish an institution independent of the Pharmaceutical Society; and this being supported by Mr. Brady, of Newcastle, received the concurrence of Mr. Schacht, although he still rather held to his original opinion. It was decided to call the association the British Pharmaceutical Conference. Its first meeting was held at Newcastle on the 2nd of September, 1863, Mr. Henry Deane occupying the chair. At this meeting the association was organized and its officers appointed. From the small gathering which met on this occasion the Conference has grown to be an important institution, from which much good work has emanated.

Concurrent with the proposition for the establishment of the Pharmaceutical Conference, and emanating to a great extent from the same source, was a design for instituting local examinations in different parts of the country, in connection with the Pharmaceutical Society. This subject was considered by the Council, but no further action was taken with reference to it.

Excise interference was a frequent source of trouble to druggists, and some new cause for such interference was continually arising. At this time it was the sale of a medicine called orange quinine wine. A case was brought under the notice of the Council which led to the following correspondence on this subject:—

"17, BLOOMSBURY SQUARE, *November* 10*th*, 1863.

" To the Honourable
    The Commissioners of the Inland Revenue.

" GENTLEMEN.—I beg very respectfully to draw your attention to, and to solicit information on, a subject of much importance to the public generally, but of especial consequence to pharmaceutical chemists and other retailers of medicine— the sale of medicated wines.

" It may be convenient that I should state that this matter has recently been brought before your honourable board by Mr. George S. Woolley, of Manchester, and that a reply has been sent to him, signed Wm. Corbett, Secretary.

" Mr. Woolley is therein informed that it is, by law, necessary that he should take out a 'sweets licence,' for the sale of his 'orange quinine wine;' but that the board will not insist on his doing so 'if the wine be sold under the patent medicine licence, and have a stamp on each bottle.'

" I cannot say whether there was any special circumstance in Mr. Woolley's case, in the wording of his label or otherwise, which made him liable to the licence or stamp, or that rendered the one avoidable by the adoption of the other; but

I beg most respectfully, on behalf of the pharmaceutical chemists of Great Britain, whom this society represents, to ask, whether the sale of medicated wines, prepared either with British or foreign wine, does really involve the necessity to the vendor to possess a licence of any kind ?

" I may submit to you that for centuries wine of various kinds has been used as a menstruum for medicinal substances, and instance as familiar examples, *aloes, antimony, colchicum, ipecacuanha, rhubarb,* and *steel,*—these are compounds of foreign wines; but more recently advantage has been taken of the acid and aromatic properties of orange wine to use it as a solvent of quinine, the particular preparation now brought in question.

" All these articles are used as medicine and *medicine only.* By the admixture of drugs they are entirely taken out of the category of *beverages,* and,—whether by special exemption or common understanding I know not,—they have always been sold without licence by chemists.

" Feeling assured that your honourable board can have no wish to throw impediments in the way of medical science, or of trade, I venture to hope that you will kindly vouchsafe me the information now sought, and subscribe myself with all respect,

" Your most obedient servant,

" George W. Sandford,

" President of the Pharmaceutical Society of Great Britain."

" Inland Revenue Office, 3rd December, 1863.

" Sir.—I am desired by the Commissioners to inform you, in reply to your letter of the 10th ult., respecting the sale of ' medicated wines,' that they are advised that whenever the articles are held out by label or advertisement as beneficial to persons suffering from any ailment affecting the human body, they can only legally be sold under a ' patent medicine licence,' and with a stamped label on each packet; and also. in strictness, under an Excise foreign or British wine licence, according to the character of the wine.

" The board, however, have instructed me to add that, except in cases where there may be reason to believe that a beverage is being sold under colour of a medicine, they will not interfere with the sale, without an Excise licence, of medicated wines of the description adverted to, provided that such medicines do not fall under the category of patent medicines.

"I am, Sir, your obedient servant,

"WM. CORBETT."

"G. W. SANDFORD, Esq."

This case serves to illustrate the way in which Excise interference is sometimes caused, for it was found, on further inquiry, although not with reference to Mr. Woolley, that orange quinine wine was sometimes sold containing so little quinine that three or four glasses of it might be taken at any time. In such instances the introduction of the quinine might be construed as a colourable pretext for evading the law.

It will be observed from the foregoing correspondence, that Mr. Sandford was now President of the Society; Mr. T. H. Hills was at the same time Vice-president. The former continued to fill the presidential chair until after the passing of the Pharmacy Act, 1868, in which he took so deep an interest.

The session of Parliament of 1863 was fertile in small attempts at the passing of laws which more or less affected pharmacy. The Bills on their way were subject to so many alterations, as was usually the case, that the committee appointed by the Council was kept in an equal state of watchfulness and uncertainty.

The Council, at a meeting specially convened on the 13th of May, to consider "A Bill to Prohibit the Sale and Use of Poisoned Grain in certain Cases," decided to petition Parliament against some of its provisions. They pointed out "that this Bill is probably intended to prevent the destruction of small birds; but your petitioners humbly submit, that in effect it will go much further, and render it penal to sell or use any poison for the destruction of rats, mice, or other vermin, or of any cat, dog, or other domestic animal which it may be desirable to destroy speedily and easily: that it will also render the advantageous and now almost universally adopted process of dressing seed-wheat (prior to sowing) with poisonous salts for the prevention of smut, at all times liable to penal misconstruction." In consequence of these and similar representations the Bill was so far modified as to render it unobjectionable, and in that form it passed.

An " Exhibition Medals Bill," for preventing fraudulent claims to distinction, in connection with public exhibitions, also passed.

A Bill for decimalizing weights and measures went through a second reading and then disappeared.

A Bill for preventing accidental poisoning was introduced by Lord Raynham ; but it came to an untimely end, being summarily rejected.

Towards the latter end of 1863, a new and very important cause of excitement arose among chemists and druggists, connected with the subject of legislation. A committee of the Medical Council had been considering the provisions of the Act under which the Medical Council was appointed, with a view to its amendment, and in their report, now presented, they recommended that application should be made to Parliament for a new Medical Act, embodying all the principal provisions of the Act of 1858, but with some material alterations and additions, involving questions of vast importance to the pharmaceutical body. It was proposed that the new Bill should include pharmacy among the departments of medical practice over which the Medical Council should exercise control. In this respect, therefore, the proposed measure would supersede part of the duty of the Pharmaceutical Society ; but while it would thus relieve the society of part of its responsibility, it would at the same time accomplish objects which the society contemplated and desired but had not been able to realize, and it would leave the society to carry out its system of education and examination under a control similar to that exercised over the medical colleges and licensing boards.

The propositions, as far as related to pharmacy, that were comprised in the draft Bill which had been prepared by the committee and sent by the Medical Council to the corporations whose interests were involved, for the purpose of obtaining an expression of opinion, were as follows :—

1. The establishment of a general system of education and examination, to be *regulated* by the Medical Council.

2. The registration of all persons qualified to practice pharmacy, as tested by such examinations.

3. The restriction of the right to dispense or compound the prescriptions of physicians or surgeons, to qualified practitioners in pharmacy, and the imposition of a penalty upon

those who should keep open shop for compounding medicines without having passed the required examination.

4. The appointment by the Medical Council of inspectors, whose duty it should be to see that the provisions of the Act, affecting pharmacy, were duly carried into effect.

5. The prohibition of the sale of all secret remedies, and the imposition of a penalty for selling any patent or quack medicine, unless a sworn certificate of the composition of such medicine were exposed for inspection in the shop or place where it was sold.

The opinion thus conveyed by the committee of the Medical Council, through their report, that further legislation was required with reference to the practice of pharmacy, and especially the indication afforded by the same high authority as to what the general nature of that legislation should be, was calculated greatly to strengthen the hands of those members of the Pharmaceutical Society and of its Council who had long been seeking the attainment of some of the objects specified. At the same time it was not likely that the proposal, as made, would be acceded to by the druggists, or that any modification of it could be effected that would satisfy both them and the Medical Council. The subject could not fail to elicit a good deal of discussion among medical men as well as chemists and druggists; and of the latter there were the two classes, one represented by the Pharmaceutical Society and the other by the United Society of Chemists and Druggists, whose opinions might not coincide. In the Medical Council itself remarks were made which showed that, although there was a general concurrence of opinion in favour of restricting the practice of pharmacy to qualified and examined men, there was a disinclination to undertake the duty of regulating the system of education and examination that should be adopted. Dr. Storrar, the representative of the University of London, said, "Nothing could certainly be more unsatisfactory than the state of pharmacy in this country; but it would be an unfortunate act of the Council to embroil itself with the druggists. The Council should drop pharmacy and encourage the Pharmaceutical Society to go on with an independent measure." Dr. Sharpey, one of the Secretaries of the Royal Society, and a member of the Council nominated by the Government, was in favour of independent legislation for

Y

pharmacy; and other members expressed a similar opinion. Dr. Christison "disapproved of any attempt to introduce pharmacy into the Medical Act. The present state of the practice of pharmacy was a disgrace to the country and to the Legislature. He hoped, however, that the Council would not meddle with the subject, except by offering its aid and influence to any body which should take up the subject of legislation in regard to pharmacy; and he thought that this could be entrusted to no better persons than the pharmaceutical chemists of the country."

The Medical Council, after an expression of opinion similar to the foregoing, which was perhaps partly caused by a little growling outside, relinquished the idea of attempting to legislate for pharmacy, but passed the following resolution:—

"That a communication be addressed to the Secretary of State for the Home Department, drawing his attention to the present defective state of the law regarding the practice of pharmacy, under which any person, however ignorant, might undertake it, and expressing the opinion of the General Medical Council, that some legislative enactment was urgently called for to ensure competency in persons keeping open shops for dispensing medicines and for the compounding of physicians' and surgeons' prescriptions."

This was the key-note to pharmaceutical legislation; but who was to undertake the leadership in the performance? The subject was left by the Medical Council in a state in which it was ripe for further action, and the Pharmaceutical Society was clearly pointed to as the most suitable body to organize and execute future proceedings.

But it soon appeared that Bloomsbury Square was not to have it all its own way. The growl to which we have alluded· as having probably helped to discourage the Medical Council from taking further action in reference to pharmacy, emanated chiefly from the United Society of Chemists and Druggists. It was not unnatural that this should be so; for to those outside the pale of the Pharmaceutical Society there was more cause for alarm than there was to registered and examined men. The Bloomsbury Society being incorporated by Royal Charter and protected by Act of Parliament, its members were comparatively safe from further interference, unless it might be that of the suggested inspectors, which all would object to.

Bloomsbury therefore maintained its equanimity, and waited the result of the decisions to be arrived at by the medical licensing bodies, and, founded on these, the decision of the Medical Council.

While this was occurring, and very soon after the report of the Committee of the Medical Council was made public, the United Society of Chemists and Druggists got up meetings in different parts of the country to oppose and prevent "the unwarrantable interference of the Medical Council with the rights of dispensing chemists."

Hitherto the United Society had not done much to justify its existence. It had an office in New Ormond Street, and an active secretary who appeared to be almost ubiquitous; but it had neither library, museum, lecture room, nor any means for imparting knowledge to, or testing the qualifications of, its members. The value of scientific qualification for the practice of pharmacy appeared indeed to be held at small account in New Ormond Street, although some qualification was found to be necessary in order to obtain recognition for the members of the Society. This fact was forced upon the attention of the United Society on the occasion of the passing of the Juries Act, when it failed to obtain for its members the exemption granted to pharmaceutical chemists; and the cause of that failure was referred to in the following resolutions passed by the Manchester committee in October, 1862.

" 1. This meeting regrets that the praiseworthy exertions made by the executive committee of the United Society of Chemists and Druggists, to get the clause exempting members of the trade from serving on juries, were not crowned with success.

" 2. That in the opinion of this committee, the principal cause of failure arose from the difficulty of defining, to the satisfaction of Her Majesty's Government, the qualifications of a chemist and druggist.

" 3. That, to obviate this difficulty, it is desirable some qualification should be named, upon which future legislation may be based; and this committee, in correspondence with the central committee, pledges itself earnestly to consider this subject before the next meeting of Parliament."

The reference thus made to "the meeting of Parliament," would seem to indicate that at that time, and arising from their experience in connection with the passing of the Juries Act, the members of the United Society felt that "some qualification," together with legislative or other recognition, was necessary to enable them to obtain the position to which they aspired. But still, no real progress was made in that direction; and after the expiration of another year, when a fresh stimulus was afforded by the proceedings in the Medical Council, we find the following resolutions passed by the Central Committee of the United Society, in August, 1863.

"1. That the proposal of the Medical Council to forcibly dispossess upwards of 30,000 chemists and druggists of their practice, to dispense medicine, is an unwarrantable interference with their civil rights and trade interests, and would be attended with danger and injustice to the entire community.

"2. That to protect the chemists and druggists from unnecessary legislative restriction, and the public from incompetent dispensers, a complete registration is necessary; and that this can best be secured by the general act of incorporation of the trade, as proposed by the United Society of Chemists and Druggists, based as it is upon a recognition of existing rights, and the inexpensive and effective mode of securing the practical knowledge required."

There was here again, as previously, a vague allusion made to the qualification contemplated by this section of the, so-called, 30,000 druggists of the country, and to "the inexpensive and effective mode" contemplated for "securing the practical knowledge required."

On the 27th of November, 1863, a meeting of the trade was convened by the United Society, and held at 20, New Ormond Street, with Mr. Alderman Dakin in the chair. This may be taken as a meeting of the United Society, for those who took part in the proceedings were men identified with that body. The following resolutions were passed:—

"1. That the chemists and druggists now assembled recognise the desirability of giving all possible encouragement to scientific and educational qualification for the trade of a chemist and druggist; but they consider themselves, in common with their brethren, quite competent to accomplish all needful reform in their own body, and repudiate the 56th and 57th clauses of the proposed Act of the Medical Council, as being unjust in principle and an unwarrantable attempt to interfere with their rights as independent citizens."

" 2. That an act of incorporation, based upon a recognition of existing rights, and subjecting every future candidate for the trade to an educational test, as suggested by the United Society of Chemists and Druggists, is most desirable ; and this meeting would urge upon the trade the necessity of a combined and determined effort for its attainment."

It might now be considered that the United Society was pledged to a course of action having for its object the incorporation of some hitherto undefined body, and the requirement of some proof of undefined qualification from all who should in future become chemists and druggists. Certainly, anything less specific than this it might have puzzled the authorities in New Ormond Street to devise or suggest.

Although the Council of the Pharmaceutical Society had taken no immediate action with reference to the proceedings in the Medical Council,—a course which might be ascribed to the strong impression entertained by them that the clauses in the proposed measure, which had created so much alarm among chemists and druggists, would never be passed in the form in which they were introduced there,—yet it could not be said that the members of the society were quite at ease on this point; in fact, there was a general feeling that something ought to be done, if not to oppose, at least to supersede legislation on pharmacy by the Medical Council. This feeling became stronger when it was found that the Medical Council was disposed to drop the subject of pharmacy, and leave pharmaceutical legislation to be worked out by pharmacists themselves.

In the early part of 1864, a requisition, signed by upwards of 300 members, was presented to the Council of the Pharmaceutical Society, to the following effect :—

" Gentlemen,—

" We, the undersigned, believing that it is highly desirable for the protection of the public that all future chemists and druggists should undergo a due professional examination before commencing business, hereby request you to convene a general meeting of the members of our society, for the purpose of considering the expediency of an immediate appli-

cation to Parliament for an amended Pharmacy Act, by which
(following the precedent of the Apothecaries' Act) *the legitimate interests of those already in business should be protected,*
and proper provision made for rendering the examinations
of future chemists by your board a compulsory instead of an
optional proceeding."

In compliance with this requisition a special general meeting of the society was held on the 17th of March, 1864.
The President, Mr. G. W. Sandford, in opening the meeting,
said, "We must all of us have observed the agitation which
has been going on of late on this subject; and we cannot shut
our eyes to the fact that the proposition of a committee of
the Medical Council to bring pharmacy within the scope, and
pharmaceutists under the control, of that Council, has tended
greatly to bring matters to a climax. I look up to the
Medical Council with all honour and respect, as the power
destined hereafter to take cognizance of all matters connected
with the medical profession; and I at once thank them for the
opinion they enunciate, that dispensing chemists, on whom
the public so much depend, and on whose ability and care
the physician must so much rely in seconding his efforts,
should be an educated body, and should not be allowed to
exercise their calling without first giving proof of their
qualification. I thank them too, for the tribute they pay to
this society, in acknowledging its certificate to be sufficient
evidence of a man's fitness to dispense; but I believe firmly
that the Medical Council have really no wish to interfere in
pharmacy." The subject was fully discussed by members from
various parts of the country; and although some thought the
time had not arrived for requiring compulsory examinations,
and an opinion even was expressed that if legislation were
required it would be the wisest course to leave it in the hands
of the Medical Council, ultimately the following resolution
was carried by a large majority :—

"That in the opinion of this meeting it is desirable for the
protection of the public, that all future chemists and druggists
should undergo a due professional examination before commencing business; and it is highly expedient that the Pharmaceutical Society make early application to Parliament for
an amended Pharmacy Act, by which the legitimate interests
of persons already in business (whether as principals or

assistants) should be protected, and proper provision made for the compulsory examination of those who intend to commence hereafter."

At a meeting of Council held 19th of April, 1864, the proposed Amended Pharmacy Bill, which had been drafted by Mr. Flux was considered, and after some discussion was ordered to be printed in the ensuing number of the *Pharmaceutical Journal*. It was again fully discussed at the Anniversary meeting in May, 1864; and the motion, " that this Bill be received and adopted," was carried unanimously, although an amendment to the effect, " that under an amended Pharmacy Act, it is desirable that the Pharmaceutical Society should include amongst its members all duly qualified dispensing chemists throughout the kingdom, and that provision for admitting such persons to membership should be made accordingly," was moved and seconded, but finally withdrawn.

At a later period in the same year the United Society also produced a Bill which was to be put in competition with that of the Pharmaceutical Society.

The two Bills, when submitted to Parliament, were called " the Chemists' and Druggists' Bills," that from the Pharmaceutical Society being No. 1, and the other No. 2. Their essential features may be thus briefly described:—

Bill No. 1 provided, that after a certain date it should be unlawful and subject to a penalty for any person to use certain titles and carry on the business of a chemist and druggist in the keeping of open shop *for the compounding of the prescriptions of duly qualified medical practitioners* in any part of Great Britain, unless such person should be a pharmaceutical chemist, or a duly registered chemist and druggist; and that no person should be registered as a chemist and druggist unless he should have been engaged in business on his own account as a chemist and druggist, or as an assistant to a chemist and druggist, before a certain date, or should have passed an examination and received a certificate of competent skill and knowledge in accordance with the regulations of the Pharmaceutical Society. And that in future the benefits of the Benevolent Fund of the Pharmaceutical Society might be applied for the relief of all distressed persons who either are or have been members or associates of the Society, and their widows and orphans.

Bill No. 2 provided that all persons, except those registered
under the Pharmacy Act, 1852, keeping shop or store for the
retailing of drugs, and all persons who should be in any
manner engaged in retailing or dispensing dangerous drugs,
simple or compound, should be required, under a penalty, to
have been examined by duly appointed examiners, and certified to possess "a competent knowledge of drugs and
medicines in general use, with their doses, and to be able
to read physicians' prescriptions with ease and accuracy,"
and to have been registered as chemists and druggists, and
to employ none but registered assistants ; but that all persons
who at the time of the Act coming into operation were engaged in business as chemists and druggists, or as assistants
or apprentices to such, and no others, might be registered
without examination ; and that no person who was required
to be registered under this Act should be entitled to recover,
in any Court of Law or Equity, any charge accruing from
the sale of any dangerous drugs or active poisons (as per
schedule), unless he should be able to prove by the production of a certificate that he was duly registered ; and further,
that in the sale of active poisons certain specified regulations
should be observed.   Moreover, all persons registered under
this Act were to be exempt from serving on juries.

Before tracing the further progress of these two Bills reference must be made to other events which occurred about this
time.

In the early part of 1864 the British Pharmacopœia was
published ; and its first appearance, as might be supposed,
attracted a great deal of attention.   Probably no similar
work had ever been looked for with so much interest as this,
or with such various anticipations of the extent to which it
would fulfil the requirements of those for whose use it was
intended.   There had been a great and unusual combination
of talent engaged in the preparation of the work, which had
induced some persons to expect a Pharmacopœia far superior
to any previously produced.   But although, in some respects,
the committees to whom the preparation of the work had
been entrusted were favourably circumstanced, in others they
laboured under great disadvantages.   Each of the three previously existing Pharmacopœias had its representatives, and
might be supposed to have had its advocates, engaged on the

new work; but these being located respectively in London, Edinburgh, and Dublin, were too far removed from each other to admit of their working thoroughly in concert; yet their concurrence in what was done was necessary, and this had involved many compromises which were unfavourable in their influence upon the character of the work. Such a result had been foreseen by many, and the predictions of a successful issue were therefore not unmixed with serious misgivings on the part of those well acquainted with the circumstances of the case.

When the book appeared, it was submitted to the criticisms of practical men in every department of medicine; and although there was evidence of a desire to bring its good rather than its bad qualities prominently into view, the general opinion formed was not favourable. That it had many good qualities was generally admitted; but unfortunately there were some serious defects both of omission and commission, which seriously affected its usefulness for the purposes of the physician. Medical men failed to find in it medicines which they were in the habit of prescribing; or, if retained there by name, such medicines were often so altered in composition and properties that new experiences of their effects were required to justify their use. The consequence was, that physicians very generally directed the medicines they prescribed to be prepared according to pre-existing pharmacopœias; and the British Pharmacopœia, which was to have superseded all others, was itself superseded and practically unused. The Medical Council were aware of the failure of this first attempt to produce a Pharmacopœia the use and authority of which could be enforced and maintained throughout the kingdom, and they decided to bring out a new edition at as early a period as possible.

Mr. Peter Squire, who had acted as representative of the Pharmaceutical Society on the London Pharmacopœia Committee of the Medical Council, almost immediately after the new Pharmacopœia appeared, brought out a book called "A Companion to the British Pharmacopœia," which proved a useful guide to medical practitioners, and acquired a great circulation.

Losses through death were still being sustained by the Pharmaceutical Society from among those who had been active workers in the Council or occupied prominent positions among its members.   Of these the following may be noticed here,—

Mr. W. H. Bucklee, of 86, New Bond Street, had been an active member of, and a regular attendant at, the Council board for thirteen years.   He died on the 3rd of October, 1863.

Mr. Thomas Herring, wholesale druggist, was one of the oldest members of the drug trade, an original promoter and a very active and zealous supporter of the Pharmaceutical Society.   He was born in Norwich, in 1785, was apprenticed to Mr. George Sothern, of that city, in 1801, came to London and entered the house of Messrs. Kirk, Hearon & Co., of Bishopsgate Street, in 1806, married, and commenced business at No. 8, Barbican, in 1808, as wholesale druggist.   His brother, Thrower Buckle Herring, having joined him, they moved in 1815 to more extensive premises, at 40, Aldersgate Street. The firm was brought prominently into notice by the introduction of vegetable and other powders of very superior quality, for the production of which they had fitted up very powerful and efficient drug-grinding apparatus.   It was a new thing at that time for a wholesale druggist to have a drug-mill on the premises, capable of producing all the vegetable and other powders on a large scale.   Such work had been invariably done by a class of men called "drug-grinders," who were not particularly noted for the production of good and genuine powders.   Herring's vegetable powders, such as rhubarb, jalap, bark, ipecacuanha, etc., while they were guaranteed to be genuine, were very different in appearance from any powders previously supplied for use in medicine.   They were fine, soft, impalpable, bright-looking powders, such as could not be produced with the pestle and mortar.   Mr. Herring was elected a member of the first Council of the Pharmaceutical Society, and continued to serve the society in that capacity up to the time of his death.   He was a regular attendant at the meetings, and took a warm interest in the proceedings.   In 1851 he was elected President of the society; and about this time he gave evidence before a Committee of the House of Commons in favour of Mr. Bell's Pharmacy Bill.   He died on the 27th of September, 1864, in his eightieth year.

Mr. John Thomas Barry was a member of the firm of

Allen, Hanburys, and Barry, of Plough Court, Lombard
Street.   He was born in 1789, and belonged to a family
several members of which were distinguished for talent.   He
entered the house in Plough Court when about fifteen years
of age, and had not been there very long before he took an
active part in the management of the business.   He introduced the method of evaporation *in vacuo* for the preparation
of medicinal extracts, having adopted a method of producing
a vacuum by means of steam.   Mr. Barry also, at an early
period, about 1814, adopted the method of using angular
bottles for keeping such poisonous substances as were required to be kept among other preparations employed in
dispensing, and of keeping the more active poisons in a com-
partment devoted exclusively to them.

When the Pharmaceutical Society was started, Mr. Barry
took an active interest in its proceedings; and although he
rarely attended the meetings, he continued to render valuable
assistance by his advice and co-operation whenever such aid
was required.   Much of his time was devoted to philanthropic
objects, and especially to that of abolishing capital punishment.   Some years before his death he retired from business and
lived a secluded life near Hornsey, where he ended his days, in
March, 1864.

Mr. Luke Howard, although never connected with the
Pharmaceutical Society, nor latterly with the practice of
pharmacy, except as a manufacturing chemist, yet, as one of
the oldest pharmacists in the country, deserves a brief notice
here.   He was originally engaged in business with William
Allen in Plough Court, Lombard Street, where, in 1796, they
attempted to bring science, such as it then was, into connection
with the preparation of medicines.   They jointly entered upon
the foundation of a laboratory for the supply of the trade at
large with the chemicals then in use.   This was first at Plaistow; but Mr. Howard, afterwards separating from Mr. Allen,
removed to Stratford, where the business of a manufacturing
chemist has been carried on ever since, by him or members
of his family, and has acquired a great reputation.   As a
scientific man, Mr. Howard devoted himself principally to the
study of meteorology.   He had long withdrawn from active
participation in commercial pursuits, when, at the great age of
92, he ended a prosperous career on the 21st of March, 1864.

A new system had recently been adopted by the Council of the Pharmaceutical Society in the appointment of local secretaries. The value of these officers of the society had long and frequently been felt, especially when there was any measure affecting pharmacy before the Legislature. But on all occasions there was much important assistance which could be rendered by the active co-operation of local secretaries in the working of the society, and it was felt to be very desirable that the appointments should be made with the concurrence of the members for whom they acted. This was the object of the new arrangement introduced in 1863, which consisted in sending, with the voting papers for the election of council, a paper requesting the voter to insert the name of a person he wished to be appointed local secretary in his district. The working of this system appeared to be satisfactory.

A new system was also adopted in 1864, in connection with the examinations for the admission of chemists and druggists already in business on their own account, as members of the Pharmaceutical Society. The door had been closed to the admission of members without examination, and yet, in the prospect of further legislation there were many chemists of long standing and good repute who had hitherto stood aloof, but would now join the society if they could do so without the necessity of going through a special course of study to prepare them for the required examination. If on no other account, many of these would object to present themselves to the ordeal together with young men of the class of their apprentices or assistants, but would submit to a separate examination if it should be of a more practical nature than that usually adopted. With the view of promoting this object, the Council, on the 6th of June, 1864, passed the following resolution :—

"That separate examinations be instituted for chemists and druggists engaged in business on their own account, provided always that such persons have either been in business for *five years*, or are *thirty years* of age.

"That the first of such examinations be held in October, and that due notice thereof be given in the Journal and Transactions."

This resolution was speedily carried into effect, and an examination was held in October of that year, when seventeen candidates presented themselves, fourteen of whom passed.

The examination comprised the following outline of proceedings :—

PRESCRIPTIONS.

1. Reading.
2. Translating.
3. Methods of dispensing the prescription.
4. Detection of unusual doses.

MATERIA MEDICA.

1. Recognition of drugs.
2. Names of plants and animals yielding them.
3. Habitats and whence imported.
4. Preparations into which they enter.
5. Indications of the commercial characters and qualities of drugs.

PHARMACY.

1. Recognition of preparations.
2. Description of their composition and proportions of active ingredients.
3. Description of pharmacopœic processes.

CHEMISTRY.

1. Recognition of chemical substances used in medicine.
2. Processes for their preparation.
3. Chemical composition and decomposition.
4. Detection of such impurities as are ordinarily met with.
5. Antidotes for poisons.
6. Nature and method of taking specific gravities.

BOTANY.

1. Recognition of important indigenous medicinal plants from fresh or dried specimens.
2. Distinctive character of roots, stems, leaves, flowers, fruits, seeds, and their parts.
3. Functions of roots, stems, and leaves.

The second meeting of the British Pharmaceutical Conference was held at Bath in September, 1864, under the presidency of Mr. Henry Deane. It was attended by about fifty members from different parts of the country; and a considerable number of papers on subjects relating to pharmacy were read.

Returning now to the progress of the two Pharmacy Bills.

On the 22nd of November, 1864, a deputation of the Council of the Pharmaceutical Society, consisting of Sandford (President) Hills (Vice-President) Hanbury (Treasurer), with Squire, Morson, Waugh, Orridge, Edwards (members of Council), Flux (Solicitor) and Bremridge (Secretary), had an interview with Sir George Grey, at the Home Office, for the purpose of explaining the provisions of the Pharmacy Bill No. 1, and, as far as possible, of enlisting the interests of the Government in its favour. No decided expression of opinion, however, was elicited from the Home Secretary; but the Council felt themselves sufficiently encouraged by opinions expressed elsewhere to induce them to proceed with their Bill. They had endeavoured, by means of the local secretaries throughout the country, to ascertain the opinions of the trade with reference to their proposed measure; and in many of the principal towns a large proportion,—in some cases all the chemists,—had signed a declaration approving of the Bill of the Pharmaceutical Society.

In these proceedings the Bloomsbury Council were in advance of the United Society, who, on subsequently pursuing a similar course, were annoyed to find that some of their members had been induced to sign the declaration in favour of Bill No. 1. A good deal of acrimonious feeling was thus engendered, which was manifested at meetings and in correspondence in the trade journals; and this, together with exaggerated statements, founded perhaps on imperfect knowledge of facts, tended to weaken the influence and the prospects of success of both parties. On one side there was too much of an assumption that all the best part of the trade was registered at Bloomsbury Square, while on the other hand there were repeated and uncorrected statements made, that the Pharmaceutical Society comprised but a very small proportion of the whole body of chemists and druggists.

In contradiction to this, an appeal had been made in the *Pharmaceutical Journal* to the census returns published by the Registrar General, from which it appeared that in 1861 the total number of persons employed in chemists' and druggists' establishments in England and Wales was 16,026, including assistants and apprentices. But of these, 3,388 were under twenty years of age, and might be taken to have been apprentices, leaving 12,638 as the number of principals and assistants. It was estimated, that probably about 6,000 would be the number of those engaged in business on their own account; and as there were upwards of 2,000 members of the Pharmaceutical Society, these would constitute about one-third of the chemists and druggists actually in business on their own account. Prominent members of the United Society had frequently stated that there were about 40,000 chemists and druggists in the country. This number was afterwards reduced to 30,000, and again, at a recent interview of a deputation of the United Society with Sir George Grey, it was put at 18,000. The interview alluded to took place in the early part of March, 1865, when a deputation, consisting of Henry Matthews (Vice-President) ; Slugg, of Manchester ; Stead, of Leeds ; Manby, of Southampton ; Toogood, of Hull ; Mayger, of Northampton ; Blain, of Bolton ; Smith, of Rye ; Barnaby, of Rochester; Miller, of Blackheath; with D'Aubney, Wade, King, Tidman, Boor, Baumgarten, Cawdell, Heppell, etc., were accompanied to the Home Office by Sir John Shelley, M.P. ; Sir Morton Peto, M.P. ; Sir Robert Clifton, M.P. ; Harvey Lewis, Esq., M.P. ; Salisbury Butler, Esq., M.P. ; William Cox, Esq., M.P. ; G. S. Beecroft, Esq., M.P. ; and Charles Forster, Esq., M.P. Sir John Shelley, in introducing the deputation, alluded to a statement, said to have been made by a deputation from the Pharmaceutical Society, to the effect that they had the support of the trade; but this, he said, the present deputation, who represented a larger society than the other, repudiated as entirely erroneous. He suggested that the Bills of both the societies should be referred to a select committee of the House of Commons. Sir George Grey, after inquiring how many members the Pharmaceutical Society had, and how many chemists there were in the United Kingdom, said the Pharmaceutical Society had obtained an interview with him some time previously, and had wished him to take charge of their Bill; but he had an idea that they did not represent all sections of the trade, and he had therefore requested them to give him some proof that they did. He had declined to take up their Bill, expecting that other interests would come forward. Finally, he promised to look over the Bill which this deputation left with him, and said he thought the course suggested by Sir John

Shelley, of referring both Bills to a select committee, a very good one.

The two Bills were now before Parliament, and they came on for second reading in the House of Commons on the 29th of March, 1865. Bill No. 1 was introduced by Sir Fitzroy Kelly, and Bill No. 2 by Sir John Shelley. The subject of the Bills was pretty fully discussed, not only by their respective movers, but also by Dr. Brady, Mr. Kinglake, Mr. Roebuck, Lord Elcho, Mr. Beecroft, and Sir George Grey. It was generally admitted that there ought to be a compulsory examination for chemists and druggists, and that such examination could not be in better hands than those of the Pharmaceutical Society. Both Bills were read a second time, and referred to a select committee.

An important report of a committee of the Medical Council on the Pharmacy Bills was opportunely issued at this time, as follows :—

"The committee appointed on April 7th, 1865, to report whether the Medical Council is charged under the Medical Act with any duty in relation to medical and surgical practice by chemists and druggists, and also to consider and report on the two Bills relating to pharmacy now before Parliament, report as follows :—

" In 1864, the General Medical Council represented to her Majesty's Government the necessity of regulating by statute the practice of pharmacy by chemists and druggists throughout the kingdom. The committee are of opinion that this necessity continues as cogent as ever, and that the Council ought to encourage and support any approved measure for effecting such legislation.

" Two Bills for the purpose have been introduced into the House of Commons during the present session, one promoted by the Pharmaceutical Society, the other by chemists and druggists not belonging to that body. The Bill of the latter is confined to England and Wales, that of the former to Great Britain.

" After carefully considering both Bills, the committee are of opinion that the preferable mode of legislation is that which adopts the Pharmaceutical Society with the Pharmacy Act of 1852 as a basis. They think the Bill promoted by the society well fitted to attain various important objects, and reasonable in its demands for powers and privileges.

"The main objects of the Bill are to form a register of legally qualified pharmaceutical chemists; to prohibit the use of certain pharmaceutic titles by persons not on the register; to confine to those registered the privilege of executing the prescriptions of medical practitioners, subject to the provisions hereinafter named, but not to restrict the sale of medicines asked for in any other manner.

"The committee desire to bring before the Council certain defects which it appears to them necessary to correct before the Bill becomes law.

"1. The Bill should be altered so as to apply to Ireland as well as to England and Scotland.   They are not aware that any state of things exists in Ireland to render the regulation of pharmacy by the State less necessary there than in Britain.

"2. The committee are of opinion that a clause should be inserted in any Pharmacy Bill, rendering it imperative on chemists and druggists to follow, in compounding prescriptions, the formularies of the British Pharmacopœia, unless otherwise directed by the prescriber.

"3. The committee consider that the promoters of the Bill, probably from a desire to disarm opposition, propose to admit, on too easy terms, into their society practising chemists and druggists not now belonging to it.   The proposal is to admit all who offer themselves for examination, or who produce a certificate from a qualified medical practitioner that they have been in the practice of dispensing medicines from the prescriptions of medical men before January 1st, 1866. The latter alternative implies a facility of entrance which will be apt to lead to abuse.   The committee are of opinion that more satisfactory evidence of qualification should be required.

"4. The last important defect in the Bill which the committee have to notice is, that no adequate provision has been made towards preventing registered pharmaceutic chemists from converting themselves into unqualified medical practitioners.

"Looking to the history of medical practice in this country the committee see great danger to the interests of the public and of the medical profession from the body which will be constituted by the Bill, should it become an Act in its present shape.   The General Medical Council, in carrying out the objects of the Medical Act, have raised, and it is hoped, may further raise, the qualifications of legally qualified medical practitioners. But their labours will be in vain should the creation of a new race of unqualified practitioners be inadvertently encouraged by an Act of Parliament. It is well known that many existing chemists and druggists, both members of the Pharmaceutical Society and others, practise medicine, although unqualified by law and not competent by education. To a limited extent this practice may be inevitable, and at all events cannot be prevented. But the existence of it gives peculiar facilities and temptations to the pharmaceutic chemist to embark largely in irregular medical practice as an unqualified practitioner.

" The committee have considered whether the danger here indicated might not be averted by extending the jurisdiction of the General Medical Council, so as to include control over pharmaceutic chemists as well as over practitioners in medicine. But they believe that such a plan is at present attended with difficulties.

" By Clause 55 of the Medical Act, chemists and druggists are expressly exempted from the provisions of the Act, so far as the ' selling, compounding, and dispensing medicines' is concerned. Nor is there any provision in the Act which gives the Medical Council any greater power to prevent chemists and druggists from practising medicine also, than the Act enables the Council to exercise over all other unqualified medical practitioners. It is plain, therefore, that the Act did not contemplate the exercise by the Medical Council of any control over chemists and druggists; and the committee consider that it would be unwise to seek to alter the existing relations between the Medical Council and chemists and druggists.

" The committee have further considered whether the danger they have pointed out might be averted by some simple provision in the Pharmacy Bill. By Section 17 of the Bill of the Pharmaceutical Society, it is declared that ' Nothing in this Act contained shall extend, or be construed to extend, to lessen or prejudice, or in any wise to interfere with, any of the rights, privileges, and immunities heretofore vested in and exercised and enjoyed by any duly qualified medical practitioner.'

" This clause sufficiently protects medical practitioners in

such right of practising pharmacy as they have hitherto
enjoyed; but it does not attempt to prevent pharmaceutic
chemists from practising medicine. Considering their peculiar temptations to practise it, however, some check seems
desirable. The committee suggest that this object may be
attained, in some measure, were the following clause to be
added to Section 17, viz.—

" 'Or to entitle any person registered under this Act to
practise medicine or surgery, or any branch of medicine or
surgery.'

" The members of the Pharmaceutic body would thus have
constantly before them the sentiments of the Legislature as to
the principles on which the Pharmacy Act was founded.

" The committee have reason to believe that the present
Council of the Pharmaceutical Society have every desire to
discourage the practice of medicine by its members. They,
therefore, apprehend that no opposition would be made to the
addition of such a clause.

" The committee call attention to the fact that the Bill
proposes to confer on the whole body of chemists and druggists the right of dispensing and selling medicines without
any control on the part of the Government, except such as is
exercised under the Pharmacy Act over registered pharmaceutical chemists. The medical profession has not been so
dealt with in the Medical Act. The Medical Council is
properly restricted in its action by the medical corporations
and Universities, and is also controlled by the Privy Council.
They submit that the whole profession of pharmacy ought to
be subjected to some control.

" The committee recommend that the above observations
should be laid by the President before the Secretary of State
for the Home Department, and the Chairman of the select
committee on the two Bills.

" Signed on behalf of the committee,

" HENRY W. ACLAND, Chairman."

At the meeting of the select committee of the House of
Commons, to which the two Pharmacy Bills were referred,
evidence was given by Dr. Alfred S. Taylor, Mr. Simon, Dr.
Quain, and Dr. Wilson, who all agreed in advocating the
necessity for an educational qualification for dispensers of
medicine, and also in commending the regulations adopted by

the Pharmaceutical Society for testing by examination the qualifications required. Evidence was also given by Mr. John Mackay, of Edinburgh, to show what the general opinion of the trade in Scotland was with reference to Bill No. 1. But as part of the evidence went strongly to favour the adoption of restrictions on the sale of poisons, and the views of the committee appeared to accord with the opinions expressed in this direction, while no provision was made in Bill No. 1 for regulating the sale of poisons, this Bill was not considered to fulfil what was required; and as Bill No. 2, although it dealt with that part of the subject, involved much that the committee was not prepared to entertain, it also was not proceeded with. Finally the committee reported as follows :—

" Your committee have examined witnesses on the general questions raised by the provisions contained in the two Bills committed to them, and have also heard evidence in support of the Chemists' and Druggists' (No. 1) Bill.

" 1. Your committee then passed the following resolutions :—

"' 1st. That no compulsory examination or registration under the Bills referred to the committee should be required of persons now carrying on the trade of chemists and druggists.'

"' 2nd. That the Bill do provide that no other person shall, after a day to be fixed by the Bill, sell certain dangerous drugs, to be scheduled in the Bill, unless he be examined and registered.'

" 2. By the adoption of the second resolution, as an amendment to a proposal that persons compounding medicines from the prescriptions of medical men should also be examined, your committee decided against the principal provision contained in the Chemists' and Druggists' (No. 1) Bill, and they accordingly resolved to proceed with the Chemists' and Druggists' (No. 2) Bill.

" 3. After several of the clauses of the Bill were passed, considerable difficulty arose in providing for the first formation of the council to which the duty of regulating the examination of chemists and druggists was to be entrusted ; and your committee, considering the advanced period of the session, were compelled to abandon the expectation of any useful result from a further consideration of the Bill.

" 4. Having therefore disposed, *pro formâ*, of the remaining clauses, they came to the following resolution :—

" 'That, inasmuch as there appears to be little prospect of any satisfactory termination to the labours of the committee in the present session, it is desirable that the evidence, so far as it has been already taken, and the proceedings of the committee, be reported to the House, accompanied by a recommendation that the Government should, early in the new Parliament, bring in a Bill on the subjects referred to the committee.'

" 5. Your committee have in conclusion to report, that, in their opinion, it is not expedient to proceed further with either of the Bills which have been committed to them."

This result could not be viewed as otherwise than a source of some mortification to the promoters of Bill No. 1 ; for while the principle of this Bill was rejected by the committee, that of Bill No. 2 was to a certain extent approved. There was some satisfaction, however, in knowing that the Bill of the Pharmaceutical Council was approved by the highest medical and other authorities, and that it comprised a principle which would have restricted the dispensing of medicines to qualified men without shackling them with burdensome conditions.

It was now the end of the session, and nearly the end of the Parliament ; therefore any further attempts at obtaining the desired legislation would have to be made under some-what altered circumstances.

The failure of their attempt at legislation was not the only trouble the pharmaceutical body had now to contend with. The proprietor of a patent for the manufacture of metallic capsules for covering the mouths of bottles, having been en-gaged for several years in expensive litigation, by which he finally established his exclusive right to the manufacture, after spending £30,000 in doing so, thought he might perhaps re-coup himself for some of his expenses by taking legal proceed-ings against the numerous class of chemists and others who were, and had for some time been, unconsciously infringing his patent. Accordingly in July, 1865, a large number of chemists in different parts of London received notice that suits in chancery were about to be commenced against them, for having infringed the patent rights of Mr. Betts, by selling articles capped with metallic capsules not made by him nor

with his sanction. This of course caused a good deal of excitement and alarm. Meetings were held, and lawyers consulted, and as several of the parties implicated were members
of the Pharmaceutical Society, the advice and assistance of the
Council and officers of the society were sought and obtained.
Previous to this, however, some of the defendants, fearful of
incurring ruinous expenses, had induced Mr. Betts' solicitor to
stop further proceedings against them by the payment of sums
of money. In one instance a widow had compromised her case
by the payment of £16, although she had never gained as
many pence by the capsules she had innocently sold attached to
proprietary articles. In another instance double that sum had
been paid under similar circumstances. At the conferences
that took place in Bloomsbury Square, and under the advice of
the society's solicitor, defendants were recommended not to
settle their cases in that way, and most of them joined in
forming a common fund, and acting together for their defence
if further proceedings should be taken. They were kept in
suspense for a long time, and a good deal of annoyance was
caused by the vacillating conduct of Mr. Betts and his agents,
but ultimately the patent died out and with it the fear of Mr.
Betts' chancery suits.

There were other sources of small troubles to chemists and
druggists, among which was the infringement of excise regulations. Several cases of this kind occurred in connection
with the sale of quinine wine. A correspondence took place
with the Inland Revenue Board as to the quantity of quinine
required to ensure the exclusion of this preparation from the
category of beverages, and keep it in that of medicines, and
the question was not completely settled until a process was
given in which the strength and composition of quinine wine
was defined in the British Pharmacopœia.

Additional attention had of late been directed to the Benevolent Fund. Hitherto only casual relief had been granted
out of the fund, and there had been an understanding that
no annuities should be granted until the invested capital had
reached the sum of £10,000. But at the time at which that
decision was come to, the subscriptions to the society were
higher than they subsequently became, and grants were then
frequently made from the funds of the society to the Benevolent Fund, which was thus steadily increasing from year to
year.

Since the subscriptions had been reduced, the income of the society had not admitted of such grants being made, and it was considered necessary to adopt some method of getting increased support for this important part of the society's objects. It was thought that the best means of increasing the capital of the fund would be to bring it into practical use, and with the view of doing so, the Council, on the 7th of June, 1865, "Resolved, that in accordance with the revised regulations for the distribution of this Fund, an election of two annuitants take place in October next, the annuities to be of the value of £30 each." In the following month a grant of one hundred guineas out of the Benevolent Fund was voted for the purpose of purchasing an admission for the orphan child of a late member into an orphan asylum. And then, on the 27th of October, at a meeting specially convened for the purpose, the first two annuitants, each to receive £30 a year from the Benevolent Fund of the Pharmaceutical Society, were elected. These active operations brought many new subscriptions and donations to the fund.

The third meeting of the British Pharmaceutical Conference was held at Birmingham, in September, 1865. There was a larger attendance of members and a greater number of papers read at this meeting than at either of the preceding ones. In fact, the Conference was assuming a very important position. Mr. Henry Deane presided at this as well as the two previous meetings.

The committee to whom the Medical Council had entrusted the preparation of a new edition of the British Pharmacopœia, having appointed Mr. Robert Warington, of Apothecaries' Hall, and Professor Redwood, of the Pharmaceutical Society, as joint editors, these gentlemen were now actively engaged in reconstructing the work in accordance with the plan which the latter had suggested in a communication read at a meeting of the Pharmaceutical Society. The discussion at meetings and in the journals, of subjects relating to the Pharmacopœia, was invited and encouraged, and many of those who on previous occasions had taken an interest in such matters, afforded valuable suggestions. Unfortunately, Mr. Warington's health became so seriously impaired shortly after his appointment, that he was obliged to relinquish active work and leave London.

The disappointment resulting from the failure of the attempts made by the two competing societies to induce the Legislature to proceed with either of the Pharmacy Bills submitted to them, greatly damped the energy previously manifested by both parties, but it was more apparent in the supporters of No. 1 than No. 2 Bill. The latter felt that they had gained a partial success, and they were anxious to turn this to the best account. Even before the select committee had completed their deliberations on the two Bills, and immediately after the first conclusion they arrived at was made known, the Executive Committee of the United Society issued the following statement addressed to the trade :—

" The Executive Committee hasten to respond to the anxious inquiry of the trade as to the progress of legislation affecting their interests.

" The select committee appointed by the House of Commons to consider the two Chemists and Druggists Bills, met on the 11th of May, and proceeded to hear evidence in favour of Bill No. 1. Dr. Alfred Swaine Taylor, throughout an examination of two hours, sustained his unswerving conviction that the sale of dangerous drugs and poisons should be subject to legislative restriction. Mr. Simon, the Medical Officer of the Privy Council, confirmed Dr. Taylor's evidence.

" On the second day's sitting, Dr. Quain gave similar evidence to that of Dr. Taylor and Mr. Simon, and emphatically denounced 'free trade' in physic as dangerous to the public. Dr. Wilson expressed his opinion to the same effect, and with equal force and clearness. Mr. Mackay, Secretary of the Pharmaceutical Society at Edinburgh, was then examined as to the general feeling of the trade in favour of Bill No. 1. The chemists and druggists of Scotland he said had petitioned for it, and those of Edinburgh were unanimously in its favour, but on the question being put to him by Sir John Shelley, whether the chemists and druggists of Glasgow were in favour of it, he was sorry to admit that Glasgow opposed it. Just at this juncture the speaker's bell rang for prayers, and the committee adjourned.

" Whilst the committee and the public were departing, Lord Elcho collected some friends of the two societies around him, and read a paper which he said he hoped would prove to be the basis of a good understanding between them. Hurried expressions of readiness to make reasonable concessions were uttered on both sides, and eventually Lord Elcho's suggestion for a conference was agreed upon. In accordance with this arrangement, Messrs. D'Aubney and Wade, with Mr. Buott, the Secretary, who were deputed on behalf of the United Society, met the President and Vice-President with the Secretary of the Pharmaceutical Society, on Wednesday, the 17th May, at the Pharmaceutical Institution in Bloomsbury Square.

" After various remarks of a preliminary character on either side, Mr. Buott observed that the object of the gentlemen representing the United Society in coming there was to hear any proposition in harmony with Lord Elcho's suggestions which the gentlemen representing the Pharmaceutical Society had to advance.   The President said, ' We are quite willing to learn what you object to in Bill No. 1, and to consider whether any alteration can be made to meet your views.'   Mr. D'Aubney replied that that would be useless, because the whole Bill was objected to as being upon a wrong basis, and Mr. Buott added, that unless the Pharmaceutical Council had some distinct proposition to make, the meeting might as well be ended.

" Mr. Hills here stated, and was confirmed in his statement by the President, that it was proposed to alter the 16th clause in Bill No. 1, so as to give all chemists registered under the Act a vote at the society's meetings.

" Mr. Wade said that would not meet the case.   Unless chemists of equal qualification were put upon an equal footing with those who were members of the Pharmaceutical Society by payment, the United Society could not support their Bill. ' You wish,' said he, ' to secure both registration and examination, and you base your claim upon the machinery you possess for such a purpose.   These are the only points at issue, and constitute the rights we claim for ourselves as independent tradesmen.   Can you suppose that we shall surrender them to a society which has failed in its objects, and whose Council represents only the dispensing interests of the trade, without an equivalent ?   Concessions must be made on both sides ; we are willing to concede even these important rights, but every man placed upon the register must have a voice in the nomination and election of the governing body.' Mr. Wade then introduced the following propositions :—

" '1. The Pharmaceutical Society to register at a certain fee all chemists and druggists in business at the time of the passing of the Act as Pharmaceutical Chemists.

" ' 2. All future candidates for registration to be examined by the examiners of the Pharmaceutical Society.

" ' 3. Those passing the minor examination to pay a fee of not more than two guineas, and to be called chemists and druggists, with the right to retail and compound articles scheduled as dangerous drugs and poisons.

" ' 4. Those passing the major examination, at a fee of not more than five guineas, to be styled pharmaceutical chemists.

" ' 5. All pharmaceutical chemists to be eligible for membership of the Pharmaceutical Society.

" ' 6. Those now to be incorporated without examination to pay a subscription of two guineas annually upon election to membership, and to be entitled to all the privileges of old members.

" ' 7. All interests to be represented on the Council, and every pharmaceutical chemist to have a vote in the election of Council.'

" The President and Mr. Hills saw no particular objection to any of these clauses except No. 1, which proposed to make common the title of Pharmaceutical Chemist, which was secured to the present members by charter.

" Mr. D'Aubney and the Secretary urged the right of representation with election; and Mr. Buott wished it to be distinctly understood that, in making the proposition, the right of nomination must be considered as a *sine quâ non*, because election without the right of nomination would be a mockery. On separating, it was agreed that the conference should be renewed on the following morning, when the parties would meet at the House of Commons. No sooner, however, had they met, than it was ascertained that the Pharmaceutical representatives were disinclined to the interpretation of clause 7, in the sense of nomination with representation; so the conference had no practical result.

" On the third day the committee consulted for more than two hours with closed doors, and having examined Mr. Mackay for a few minutes, they ordered the room again to be cleared. On our readmission the chairman read the following resolutions :—

"'1. That no compulsory examination or registration should be required of persons now carrying on the business of chemists and druggists.

"'2. That no other person shall, after a day to be fixed, sell certain dangerous drugs to be scheduled in the Bill, unless he be examined and registered.

"'3. That the committee do proceed on this day week with Chemists and Druggists Bill No. 2.'

"Not one of these three simple, brief, but conclusive resolutions touched a single object aimed at by Bill No. 1, to give it legislative life; so, in parliamentary phraseology, the Bill was thrown out.

"The day on which the above resolutions were adopted was Thursday, the 18th May.

"Considerable excitement prevailed amongst the Metropolitan chemists when the news, that the Bill of the Pharmaceutical Council was lost, became known, each expressing his joy or regret according to his individual bias.

"On the following Tuesday the members of the select committee had a private consultation, and agreed to further adjourn the consideration of Bill No. 2, from Thursday, the 25th May, to Thursday, the 1st June.

"The interest which had been excited by the announcement of the Bill of the Pharmaceutical Council being thrown out, might be supposed to have been almost extinguished by this unexpected adjournment; but at twelve o'clock on the 1st of June, it was evident, from the crowded appearance of the corridor of the House of Commons leading to Committee Room No. 16, that something very much like a sensation had been created amongst the chemists and druggists of London, who, anxiously and patiently, but cheerfully and hopefully, waited on the outside of the Committee Room from twelve till half-past two o'clock, when all hopes and fears were alike set at rest by the advent of Sir Fitzroy Kelly and Sir John Shelley, who explained to their respective adherents the result of the long deliberation which had taken place. Sir John Shelley stated that the committee had agreed to the preamble and first three clauses of the Bill No. 2, and recommended that the Council of the Pharmaceutical Society and the Executive Committee of the United Society should each give in the names of ten gentlemen, who, together with three gentlemen to be nominated by Government, should be appointed under the Act to carry out its provisions.

"The Executive Committee furnish this simple narrative of a long protracted and arduous struggle for independence, without any comment of their own, believing that every incident it records will prove of interest, not only to the chemists and druggists now in business, but also to their successors, and stand upon the page of history in bright testimony to the persevering efforts which have been made to elevate the trade, and to place their rights and privileges upon a sound legislative basis for the future.

"By order of the Executive Committee,

"CYRUS BUOTT,

"*Secretary*.

"United Society of Chemists and Druggists,

"20, New Ormond Street, W.C.,

"*June* 10*th*, 1865."

The concluding report of the select committee (page 340), the purport of which slightly differs in one respect from the the foregoing, is not alluded to in Mr. Buott's statement, and, no doubt, was not found to be quite so satisfactory to the executives of the United Society as they expected it to be. There was a good deal of discussion on the subject both in London and throughout the country. At the discussions in London, disagreements arose among leading members of the United Society. Unseemly disputes occurred with the Secretary at public and committee meetings. The President, Alderman Dakin, resigned his appointment, and symptoms in several respects of disorganization were manifested. But in some of the provincial towns, and especially at Manchester, more unanimity and a better spirit appeared to prevail. It was at first proposed to make Alderman Bowker, of Manchester, the new President, but as he did not respond to the invitation, Mr. Henry Matthews, of Gower Street, an analytical chemist, unconnected with pharmacy, was elected to the somewhat difficult office of presiding over the disunited members of the United Society. The advantage possessed by a well organized and incorporated institution, such as the Pharmaceutical Society, was seen and admitted by all; and although members of the United Society were disposed to exult over their neighbours in Bloomsbury, on the ground of the better

success of Bill No. 2 than that of No. 1, they could not fail
to perceive that the greater amount of influence and better
chance of success would lie on the side of any measure
introduced by the promoters of the latter.

The advantage of having a journal devoted to the interests
of the promoting body was also felt, and a proposition was
made for establishing a new journal to represent the United
Society, but this was not carried out. The proceedings of
the society had, from their commencement, been reported in
the *Chemist and Druggist*, a trade journal, which had started
some years previously in a small way, but was at this time
expanding to larger dimensions, and ultimately became a
popular, widely circulated, and influential publication. The
independent spirit manifested by this journal sometimes gave
offence to the leaders of the United Society, but no sufficient
grounds were adduced for discrediting its reports and comments, which on the whole appeared to be true and fair.

It was evident to all candid observers that the only chance
of carrying a Pharmacy Bill through Parliament, would be
for the two societies to agree upon some measure, and direct
their united efforts towards getting it passed.

At a meeting of the Council in Bloomsbury Square on the
3rd January, 1866, a letter was read from Mr. Buott, enclosing
a resolution which had been passed at the Annual Meeting of
the United Society, on the 23rd November, 1865, and which
the meeting had directed to be sent to the Pharmaceutical
Council, as follows:—

"That this annual meeting confirm the recommendation
of the Provincial Associations at Liverpool, Manchester,
Sheffield, Leeds, Hull, Bradford, Bristol, Oxford, Bolton,
Newcastle-on-Tyne, etc., to make the first seven clauses of
the Chemists and Druggists Bill No. 2, as approved by the
select committee of the House of Commons *—the basis of
any future proceeding in the name of the United Society, in
case the Pharmaceutical Society decline to co-operate upon

---

* These clauses merely related to the proposed title of the Act, the
date at which it should take effect, and the constitution and mode of
election of the governing body or council. The next succeeding clauses
related to the incorporation of a constituency, which, the committee
say, presented considerable difficulty, on which account they relinquished the further consideration of the Bill.

the condition of the self-government of the trade being secured by representative election."

The communication having been considered, the Secretary was instructed to forward to the Executive Committee a copy of the following resolution :—

"That the Council of the Pharmaceutical Society have no idea of recommending any measure to Government for the regulation of chemists and druggists which shall not give to all registered chemists and druggists a voice in the election of the governing body."

At a later date, in March, a correspondence took place between the Presidents of the two societies. A resolution had been passed by the Executive Committee of the United Society, "That the President be requested to call upon or write to the President of the Pharmaceutical Society, to ascertain whether it is his opinion that the Council of that society would be ,'willing to co-operate with the Executive Committee of the United Society in urging and assisting the Government to introduce a Chemists and Druggists Bill into Parliament, based upon the recommendations of the select committee, and submitted to the Government at the close of the last session."

To this Mr. Sandford replied as follows :—

" 47, PICCADILLY, *March* 17*th*, 1866.

" Sir,—In reply to your note of the 16th inst., asking my opinion as to the willingness of the Pharmaceutical Society to co-operate with your society in urging and assisting the Government to introduce a Chemists and Druggists Bill into Parliament, based upon the recommendation of the select committee of last year, I beg to say that it is the unanimous opinion of the Council of the Pharmaceutical Society, that urging the Government at this time would be useless, unwise and impolitic. The great press of matter before Parliament just now, connected with reform, rinderpest, and Fenianism, renders it almost certain that the ministry will not adopt the recommendation of the select committee to introduce a Bill on the subjects in which we are interested during the present session. Should this expectation of delay, however, be incorrect (and, for myself, I should much rejoice to find it so), our Council will always be ready to assist the Government in arranging an efficient, and yet liberal, measure for the settlement of the question.

" I say ' *an efficient measure*,' and I think you will agree with me that a mere Poison Bill, fettering us with registration of sales and attendance of witnesses, prescribing a particular form of bottle in which poisons might be kept and sold, and a particular corner in our shops in which they should be placed, would be only an encumbrance to the statute-book, inoperative as regards the public, and especially objectionable to men who, if they be properly qualified to deal in dangerous articles, will each, according to the special circumstances of his case, adopt precautions far more conducive to the public safety.

"I have said also a '*liberal measure*,' and on this point I may add, that the Home Secretary is already in possession of the views entertained by the Pharmaceutical Society, and I believe no chemist and druggist, properly so called, could, whether he be now a member of our society or not, fairly object to those views.   Our desire is to make the compulsory parts of the Bill entirely prospective, and to give all persons registered under it equally easy means of access to the society which should regulate the examinations, etc.   To suppose that there will ever be two societies for the same object established by law requires a stretch of imagination to which I am not yet equal, and is a thing, I believe, entirely beyond the hope—nay even the desire—of the best members of your society.

" I fully recognise the right of all persons ' *governed* '—(but mind, I think ' *governed* ' is a strong expression for the present case)—to have a voice in the governing body, and I would for this reason carry the provisions of the Bill a little further than I have yet stated.

" You know the select committee resolved that there should be no compulsory registration for men already in business.   I would nevertheless have a voluntary registration; and all able to bring 'the required certificate of their having been chemists, properly so called, should be entitled to that registration, and so have the same easy access I have mentioned before to the society.

" These men would be in no way interfered with by the proposed legislation, but, being engaged in the same trade, I know many of them would like such a provision ; and beyond that, I regard the union of all men of our calling as an important means for elevating the standing of the whole body.

" I have written rather fully on this matter, because I am anxious to assure you that there is really no foundation for the oft-repeated charge made against the society, over which I have the honour to preside, of a desire to subjugate all chemists and druggists throughout the country to their authority; and I trust you will agree with me in thinking that the measure we desire to pass is one which would be beneficial, and ought to be supported by the whole trade.

"I have the honour to be, Sir,

"Your obedient servant,

"GEORGE W. SANDFORD.

" To HENRY MATTHEWS, Esq.,

"President of the United Society of Chemists and Druggists."

In the discussion which took place at the reading of this letter before the Executive Committee of the United Society, some exception was taken to the absence of information on the point with reference to which a question had been asked, and a resolution was passed,—" That this meeting, while acknowledging the courtesy with which the President of the Pharmaceutical Society has answered the letter addressed to him, regrets that he does not give any definite reply to the question : ' Whether the Pharmaceutical Society would be willing to co-operate with the United Society in urging Government to pass a Bill *for the incorporation of the trade,* based upon the recommendations of the Parliamentary Select Committee ? ' "

With reference to this resolution, Mr. Sandford addressed the following letter,—

" To the Editor of *The Chemist and Druggist.*

" Sir,—On page 52 of the last number of your paper, in the transactions of the United Society of Chemists and Druggists, you publish a letter which was addressed by me to Mr. Matthews, and on page 53 a resolution of the Executive Committee of the society appears, professing to state the question to which my letter was a reply.

" It runs thus—' Whether the Pharmaceutical Society

would be willing to co-operate with the United Society in urging Government to pass a Bill *for the incorporation of the trade,* based upon the recommendations of the Parliamentary Select Committee?'

" The question actually put to me, as I find by a reference to Mr. Matthews' letter, and you may see in your March number, was, whether in my opinion the Council ' would be willing to co-operate with the Executive Committee of the United Society in urging and assisting the Government to introduce a Chemists' and Druggists' Bill into Parliament, based upon the recommendations of the select committee, and submitted to Government at the close of the last session ? '

" Now I think I have some reason to complain of the introduction of the words, ' for the incorporation of the trade,' to the question, after my answer had been considered; inasmuch as the expression in the last paragraph but one of my letter, ' *that I regard the union of all men of our calling as an important means for elevating the standing of the whole body,*' was neither caused by anything which occurred in the question put to me, nor by the recommendations of the Select Committee of the House of Commons, which contains no mention whatever of such an incorporation, but simply from an opinion I have always held, and continue to hold, in common, I believe, with all members of the society over which I have the honour to preside.

"I have the honour to be, Sir,

" Your obedient servant,

" GEORGE W. SANDFORD.

" 47, Piccadilly, *May* 10*th*, 1866."

At nearly the same time the Secretary of the United Society, under instructions from his Committee, sent the following letter,—

" 20, New Ormond Street, W.C.

" London, *May* 5*th*, 1866.

" Sir,—At a meeting of the Executive Committee of this society, held here yesterday, reference was made to a letter of the President of the Pharmaceutical Society, dated March 17th, 1866, and addressed to the President of the United Society of Chemists and Druggists, in which the President of the Pharmaceutical Society says,—' I regard the union of all men of our calling as an important means for elevating the standing of the whole body;' and in the *Pharmaceutical Journal* for this month, in which this letter is printed, a hope is expressed ' that those equally and alike interested in the result of legislation will not be found acting in opposition to each other.'

" The sentiments thus expressed were reciprocated by the meeting, and led to the unanimous adoption of the accompanying resolution.

" Waiting the reply of the Pharmaceutical Council to the inquiry therein embodied,

"I am, Sir, your obedient servant,

" CYRUS BUOTT, Secretary.

"To ELIAS BREMRIDGE, Secretary.

"Resolution, That the Secretary be instructed to write to the Council of the Pharmaceutical Society, requesting a reply to the question, Will the Council of the Pharmaceutical Society co-operate with the Executive Committee of the United Society in promoting a Bill for the incorporation of the trade, based upon the recommendation of the Select Committee of the House of Commons ?

" CYRUS BUOTT, Secretary."

In reply to this communication, the Secretary was instructed to forward a copy of the following resolutions :—

" 1. That the Council cannot find any expression referring to the incorporation of the trade in the recommendation of the Select Committee of the House of Commons on the Chemists' and Druggists' Bills.

" 2. That the Council do not think it wise to take any immediate steps towards legislation, but intend at present to await the action of Government.

" 3. That whenever a Bill shall be brought into Parliament affecting the interests of chemists and druggists, the Council of the Pharmaceutical Society will be very glad to have the co-operation of all concerned, whether of the Pharmaceutical Society, the United Society, or the large number who are not connected with either, to obtain a satisfactory and liberal settlement of the question."

The United Society at this time had ceased to justify

its name. It had fallen into what the *Chemist and Druggist* called an "incoherent state," in which "deplorable dissension" prevailed at the committee and other meetings. The Secretary, a clever man with much persevering energy, attempted to rule the proceedings in opposition to the President and a majority of the Executive Committee; and, backed by country members, he succeeded at the anniversary meeting in carrying his point, thus contributing to split up the society and weaken its power for any effective work. It would be a profitless task to attempt to follow this controversy through all its details, which extended over many months and resulted in some of the most influential members of the United Society seceding, and either joining the Pharmaceutical Society or holding themselves aloof from both societies.

The Bloomsbury Council considered that the time had not yet come at which they could, with good effect, renew their efforts in seeking legislation by any active means; but with the view of keeping the subject under the notice of the Government, the Council in the early part of 1866 had sent to the Home Office a brief outline of such a measure as they thought would accord with the recommendation of the Select Committee of the House of Commons, and at the same time meet the views of the body of chemists and druggists. It was to the following effect :—

" 1. That in future all persons, before assuming the name or title of Chemist and Druggist, or keeping open shop for the compounding of medicines under physicians' and surgeons' prescriptions, or for vending, dispensing or compounding certain dangerous drugs, chemicals, and other poisonous substances to be enumerated in a schedule, should undergo an examination and be registered as Pharmaceutical Chemists, or Chemists and Druggists.

" 2. The examination for Pharmaceutical Chemists should be, as heretofore, that which is known as the major examination of the Pharmaceutical Society.

" 3. The examination for Chemists and Druggists should be that which is known as the minor examination, and to which persons hitherto registered as Assistants have been subjected.

" 4. That all persons registered as Chemists and Druggists should be eligible for election to membership of the Pharma‚

ceutical Society, under the bye-laws thereof; but they should not by virtue of that membership be entitled to registration as Pharmaceutical Chemists, that title being strictly kept for those only who pass the major examination. They should have the right of nominating and voting for members of Council, but the Council should consist only of members who are Pharmaceutical Chemists.

" 5. All persons registered under the Bill as Chemists and Druggists to be exempt from serving on juries.

" 6. Nothing in the Bill to interfere with, or curtail the rights of, chemists already in business, or of persons of the full age of twenty-one years who should, at a given date, be assistants to chemists and druggists. Other necessary exemptions to be made for apothecaries, veterinary surgeons, wholesale dealers, etc.

" 7. That chemists and druggists already in business may, if they choose, be placed on the register of chemists and druggists, if within a certain time after the passing of the Bill they make application, and produce to the Registrar satisfactory evidence that they were actually in business on their own account, and engaged in the compounding and dispensing of medicines under physicians' and surgeons' prescriptions, and vending, compounding, and dispensing the dangerous poisons as per schedule, prior to that date."

Having thus intimated their views and wishes to the Government, the Pharmaceutical Society took no further immediate action with regard to legislation, but they were fully sensible of the importance of inducing, and anxious to bring about, a union of the power and influence which could be brought to bear in the interests of Pharmacy, when it should be found practicable and expedient to make a fresh appeal to Parliament.

A very successful meeting of the British Pharmaceutical Conference was held at Nottingham this year, under the presidency of Professor Bentley. The papers read were numerous and interesting. One especially on Pharmaceutical Ethics, by Mr. Joseph Ince, attracted considerable attention both then and subsequently. There was a new feature introduced into this Conference meeting which consisted of an exhibition of objects relating to pharmacy.

Attempts were still being made to obtain increased support

for, and to extend the benefits of, the Benevolent Fund. This was neutral ground on which all parties could meet; and while they were engaged in furthering the objects of the fund by which charity was extended to others, there was room and a fitting opportunity for the cultivation of a similar sentiment among themselves. It was proposed to have a dinner in support of the Fund, and this was promoted by many of those called outsiders, who were now manifesting a disposition to co-operate with Bloomsbury Square in furthering such objects as could be mutually agreed to.

The Benevolent Fund dinner took place at Willis's Rooms, on Wednesday, the 20th of February, 1867, and proved a great success. It was the largest gathering of our pharmacists which had ever met at a festive board. In all 264 sat down to dinner, and subscriptions amounting to upwards of fifteen hundred pounds were collected.

Scarcely less important in its beneficial influence was another gathering of a social character which occurred in the previous month, on the 30th of January, when 247 ladies and gentlemen inaugurated the series of Chemists' Balls, which have subsequently been kept up annually in the same rooms, and have contributed to the promotion of friendly intercourse and good feeling among those engaged in the same occupation. The Chemists' Ball originated in a praiseworthy desire of a number of the younger followers of pharmacy, most of whom were unconnected with the Pharmaceutical Society, to do something which should show their sympathy in the objects of the Benevolent Fund. On this occasion there was a surplus of receipts beyond the expenditure amounting to £29 10s. 6d., which was given to the Benevolent Fund.

We have now entered upon the year 1867, when increased activity was again manifested by the Bloomsbury Council with regard to legislation. To some extent this was promoted by external conditions and influences.

On the 2nd January, 1867, a communication was received through Mr. Buott, acting for the Executive Committee of the United Society of Chemists and Druggists, enclosing resolutions passed at a public meeting held at the Clarence Hotel, Manchester, November 23rd, 1866, Wm. Bowker, Esq., Ex-Mayor of Manchester, in the chair. These resolutions were in accordance with the general views which had been expressed by the Council in the paper left at the Home Office in February, 1866, and the Secretary was therefore desired to send a copy of that paper to the Executive Committee of the United Society, with a request that it might be transmitted to the Chairman of the Manchester meeting. The *Pharmaceutical Journal*, in publishing the Manchester resolutions, remarked : " Looking to the year that has just departed, we find there has been a lull in the action of our society in the work which they promoted so earnestly in the preceding year. We do not mean to imply that the Council has fallen off from its duty, or failed to promote the great object commenced by our founders ; but for certain reasons, which were set forth some months ago in this Journal, 1866 was deemed an unfavourable season for intruding pharmaceutical legislation on a pre-occupied House of Commons."

A letter appeared in the *Chemist and Druggist*, signed by Edmund Holt, Hon. Sec. United Society of Chemists and Druggists, Manchester District, dated January 9th, 1867, which was written in a very different spirit from that which pervaded the Manchester resolutions alluded to. It discredited, in every possible way the proposals and suggestions put into the hands of the Government by the Pharmaceutical Society. The discrepancy between this letter and the resolutions previously received was so great and unaccountable that inquiry was made into the matter, and it was found that the first communication was a notice of resolutions passed at an independent meeting of members of the trade in Manchester and the districts for many miles round. These resolutions had been sent to the United Society as the best parties to represent them to the Pharmaceutical Board, as they had already communicated with that society. Since that they had never seen the reply sent by the Council, although it had been sent to the Local Committee for transmission. The hostile resolutions were drawn up by the District Committee of the United Society on their own responsibility.

At an adjourned meeting of the Council of the Pharmaceutical Society, held 9th January, 1867, Mr. Sandford, President, in the chair, it was resolved that the Parliamentary Committee be requested to confer with the Home Secretary on the subject of legislation as regards an amended Pharmacy Act. An interview accordingly took place with the Under Secretary, Earl Belmore, at the Home Office, on the 16th January.

On the 24th of January a public meeting of the trade was held at the London Coffee House, Ludgate Hill, to receive and consider certain resolutions which the Executive Committee of the United Society had agreed to at a meeting held by them on the 17th of that month. The President, Mr. Henry Matthews was in the chair, and there were about sixty persons present.

The Secretary, Mr. Cyrus Buott, having read the circular convening the meeting, Mr. Anderson moved the first resolution, "That in relation to the first clause of the suggestions of the Pharmaceutical Council for the incorporation of the trade, viz., 'That in future all persons, before assuming the name or title of Chemist and Druggist, or keeping open shop for the compounding of medicines under physicians' and surgeons' prescriptions, or for vending, dispensing, or compounding certain dangerous drugs, chemicals, and other poisonous substances to be enumerated in a schedule, should undergo an examination, and be registered as Pharmaceutical Chemists, or Chemists and Druggists :' This meeting has much pleasure in according its concurrence therewith, and hopes that the compulsory examination it sets forth, desired as it is by the entire body of chemists and druggists, sanctioned by the medical profession, and recommended by the Select Committee of the House of Commons, will effectually secure the public against the practice of incompetent druggists, and greatly elevate and benefit the trade." The mover of the resolution said they could adopt the suggestions of the Pharmaceutical Society, as they were based upon the most liberal principles so far as the trade was concerned. It was carried unanimously. The second resolution, which was also carried unanimously, was, "That as to the system of examination specified in the 2nd and 3rd clauses, to the effect, 'that the examination for Pharmaceutical Chemists should be, as heretofore, that which is known as the major examination of the Pharmaceutical Society, and the examination for Chemists and Druggists should be that which is known as the minor examination, to which persons hitherto registered as assistants have been subjected, this meeting takes no exception to it."

The third resolution was the point of departure from concurrence with the recommendations of the Pharmaceutical Society. It was to the following effect: "This meeting concurs in the desirability of limiting the title of Pharmaceutical Chemist to those who may pass their major examination; but it is decidedly opposed to registered chemists and druggists being subjected to election by the Pharmaceutical Council as a condition for the exercise of their right to vote upon the election of the members of that Council; and it is equally and decidedly opposed to the Council of so large a body as the chemists and druggists will be under an Act of general incorporation being limited to those who are now, or may be hereafter, Pharmaceutical Chemists."

Mr. Betty then moved the following resolution :—

"That, as among the interests influencing the entire trade of chemists and druggists, two elements, the educational and the commercial, are inseparably connected, and as it is of vital importance in maturing any form of government for the whole trade that these two interests should, so far as practicable, be blended, this meeting cherishes the hope that from the resolutions it has adopted, the advantages of a mutual understanding and combined action may be brought into operation, and authorizes a deputation of the trade to wait in this spirit upon the Pharmaceutical Council." This resolution was also passed unanimously. For the purpose of carrying it into effect, Mr. Wade moved :—" That the deputation or committee consist of twenty-one unincorporated chemists and druggists, comprising ten members of the United Society and the President, and ten unconnected with either society; and that they be empowered to confer with the Council of the Pharmaceutical Society for the purpose of framing an Act of incorporation, based upon the foregoing resolutions." This raised a complete storm, and great indignation was expressed at the proposal to take the performance of this duty out of the hands of the Executive Committee, which, it was said, had been in existence for seven years, and had worked hard for the good of the trade. Finally it was decided, "That the deputation should consist of the Executive Committee of the United Society of Chemists and Druggists, and any other gentlemen willing to join them."

Application was made to the Pharmaceutical Council by the

President of the United Society, requesting them to receive the deputation appointed at the London Coffee House; and a separate application for an interview was made by Mr. Wade, on behalf of himself and other members of the trade not acting with the United Society. Arrangements were made for receiving these deputations on the 19th of February. The first to arrive was that headed and introduced by Mr. Henry Matthews, the President of the United Society. Mr. Betty opened the business of the deputation, and asked the Council to take into consideration the conclusions arrived at by the chemists and druggists at the London Coffee House. He trusted some understanding would be come to by which the trade would attain its proper influence, and keep pace with the increasing educational requirements of the age. Messrs. Anderson, Salter, Pass and Mercer, followed in a similar strain, and explained the purport of the resolutions which had been passed at their meeting, pointing out the objection which had been taken to the constitution of the society and its Council as suggested by the Pharmaceutical Society.

Mr. Sandford explained that as to the constitution of the Society the mode of electing members hitherto in use was the most simple; that there was no reason to apprehend any opposition to their admission, but that on the contrary it must be the interest of the society to enlarge its borders and embrace if possible the whole trade; that a man being *eligible* had a positive right to admission, presuming always that there was no disqualifying circumstance attaching to him, which the Court of Queen's Bench as well as the Pharmaceutical Society would recognise.

Mr. Betty.—Do you object to substitute for the term ' eligible,' the words ' shall have the right '?

Mr. Sandford.—Certainly not.

Then with regard to the constitution of the Council; it was necessary in order to retain the confidence of the public that the society and its Council should be kept up to a proper standard, and therefore it had been proposed to limit the Council to Pharmaceutical Chemists, by which means not only would the character of the Council be maintained, but a greater inducement would be held out for passing the major examination. That was the chief reason for the restriction, but there might be other reasons, such as the accumulation of a large amount of property by the society, and the expenditure of more than £100,000, collected entirely from members of the society during a quarter of a century of subscription, and very hard work on the part of the Council. Still, remembering that the Pharmaceutical Society was established to embrace all chemists and druggists in Great Britain, the Council, animated by the desire that it should do so, proposed that in the event of obtaining an Act of Parliament to compel the examination of all men entering the trade in future, those chemists in business at the time of the passing of that Act, who might choose to become members of the society, should be eligible for the Council, but that three-fourths, or two-thirds, of the Council should always consist of Pharmaceutical Chemists. This would certainly give all the opportunity for a fair representation, and the votes of the members would regulate it.

Mr. Anderson expressed his entire satisfaction with the explanations afforded by the Council, and proposed to take a show of hands from the deputation as to whether they were not all satisfied.

The Council retired from the room, and Mr. Matthews having put the question, it was answered unanimously in the affirmative.

Mr. Matthews and his friends having withdrawn, the second deputation, consisting of chemists and druggists unrepresented by any organized society, and therefore actual outsiders, was introduced by Mr. Wade, when, after discussing the subject, a satisfactory understanding was arrived at.

The differences of opinion and opposition of parties which had hitherto existed in the trade, and had prevented the carrying of any measure of pharmaceutical legislation, being now happily removed, there appeared to be no further difficulty in appealing to the Government as a united body. The Council therefore, at their meeting on the 3rd of April, resolved "that the Parliamentary Committee be requested forthwith to take the necessary steps to introduce the proposed Amended Pharmacy Bill into Parliament." But it was soon found that there was still another party to some of the questions which had arisen. A correspondence sprang up regarding the concessions which had been made by the Council to those outside the society, which were thought to be scarcely fair to examined men. The Council, viewed as trustees, had no easy task to perform, and their difficulties were by no means over.

At a special meeting of the Council, held on the 24th of April, 1867, a requisition was received to the following effect:—

"To the Secretary of the Pharmaceutical Society of Great Britain.

" We, the undersigned members of the Pharmaceutical Society of Great Britain, being of opinion that the proposed ' Amended Pharmacy Act,' in reference to at least the 19th clause, will operate unfairly towards present members, and be inimical to the interests of the public, do hereby request that the President of the said society be asked to convene a *special general meeting* of the members, to be held at the society's house in Bloomsbury Square, on some day between the 6th and 11th of May next, for the purpose of taking into consideration and the general discussion of the said Bill; and that the Council be requested to take no further steps with regard to the said Bill until it has received, either in its present or some amended form, the sanction of the members then assembled."

In compliance with this requisition a meeting was convened, to be held on the 15th of May, at two o'clock p.m., the day of the anniversary meeting.

The appearance of the requisition and notice of meeting drew forth a counterstatement, which was published in the *Pharmaceutical Journal* for May, 1867, as follows:—

" To the Editor of the *Pharmaceutical Journal.*

" Sir,—We understand that a circular has been forwarded to some of our examined members, urging them to sign a requisition to the Council to convene a special meeting for the purpose of opposing that clause of the new Bill by which *' chemists and druggists in business at the time of the passing of the Act are made eligible for admission as members of the society, under the bye-laws thereof,'* but are *not* to use the title of Pharmaceutical Chemist. The circular professes to represent the examined members as indignant at what is considered the injustice which will be done them if this Act becomes law.

"We, the undersigned members of the Pharmaceutical Society, Pharmaceutical Chemists by examination, beg to protest against the views enunciated in this circular, and to express our cordial approval of the liberal policy adopted by the Council towards all chemists and druggists. Considering the difficulties that have hitherto existed in the matter of trade legislation, we believe the Bill framed by the Council to be the best compromise that could have been effected under the circumstances. We feel convinced that the sincere desire of the vast majority of our members, whether examined or not, is to consummate the wishes of the founder, and to fulfil the object he had in view when the society was formed, namely, *the amalgamation of the whole trade, and the compulsory examination of all persons entering it after a given time.*

"Our firm belief is, that this Bill will effectually accomplish both these objects; and we trust the Council will spare no effort to pass it into law at the earliest possible opportunity.

"We are, Sir, yours respectfully,

CHARLES BOORNE, *Bristol.*
JOHN BOUCHER, *Bristol.*
ISAIAH BOURDAS, jun., *London.*
W. H. BELL, *London.*
H. B. BRADY, *Newcastle.*
M. CARTEIGHE, *London.*
ROBERT ELLIOTT, *Gateshead.*
H. S. EVANS, *Liverpool.*
SAMUEL GALE, *London.*
R. W. GILES, *Clifton.*
W. H. HOLROYD, *London.*
WALTER HOLGATE, *Liverpool.*

JOSEPH INCE, *London.*
JOHN MAYFIELD, *Leeds.*
C. R. QUILLER, *London.*
RICHARD REYNOLDS, *Leeds.*
J. ROBBINS, *London.*
G. F. SCHACHT, *Clifton.*
W. SMEETON, *Leeds.*
C. SYMES, *Birkenhead.*
F. TIBBS, *London.*
CHARLES UMNEY, *London.*
ALFRED UTLEY, *Liverpool.*
EDWIN B. VIZER, *London.*"

In the discussion of the subject at the special meeting, a resolution was moved by Mr. Abraham, of Liverpool, and seconded by Mr. Boyce, of Chertsey: "That the indiscriminate admission of chemists and druggists to the membership of the Pharmaceutical Society would destroy the value of the title 'Pharmaceutical Chemist'; that the chemists and druggists, having had no part in gaining for the society the reputation which it enjoys, have no claim to its honours; and

that it is not expedient to depart from the test of examination
which has so long prevailed in the admission of members of
the society."

To this an amendment was moved by Mr. J. R. Collins,
and seconded by Mr. Vizer, both of London : " That, in the
opinion of this meeting, the proposed amendment of the
Pharmacy Act is both wise and expedient, as by enlisting the
support of those members of the trade outside the pale of the
society the way is cleared for carrying into effect the primary
objects of the founders of the society, viz., the consolidation
of the whole trade, and legislative provision for the compulsory examination of all persons entering the same after a
given time. This meeting would further express its entire
approval of the action taken by the Council, and pledges itself
to support by all possible means the passage of the Bill
through Parliament."

Both propositions were temperately and fairly advocated,
and finally the amendment was carried by a large majority.

A further resolution was then moved by Mr. Michael
Carteighe, seconded by Mr. Joseph Ince, and carried unanimously : " That it be a recommendation to the Council that
they arrange, if practicable, for assistants and apprentices at
the time of the passing of the Act not being made eligible for
membership without passing the minor examination."

The result of this meeting, and the conciliatory tone which
had pervaded its proceedings, were satisfactory to the promoters of the Bill, which there was reason to believe all
chemists and druggists would either support or at least would
not actively oppose. The difficulties which stood in the way
of this Bill a month or two previously, were now apparently
removed, and if no fresh obstacles should arise, there seemed
a fair prospect of carrying such a legislative measure as would
satisfy all parties concerned.

The success which had thus far attended the efforts of the
Council in the pursuit of this object was mainly due to the
firm yet liberal and wise policy which had been adopted
throughout a lengthened controversy, and there was still
occasion for a continuance of the same judicious course of
proceedings while the consummation of the object remained
to be accomplished.

The Pharmaceutical Council were fully sensible of the

importance of consistently maintaining the same policy they
had hitherto adopted, and with a view to its realization, at
their meeting on the 5th of June, when the officers for the
ensuing year were to be appointed, a paper was signed by
every member present, to the following effect: "That in
unanimously requesting Mr. George Webb Sandford to continue the onerous duties of President for another year, the
Council desire most earnestly to express their thanks for his
past services. They are conscious of the encroachment upon
his time that is necessitated by the appointment, but believing
that his continuance as President is important to the well-
being of the Pharmaceutical Society, request him again to
accept the office."

Mr. Sandford had already occupied the position for four
consecutive years, during which he had been the leader and
prime-mover in what had been done in the direction of legislation. He had become indeed so identified with the proceedings of the Council in this matter, was so familiar with all
the details of the business, and so well acquainted with
Members of Parliament and the Government, whose interest
and influence it would be necessary to have, that it was felt a
change of presidency at this time would have seriously
weakened the prospects of success.

After appointing Sandford *President*, and Hills *Vice-President*, the Council received a deputation of members of the
trade residing at Stamford, Sleaford, Lincoln, Peterborough,
Norwich, and Gainsborough, with reference to the schedule
of poisons in the proposed Pharmacy Bill.

Members, examined and unexamined, continued to discuss
some of the provisions of the Bill, and especially the one for
admitting chemists and druggists as members of the Pharmaceutical Society without examination. Gradually, however,
the objection to this provision was disappearing. The Bill
had been prepared, but there was no prospect of its being
introduced into Parliament during this session which was now
far advanced.

The United Society of Chemists and Druggists, having
obtained certain concessions from the Pharmaceutical Society,
had not only withdrawn opposition from the proposed Pharmacy Bill of the latter, but were prepared to co-operate with
them in promoting its acceptance by the Legislature. The

annual festival of the United Society, for 1867, was transferred from London to Manchester, where it was held at the
Clarence Hotel, on the 26th of June, with Mr. Alderman
Bowker in the chair. It was stated in the official circular
convening this meeting, that it would "be specially devoted
to a commemoration of the good understanding now happily
established between the United Society and the Pharmaceutical Society for the union of the trade by means of an
amended Pharmacy Bill." At the annual meeting, held at
the same place on the following day, Mr. E. P. Hornby, of
Sheffield, was elected President of the United Society, in the
place of Mr. Henry Matthews.

The new edition of the British Pharmacopœia (1867) had
now come into circulation, and was favourably received. The
Pharmaceutical Journal of July, 1867, referring to it, says:
" Very strong testimony has been borne to the fact, that the
work has been carefully and well prepared, and that it is, on
the whole, a decided success. The testimony to this effect,
which has been given by the Medical Council, the Medical
Journals, and members both of the medical and pharmaceutical professions, whose qualifications to judge are above
suspicion, stands unchallenged, as far as we know, by any
adverse opinions."

The fifth meeting (fourth annual meeting) of the British
Pharmaceutical Conference was held in September, 1867, at
Dundee; Professor Bentley again presided at this meeting,
which proved no less successful than its predecessors.

An Act was passed, which came into operation on the 1st
October, 1867, by which the licence for the sale by retail of
methylated spirit was reduced from two guineas to ten
shillings a year.

Mr. Daniel Bell Hanbury, having resigned his office of
Treasurer of the Pharmaceutical Society, Mr. Thomas Hyde
Hills, the Vice-President, was appointed Treasurer, and Mr.
Henry Sugden Evans was elected Vice-President.

As another session of Parliament was approaching, the
Pharmaceutical Council, sensible of the duty they had to
perform, resolved, at a meeting held on the 6th of November,
1867, "That steps be immediately taken to introduce into
Parliament an amended Pharmacy Bill, and that the Parliamentary Committee be instructed accordingly."

368 THE HOME SECRETARY ON PHARMACEUTICAL LEGISLATION.

The Executive Committee of the United Society also, at a meeting held on the 5th of December, resolved, "That the Parliamentary Committee of the United Society of Chemists and Druggists be at once re-appointed, to work in union with the Parliamentary Committee of the Pharmaceutical Society, with similar power to act in order to secure an amended Pharmacy Bill upon the basis already agreed upon."

As soon as Parliament met for the despatch of business, application was made to the Home Secretary, Mr. Gathorne Hardy, who consented to receive a deputation of members of the Council of the Pharmaceutical Society, with whom were associated the President of the United Society, and two other gentlemen not belonging to the Pharmaceutical Society. A copy of the Bill in the form agreed upon had been previously left at the Home Office for consideration. The result of this interview was highly satisfactory. The Home Secretary said that personally he approved of the propositions submitted to him; he entirely concurred in the necessity for an educational qualification in persons who were entrusted to compound medicines; but that he saw no chance of proceeding with legislation on the subject before Easter, and that he could not, without consulting his colleagues, say whether or not the Government would introduce a measure on the question.

The President had several interviews with Mr. Hardy afterwards, and on the 18th of February he received the following letter :—

"*February* 18*th*, 1868.

" To G. W. SANDFORD, Esq.

" Sir,—I am not unwilling to support a Bill restricting the title of ' Chemists and Druggists ' to

" 1. Those now in business as such.

" 2. Those to be examined for the future and passed by proper examiners.

" 3. Pharmaceutical Chemists.

" 4. Medical practitioners under the Medical Act.

" No others to be allowed to sell certain drugs, etc., named. I think this will be sufficient.

" Yours faithfully,

" GATHORNE HARDY."

As there appeared to be some doubt whether the word

" sell," as used above, was intended to include dispensing and compounding drugs, Mr. Sandford communicated with the Under Secretary, Sir James Fergusson, on this point, and received the following reply :—

" Home Office,

" 19th February, 1868.

" Dear Sir,—In answer to your question, whether the words used by Mr. Hardy in his of the 18th February, ' no other person to be allowed to sell certain drugs, etc., named,' includes dispensing and compounding, and whether Mr. Hardy will accept the words in the first clause of the draft Bill, ' it shall be unlawful for any person to keep open shop for the purpose of retailing, dispensing, or compounding poisons '; I beg to inform you that Mr. Hardy does intend the prohibition of selling dangerous drugs by unauthorized persons, to include also dispensing or compounding for payment such drugs as may be specified as ' dangerous ' or ' poisonous.'

" Believe me, yours faithfully,

" JAMES FERGUSSON.

" G. W. SANDFORD, Esq."

The Bill referred to in this correspondence, which had been agreed to by the Pharmaceutical Society, the United Society, and others, and which was shortly afterwards submitted to Parliament, was as follows :—

A BILL TO REGULATE THE SALE OF POISONS AND ALTER AND AMEND THE PHARMACY ACT, 1852.

(As introduced in the House of Lords on the 11th of May, 1868.)

Whereas it is expedient for the safety of the public that persons keeping open shop for the retailing, dispensing, or compounding of poisons, and persons known as Chemists and Druggists, should possess a competent practical knowledge of their business, and to that end, that from and after the day herein named all persons not already engaged in such business should, before commencing such business, be duly examined as to their practical knowledge, and that a register should be kept as herein provided, and also that the Act passed in the 15th and 16th years of the reign of her present Majesty, intituled An Act for Regulating the Qualification of Pharmaceutical Chemists, hereinafter described as the Pharmacy Act, should be amended: be it enacted, by the Queen's Most Excellent Majesty, by and with the advice and consent of the Lords Spiritual and Temporal and Commons in this present Parliament assembled, and by authority of the same, as follows:

1. From and after the 31st day of December, 1868, it shall be unlawful for any person to keep open shop for retailing, dispensing, or compounding poisons, or to assume or use the title "Chemist and Druggist" or Chemist or Druggist in any part of Great Britain unless such person shall be a Pharmaceutical Chemist, or a Chemist and Druggist within the meaning of this Act.

2. The several articles named or described in the Schedule A shall be deemed to be Poisons within the meaning of this Act, and the Council of the Pharmaceutical Society of Great Britain (hereinafter referred to as the Pharmaceutical Society) may, from time to time, by resolution, declare that any article in such resolution named ought to be deemed a poison within the meaning of this Act; and thereupon the Registrar hereinafter named shall submit such resolution to the Medical Council, and if the Medical Council shall resolve that such resolution ought to be confirmed, the said Registrar shall then submit the same for the approval of one of her Majesty's Principal Secretaries of State, and if such approval shall be given, then such resolution, confirmation, and approval shall be advertised in the *London Gazette*, and on the expiration of one month from such advertisement, the article named in such resolution shall be deemed to be a poison within the meaning of this Act.

3. Chemists and Druggists within the meaning of this Act shall consist of all persons who, at any time heretofore, have carried on, in Great Britain, the business of a Chemist and Druggist, in the keeping of open shop for the compounding of the prescriptions of duly qualified medical practitioners, also of all Assistants and Associates duly registered under or according to the provisions of the Pharmacy Act, and also of all such persons as may be duly registered under this Act.

4. Any person who, for two years prior to the time of passing this Act, shall have been apprenticed to, or who, at

the time of the passing of this Act, shall be of full age and shall have been actually engaged and employed in dispensing and compounding prescriptions, as assistant to any Pharmaceutical Chemist, or any such Chemist and Druggist as defined by clause 3 hereof, may, on transmitting to the Registrar, before the 31st day of December, 1870, certificates, according to the Schedule E to this Act, be registered under this Act.

5. Such of the Chemists and Druggists, defined by clause 3, as may, on or before the 31st day of December, 1870, by notice in writing, signed by them, and given to the Registrar, request to be registered under this Act, shall, on production of certificates according to the Schedules C and D to this Act, be registered accordingly.

6. All such persons as shall from time to time have been appointed to conduct examinations under the Pharmacy Act, shall be, and are hereby declared to be examiners for the purposes of this Act, and are hereby empowered and required to examine all such persons as shall tender themselves for examination under the provisions of this Act, and every person who shall have been examined by such examiners, and shall have obtained from them a certificate of competent skill and knowledge and qualification, shall be entitled to be registered as a Chemist and Druggist under this Act, and the examination aforesaid shall be such as is provided under the Pharmacy Act for the purposes of a qualification to be registered as Assistant under that Act, or as the same may be varied from time to time by any bye-law to be made in accordance with the Pharmacy Act, with the approbation of one of her Majesty's Principal Secretaries of State.

7. Such fees shall be payable upon every such examination and registration as aforesaid, as shall from time to time be fixed and determined by any bye-law, to be made in accordance with the Pharmacy Act, with the approbation of one of her Majesty's principal Secretaries of State, and shall be paid to the Treasurer of the said society, for the purposes of the said society.

8. The Registrar appointed, or to be appointed, under or by virtue of the Pharmacy Act, shall be Registrar for the purposes of this Act.

9. The Council of the Pharmaceutical Society shall, with

all convenient speed, after the passing of this Act, and from time to time, as occasion may require, make orders or regulations for regulating the register, to be kept under this Act as nearly as conveniently may be in accordance with the form set forth in the Schedule B to this Act, or to the like effect, and such register shall be called the Register of Chemists and Druggists.

10. It shall be the duty of the Registrar to make and keep a correct register, in accordance with the provisions of this Act, of all persons who shall be entitled to be registered under this Act, and to erase the names of all registered persons who shall have died, and from time to time to make the necessary alterations in the addresses of the persons registered under this Act; to enable the Registrar duly to fulfil the duties imposed upon him, it shall be lawful for the Registrar to write a letter to any registered person, addressed to him according to his address on the register, to inquire whether he has ceased to carry on business or has changed his residence, such letter to be forwarded by post as a registered letter, according to the Post-Office regulations for the time being, and if no answer shall be returned to such letter within the period of six months from the sending of the letter, a second, of similar purport, shall be sent in like manner, and if no answer be given thereto within three months from the date thereof, it shall be lawful to erase the name of such person from the register, provided always that the same may be restored by direction of the Council of the Pharmaceutical Society, should they think fit to make an order to that effect.

11. Every Registrar of Deaths in Great Britain, on receiving notice of the death of any Pharmaceutical Chemist, or Chemist and Druggist, shall forthwith transmit, by post, to the Registrar under the Pharmacy Act, a certificate, under his own hand, of such death, with the particulars of the time and place of death, and on the receipt of such certificate, the said Registrar under the Pharmacy Act shall erase the name of such deceased Pharmaceutical Chemist, or Chemist and Druggist, from the register, and shall transmit to the said Registrar of Deaths the cost of such certificate and transmission, and may charge the cost thereof as an expense of his office.

12. No name shall be entered in the register, unless the Registrar be satisfied by the proper evidence, that the person claiming is entitled to be registered ; and any appeal from the decision of the Registrar may be decided by the Council of the Pharmaceutical Society ; and any entry which shall be proved to the satisfaction of such Council to have been fraudulently or incorrectly made, may be erased from or amended in the register, by order, in writing, of such Council.

13. The Registrar shall, in every year, cause to be printed, published, and sold, a correct register of the names of all Pharmaceutical Chemists, and a correct register of all persons registered as Chemists and Druggists, and in such registers, respectively, the names shall be in alphabetical order, according to the surnames, with the respective residences, in the form set forth in Schedule B to this Act, or to the like effect, of all persons appearing on the Register of Pharmaceutical Chemists, and on the Register of Chemists and Druggists on the 31st day of December last preceding, and such printed registers shall be called " The Registers of Pharmaceutical Chemists and Chemists and Druggists," and a printed copy of such registers for the time being, purporting to be so printed and published as aforesaid, or any certificate under the hand of the said Registrar, and countersigned by the President or two Members of the Council of the Pharmaceutical Society, shall be evidence in all Courts and before all Justices of the Peace and others, that the persons therein specified are registered according to the provisions of the Pharmacy Act or of this Act, as the case may be, and the absence of the name of any person from such printed register shall be evidence, until the contrary shall be made to appear, that such person is not registered according to the provisions of the Pharmacy Act or of this Act.

14. Any Registrar who shall wilfully make or cause to be made any falsification in any matter relating to the said registers, and any person who shall wilfully procure or attempt to procure himself to be registered under the Pharmacy Act or under this Act, by making or producing, or causing to be made or produced, any false or fraudulent representation or declaration, either verbally or in writing, and any person aiding or assisting him therein, shall be deemed guilty of a misdemeanour in England, and in Scotland, of a crime or offence

punishable by fine or imprisonment, and shall on conviction thereof be sentenced to be imprisoned for any term not exceeding twelve months.

15. From and after the 31st day of December, 1868, any person keeping an open shop for the retailing, dispensing, or compounding poisons, or who shall take, use, or exhibit the name or title of Chemist and Druggist or Chemist or Druggist, not being a duly qualified Pharmaceutical Chemist or a Chemist and Druggist, or who shall take, use, or exhibit, the name or title Pharmaceutical Chemist or Pharmaceutist or Pharmacist, not being a Pharmaceutical Chemist, shall, for every such offence, be liable to pay a penalty or sum of £5, and the same may be sued for, recovered, and dealt with in the manner provided by the Pharmacy Act for the recovery of penalties under that Act.

16. Nothing herein before contained shall extend to or interfere with the business of any duly qualified medical practitioner or of any member of the Royal College of Veterinary Surgeons of Great Britain, nor with the making or dealing in patent medicines, nor with the business of wholesale dealers in supplying poisons in the ordinary course of wholesale dealing, nor with the retailing of arsenic, oxalic acid, cyanide of potassium, or corrosive sublimate, for use in manufactures or photography ; and upon the decease of any Pharmaceutical Chemist or Chemist and Druggist actually in business at the time of his death, it shall be lawful for any executor, administrator, or trustee of the estate of such Pharmaceutical Chemist or Chemist and Druggist to continue such business if and so long only as such business shall be *bonâ fide* conducted by a duly qualified assistant, and a duly qualified assistant, within the meaning of this clause, shall be a Pharmaceutical Chemist or a Chemist and Druggist registered by the Registrar under the Pharmacy Act or this Act.

17. It shall not be lawful to sell any poison, either wholesale or by retail, unless the box, bottle, vessel, wrapper, or cover in which such poison is contained be distinctly labelled with the name of the article and the word poison, and with the name and address of the seller of the poison; and any seller of any poison not so distinctly labelled shall, upon a summary conviction before two Justices of the Peace in England or the Sheriff in Scotland, be liable to a penalty not

exceeding £5 for the first offence, and to a penalty not exceeding £10 for the second offence, and for the purpose of
this clause the person on whose behalf any sale is made by any
apprentice or servant shall be deemed to be the seller, but the
provisions of this clause, so far as regards the name and address of the seller, shall not apply to articles to be exported
from Great Britain by wholesale dealers, and nothing in this
Act contained shall repeal or affect any of the provisions of
an Act of the Sessions holden in the fourteenth and fifteenth
years of the reign of her present Majesty, intituled "An Act
to regulate the Sale of Arsenic."

18. Chemists and Druggists registered under this Act shall
be deemed to be within the provisions of the second section of
the Juries Act, 1862, in relation to the exemption from service
on juries.

19. Every person who, at the time of the passing of this
Act, is or has been in business on his own account as a Chemist and Druggist as aforesaid, and who shall be registered as a
Chemist and Druggist, shall be eligible to be elected and continue a member of the Pharmaceutical Society according to the
bye-laws thereof ; but no person shall, in right of membership
acquired pursuant to this clause, be placed on the register of
Pharmaceutical Chemists, nor, save as is hereinafter expressly
provided, be eligible for election to the Council of the Pharmaceutical Society.

20. Every person who is or has been in business on his own
account as a Chemist and Druggist as aforesaid at the time of
the passing of this Act, and who shall become a member of the
Pharmaceutical Society, shall be eligible for election to the
Council of the Pharmaceutical Society; but the said Council
shall not at any time contain more than seven members who
are not on the register of Pharmaceutical Chemists, nor more
than seven members who shall not at the time of election *bonâ
fide* reside within twelve miles by highway or road from the
General Post Office in St. Martin's-le-Grand.

21. Every Apprentice and Assistant, as described in Clause 4
of this Act, who shall cause his name to be registered as provided in that clause, and every person who shall have been
registered as a Chemist and Druggist under this Act, by reason
of having obtained a certificate of qualification from the Board
of Examiners, as provided in Clause 6 of this Act, shall be eligi-

ble to be elected an Associate of the Pharmaceutical Society, and every such person so elected and continuing as such Associate, being in business on his own account, shall have the privilege of attending all meetings of the said society and of voting thereat, and otherwise taking part in the proceedings of such meetings, in the same manner as Members of the said society, provided always that such Associates contribute to the funds of the said society the same fees or subscriptions as Members contribute for the time being under the bye-laws thereof.

22. At all meetings of the Pharmaceutical Society at which votes shall be given for the election of officers, all or any of the votes may be given either personally or by voting papers, in a form to be defined in the bye-laws of the said society, or in a form to the like effect, such voting papers being transmitted under cover to the Secretary, not less than one clear day prior to the day on which the election is to take place.

23. And whereas, by the Charter of Incorporation of the said Pharmaceutical Society, it is provided that the Council of the said society shall have the sole control and management of the real and personal property of the said society, subject to the bye-laws thereof, and shall make provision thereout, or out of such part thereof as they shall think proper, for the relief of the distressed Members or Associates of the said society, and their widows and orphans, subject to the regulations and bye-laws of the said society : And whereas, for extending the benefits which have resulted from the said provision in the said Charter of Incorporation, it is desirable that additional power should be granted to the said Council : Be it enacted, that from and after the passing of this Act, the said Council may make provision out of the real and personal property aforesaid, and out of any special fund, known as the Benevolent Fund, not only for the relief of the distressed Members or Associates of the said society and their widows and orphans, subject to the said regulations and bye-laws, but also for all persons who may have been and have ceased to be Members or Associates of the said society, or who may be or have been duly registered as " Pharmaceutical Chemists " or " Chemists and Druggists," and the widows and orphans of such persons, subject to the regulations and bye-laws of the said society.

24. Persons registered under "The Medical Act" shall not be or continue to be registered under this Act.

25. This Act may be cited as the Pharmacy Act, 1868.

SCHEDULE A.

Arsenic and its preparations.

Oxalic Acid.

Prussic Acid.

Chloroform.

Cyanides of Potassium and Mercury,

Strychnine, and all poisonous vegetable alkaloids and their salts.

Aconite and its preparations.

Emetic Tartar.

Corrosive Sublimate.

Belladonna and its preparations.

Essential Oil of Almonds, unless deprived of its Prussic Acid.

Cantharides.

Savin and its oil.

SCHEDULE B.

Name.	Residence.	Qualification.
A. B.	Oxford Street, London.	In business prior to Pharmacy Act, 1868.
C. D.	George Street, Edinburgh.	Examined and certified.
E. F.	Cheapside, London.	Apprentice or Assistant prior to Pharmacy Act, 1868.

SCHEDULE C.

Declaration by a person who was in business as a Chemist and Druggist in Great Britain before the Pharmacy Act, 1868.

To the Registrar of the Pharmaceutical Society of Great Britain.

I,   residing at   , in the county of
hereby declare that I was in business as a Chemist and Drug-

gist in the keeping of open shop for the compounding of the
prescriptions of duly qualified medical practitioners at   ,
in the county of   , on or before the   'day of
            , 186 .

                                   Signed (Name.)
      Dated this   day of   , 18 .

SCHEDULE' D.

*Declaration to be signed by a duly qualified Medical Practitioner,
or Magistrate, respecting a person who was in business as a
Chemist and Druggist in Great Britain before the Pharmacy
Act, 1868.*

To the Registrar of the Pharmaceutical Society of Great
                          Britain.

      I   residing at   , in the county of
            , hereby declare that I am a duly qualified
Medical Practitioner [*or* Magistrate], and that to my knowledge   , residing at   in the county
of   , was in business as a Chemist and Druggist,
in the keeping of open shop for the compounding of the prescriptions of duly qualified medical practitioners, before the
                  day of   , 186 .
                                   (*Signed*)

SCHEDULE E.

*Declarations to be signed by and on behalf of any Apprentice
or Assistant claiming to be registered under the Pharmacy
Act, 1868.*

To the Registrar of the Pharmaceutical Society of Great
                          Britain.

      I hereby declare that the undersigned   ,
residing at   , in the county of   ,
had, before the passing of the Pharmacy Act, 1868, been employed in dispensing and compounding prescriptions, as an
Assistant to a Pharmaceutical Chemist or Chemist and Druggist, and attained the age of twenty-one years [*or* had been

apprenticed to a Pharmaceutical Chemist or Chemist and Druggist, keeping open shop for the compounding of prescriptions of duly qualified medical men].

As witness my hand, this   day of   186 .

        A. B., duly qualified Medical Practitioner.

        C. D., Pharmaceutical Chemist.

        E. F., Chemist and Druggist.

        G. H., Magistrate.

(*To be signed by one of the four parties named.*)

I hereby declare that I was an Apprentice to

of   in the county of   in the year

        L. M., Apprentice.

I hereby declare that I was an Assistant to   of

     in the county of   in the year   ,

and was actually engaged in dispensing and compounding prescriptions, and that I had attained the full age of twenty-one years at the time of the passing of the Pharmacy Act, 1868.

        N. O., Assistant.

This Bill was drawn in accordance with the recommendation of the Select Committee of 1865, and as all parties were agreed in assenting to the principles comprised in its provisions, it was considered undesirable to endanger the chance of its passing, by including other provisions which might be wished for if attainable, but which were not equally easy of attainment.

The suggestion of the Committee of the Medical Council had been, to restrict *the dispensing or compounding of all prescriptions of physicians or surgeons* to examined and qualified chemists and druggists, and this had been made the basis of the Bill adopted by the Pharmaceutical Council in 1865; but the Select Committee of the House of Commons had rejected that principle and proposed to limit the restriction only to the sale or dispensing of poisonous substances. It was afterwards thought by the Council that with the view of giving a broader basis to the proposed legislation both principles might be included, and a Bill was drafted,* the first clause of which provided that " it shall be unlawful for any person to keep open shop for retailing, dispensing or compounding poisons, *or for compounding the prescriptions of duly qualified medical practitioners, etc.,*" " unless, etc.," but this was not persevered with, for the reason already stated.

It was not until the 11th of May, 1868, that the Council succeeded in getting their Bill into Parliament, but it was then introduced under very favourable circumstances, and there seemed a fair chance of its being carried.   The Government were not opposed to it ; in fact, the Home Secretary was only deterred from taking charge of it by press of other occupations ; and while no obstruction was therefore likely to arise in that quarter, a leading member of the opposite party, Earl Granville, undertook the duty of submitting the Bill to the House of Lords, where it passed a second reading on the 28th of May, without opposition or even discussion. On the 15th of June it passed through committee and was discussed, but the only alterations suggested were, that it should be extended to Ireland, and that provision should be made for the use of angular bottles in dealing with poisons. This latter proposition, although not pressed to a division on that occasion, was renewed, but rejected, at the third reading of the Bill on the 18th of June, when the measure was passed by the Lords without alteration.   In the Commons it met with rougher treatment, but still no important alteration was made, except that the clause by which it was proposed that chemists and druggists should be exempted from serving on juries was expunged.

The Bill passed through several hands in the House of Commons : first, it was in charge of Mr. Headlam, but as he was obliged to leave town before it had reached its final stage, it was transferred to Lord Elcho ; and afterwards, as his lordship was also called away, it was taken up by Mr. Ayrton, under whose charge it finally received the sanction of both Houses of Parliament, and became law on the 31st of July, 1868.

The passing of this Act was the fulfilment of one of the

---

* *Pharmaceutical Journal,* vol. ix. N.S. 435.

prominent objects of ambition which had dwelt in the minds and stimulated the exertions of those who for a quarter of a century had been contributing, through the operations of the Pharmaceutical Society, to render its realization possible. For the future the chemists and druggists of Great Britain would be a definable and recognised body. At no very distant period they would all be examined and qualified members of a fraternity possessing rights and privileges of acknowledged value, which had been eagerly sought after, but which were also accompanied by duties and responsibilities which some-what detracted from the importance of the advantage gained. This was especially the case with regard to the regulations required to be observed in the keeping and sale of poisons, for the carrying out of which, as well as for other purposes connected with the application of the law, a new set of bye-aws of the Pharmaceutical Society was required. Much work, involving the exercise of considerable judgment, had yet to be done by the Pharmaceutical Council, not only in carrying out the letter of the law the execution of which had been entrusted to them, but also in justifying the confidence reposed in them by the Legislature, which had left to their discretion the adoption or suggestion of any further required regulations connected with the keeping and sale of poisons. This was an anxious duty in the performance of which it soon became evident that much diversity of opinion and warmth of sentiment were likely to be elicited.

The fifth annual meeting of the British Pharmaceutical Conference was held at Norwich, in August of this year, under the presidency of Mr. Daniel Hanbury, F.R.S. Several interesting papers were read, and among the prominent subjects of conversation which the assembled pharmacists engaged in was that of the recently passed Pharmacy Act which so intimately affected their interests. This was in fact the first subject publicly discussed at the opening meeting, after the President's address had been delivered, and the following resolutions were passed unanimously:—

" 1. That the cordial thanks of this Conference and the whole profession, are due and hereby tendered to the President of the Pharmaceutical Society, and those who laboured with him, for those exertions in the cause of pharmaceutical education which have resulted in the Pharmacy Act of 1868.

" 2. That it is desirable there should be some public recognition of the services rendered to the cause of pharmaceutical education, and the improvement of the status of the profession, by Mr. George Webb Sandford, President of the Pharmaceutical Society, to whose careful and constant devotion the passing of the Pharmacy Act of 1868 is in great measure due.

" 3. That the President of the Conference be requested to address the Council of the Pharmaceutical Society, requesting the use of the Society's house for the purpose of holding a meeting on Tuesday, the 6th of October next, with a view to the carrying out of the foregoing resolutions."

Mr. Hanbury's letter embodying the above request was laid before the Council at their meeting on the 2nd of September, and the desired permission was at once granted.

The meeting was held at 17, Bloomsbury Square, on the 6th of October, Mr. Daniel Hanbury, F.R.S., in the chair, when it was resolved :—

" 1. That it is eminently desirable that a testimonial be presented to Mr. George Webb Sandford, President of the Pharmaceutical Society, for his able and unremitting services in promoting the passing of the Amended Pharmacy Act.

" 2. That the gentlemen now present do constitute a General Committee for the purpose of carrying out the foregoing resolution, with power to add to their number.

" 3. That Mr. Frederick Barron, of the firm of Drew, Barron & Co., Bush Lane, be requested to act as Chairman of the General Committee.

" 4. That Mr. Benjamin Brogden Orridge be requested to accept the office of Treasurer, and that Mr. Michael Carteighe, Mr. John Mackay (Edinburgh), and Mr. Henry Matthews, be requested to act as Honorary Secretaries."

At a meeting of the Committee, held on the 13th of October, 1868, it was decided that the testimonial should be both *personal* and *commemorative*, and that subscriptions should be at once solicited for the " Sandford Testimonial Fund."

A meeting of the Committee was held again on the 19th of April, 1869, to decide on the manner of applying the amount which had been raised. It had been previously arranged, in the event of the fund being sufficient, that the testimonial should consist of a portrait of Mr. Sandford,

President of the Pharmaceutical Society, and a service of plate, to be presented as a mark of the high appreciation which had been formed of the valuable services which he had rendered to the Society.   The amount of the subscriptions was found to be ample for the accomplishment of those two objects, and a committee was therefore appointed to carry them into effect at as early a period as possible.

On the 19th of May, 1869, after the anniversary meeting of the Pharmaceutical Society, which was held on that day, the subscribers to the " Sandford Testimonial Fund " met in the lecture hall of the Society, for the purpose of present- ing to Mr. Sandford the first part of the testimonial, consisting of an elegant assortment of plate, of the value of 200 guineas. The remainder of the fund, which amounted in the whole to upwards of £500, was devoted to the painting of a portrait of Mr. Sandford, by J. P. Knight, R.A., Secretary to the Royal Academy, which is suspended in the Council room of the Pharmaceutical Society.   In the evening a complimentary dinner was given to Mr. Sandford at the Freemasons' Tavern. On both these occasions Mr. Frederick Barron presided, and conveyed in most appropriate terms the sentiments not only of those who were present, but of all who participated in the prospective benefits of the Act which had been so long sought for, and the attainment of which was largely due to the firm, consistent, and persevering efforts of the President of the Pharmaceutical Society.

This festival formed an appropriate sequel to a labour which had thus far terminated successfully for the cause of pharmaceutical progression.   Henceforth we enter upon a new era in Pharmacy.

INDEX.

A.

B.

C.

D.

Dispensers for the Army, 305, 306.
Ditto, Qualifications, 306.
Crimean War, 250.
Dispensers of Medicine, Education of, 247.
Dispensing in the Army, 250.
Distillation, Illicit, 177.
Donovan, Professor.
(Dublin Pharmacopœia), 136.
Dove, William (Leeds), (Strychnia case), 244.
Druggist Dispensers, 45.
Druggists, Denunciation of, 35.
Franchise, 312.
Increase of, 38.
Prescribing, 39.

Druggists—
Non-professional Standing, 156.
Dublin College.
Angular Poison Bottles, 248, 249.
Pharmacopœia, 75, 136, 205.
Weights adopted, 205.
Weights and Measures, 273.
Dumas, M. (Alchemy), 12.
Philosophie Chimique (1837), 12.
Duncan, Dr., Dispensatory, 30.
Dundee, British Pharmaceutical Conference (1867), 367.
Duty on Glass (1812), 45.

E.

Early Closing Movement, 85, 86, 173.
Editio Altera (1815), 207.
Remarks on (Phillips), 44.
Edinburgh College of Physicians, (Pharmacopœia), 267.
Education of Dispensers of Medicine and Sale of Poisons, 247.
Pharmaceutical, 163, 184, 185.
Wilson, Dr. George, 184.
Provincial, 158.
Elcho, Lord (Medical Bill), 253.

Elements of Materia Medica (Pereira), 225, 226.
"Eligible," the word, 361.
Emigrant Vessels, Supply of Medicines, 223.
Emigration and Land Commissioners, 223.
Empirics, 4–6.
Anthony, Francis (1602), 5.
Booffeat, John (1583), 4.
Briscoe, Mr. (1634), 6.
Buck, Paul (1593), 5.
Fairfax, Paul (1588), 5.
Grig (1552), 4.
Kennix, Margaret (1581), 4.

F.

G.

H.

I.

J.

James, Dr. (1747), 30.
  Pharmacopœia Universalis, 31.
Jesuits' Bark (Evelyn), 32.
Journal, Chemist and Druggist, 349.
  Pharmaceutical, 113, 114, 138.
    Originated, 151.
    Special Editors, 294.

Journal, Pharmaceutical—
  Transfer of Copyright, 291.
Juries Bill, 308–312.
  Claim for Exemption, 308
  Secretary, Valuable Aid of, in obtaining, 311, 312.
  Ultimate Success of Pharmaceutical Chemists, 311.

K.

Kennix, Margaret (1581), 4.
Kerrison, Robert Masters, Inquiry, 47.

King's Evil, 123.
Knight, J. P., R.A., Portrait of Mr. G. W. Sandford, 383.

L.

Laboratory, Apothecaries' Hall, 13, 81, 82.
  Bell's, 190.
  Birkbeck, 175, 186.
  College of Chemistry, 186.
  Godfrey's, 11.
  Pharmaceutical, 167, 175.
    Enlargement, 307.
    New Erection, 293.
Laboratory and Lectures, 307.
Lancet Journal, The, 164.
  Adulteration of Food and Drugs, 222.
  Druggists' Franchise, 312.
Land and Emigration Commissioners, 223.

Laws of the Society, Original Draft, 103.
Lectures at Bloomsbury Square, 163.
  Evening, 153.
  Polarized Light, Pereira, 162.
Lee and Vallance, Brandy and Salt, 124.
Legislation, Medical, 262.
  Pharmaceutical, Home Secretary on, 368, 369.
  Pharmaceutical, Report on, by United Society, 344–348.
  Pharmaceutical and Medical, 187.

M.

N.

O.

P.

S.

T.

U

V.

W.

Butler & Tanner, The Selwood Printing Works, Frome, and London.

Printed in the United States
By Bookmasters